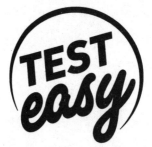

NURSING
Entrance Exams

By Dr. Maryanne Baudo DNP, NP-C, MSN, RN, and Robin Kavanagh, MA
Illustrated by Kara LaFrance

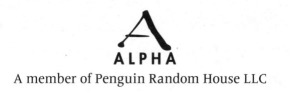

ALPHA
A member of Penguin Random House LLC

DK | Penguin Random House

Publisher: Mike Sanders
Senior Acquisitions Editor: Janette Lynn
Cover Designer: William Thomas
Book Designer/Layout: Ayanna Lacey
Copy Editor: Monica Stone
Indexer: Celia McCoy
Proofreader: Laura Caddell

To my husband and my family for their constant support of my career and my every endeavor.
—Maryanne Baudo

To my loved ones who are nurses and share both their hearts and knowledge to help people heal daily. Also, to my family, who has always been behind me in this crazy journey of life.
—Robin Kavanagh

Published by Penguin Random House LLC
001-309803-MAR2019.
Copyright © 2019 by Maryanne Baudo and Robin Kavanagh

All rights reserved. No part of this book may be reproduced, scanned, or distributed in any printed or electronic form without permission. Please do not participate in or encourage piracy of copyrighted materials in violation of the authors' rights. Purchase only authorized editions. No patent liability is assumed with respect to the use of the information contained herein. Although every precaution has been taken in the preparation of this book, the publisher and authors assume no responsibility for errors or omissions. Neither is any liability assumed for damages resulting from the use of information contained herein. For information, address Alpha Books, 6081 E. 82nd Street, Indianapolis, IN 46250.

International Standard Book Number: 978-1-46547-349-3
Library of Congress Catalog Card Number: 2018958034

21 20 19   10 9 8 7 6 5 4 3 2 1

Interpretation of the printing code: The rightmost number of the first series of numbers is the year of the book's printing; the rightmost number of the second series of numbers is the number of the book's printing. For example, a printing code of 19-1 shows that the first printing occurred in 2019.

Printed in the United States of America

Note: This publication contains the opinions and ideas of its authors. It is intended to provide helpful and informative material on the subject matter covered. It is sold with the understanding that the authors and publisher are not engaged in rendering professional services in the book. If the reader requires personal assistance or advice, a competent professional should be consulted. The authors and publisher specifically disclaim any responsibility for any liability, loss, or risk, personal or otherwise, which is incurred as a consequence, directly or indirectly, of the use and application of any of the contents of this book.

Most Alpha books are available at special quantity discounts for bulk purchases for sales promotions, premiums, fund-raising, or educational use. Special books, or book excerpts, can also be created to fit specific needs. For details, write: Special Markets, Alpha Books, 345 Hudson Street, New York, NY 10014.

Trademarks: All terms mentioned in this book that are known to be or are suspected of being trademarks or service marks have been appropriately capitalized. Alpha Books and Penguin Random House LLC cannot attest to the accuracy of this information. Use of a term in this book should not be regarded as affecting the validity of any trademark or service mark.

Reprinted from *The Complete Idiot's Guide to the Nursing Entrance Exams*

Contents

Introduction

"I want to be a nurse when I grow up!" This phrase is uttered by countless children every day and for good reason. Nursing is a noble profession that is not only personally fulfilling but is also one of the fastest-growing health-care specializations in the country.

According to 2018 projections from the U.S. Bureau of Labor Statistics' Occupational Outlook Handbook, employment opportunities for registered nurses is expected to increase 15 percent by 2026, particularly in long-term care facilities, outpatient care centers, and home-based care. This growth is estimated to be much faster than average, when compared with other professions. And with a current median salary of $70,000 a year, or $33.65 per hour, now is a great time to consider nursing school.

But deciding to become a nurse is only the first step you need to take in the journey to reach your goal. Another step may be passing a standardized entrance examination. There are currently a handful of exams that most two-year and four-year schools require as part of a nursing program admission. These can vary from semester to semester, as well as from school to school.

We offer this book as a general guide to help you decide which program is right for you and prepare you for the various exams that are used to determine eligibility for nursing school programs. Within the pages that follow, you'll find reviews in the disciplines that are most frequently tested, tons of practice questions to help strengthen your knowledge, and test-taking tips that will help you get through any kind of standardized exam.

You may not agree with all of our advice, and some of what we have to say may not work for you as an individual. That's okay. No piece of advice is right for every person. We encourage you to make your test-prep experience your own and pursue whatever works best for you.

When you're using this book, keep in mind that we are giving advice based on our extensive research and personal experience with this subject. The information we provide is the most current that we can offer as of the date that this book was written, and we have made every effort to ensure the accuracy of the information provided.

When in doubt, though, communicate with the program or programs you're applying to in order to get the best advice and information relevant to your goals. They are your first and best source for guidance.

How to Use This Book

Everyone has their own learning style and academic strengths. When you're preparing for tests like those for nursing school entrance, you need to play to those strengths and focus on improving in the areas that are challenging you.

Purchasing this book is a great way to start preparing for your exam. We've tried to make reading and using this book as easy for you as possible. We break down all of the information you need into five main sections, so you can pick and choose what you want to read and when.

Part 1, Decision Diagnosis, describes the many different types of nursing careers. It shows you how the path you choose affects which exams you'll take, the most commonly used exams, what to expect, and how to prepare for and take your test.

Part 2, Say It Right: Verbal Review, discusses reading, writing, vocabulary, spelling, and grammar—all skills that nursing school entrance exams want to assess in potential students. We walk you through the different skills that are tested and provide review and practice that will help you understand and apply these concepts.

Part 3, Math Matters, shows you why mathematics is an extremely important skill for nurses to master and why all of the nursing school entrance exams include at least one math section. This part will help you brush up on your basic arithmetic, algebra, and geometry in preparation for any of these exams.

Part 4, Scientific Method, provides a comprehensive review of earth and life sciences, biology, anatomy and physiology, chemistry, and physics concepts to help you through the scientific sections of your test. Be sure to check out the practice questions at the end of each chapter to test yourself on what you learned.

Part 5, Strength Training: Test Your Skills, gives you a chance to challenge yourself with two sample tests featuring the types of questions often seen on the different types of nursing school entrance exams. We also give you detailed answers and explanations to help you practice your skills and learn from your mistakes.

If you're still thirsty for more, check out the info-packed Resources appendix, which includes a listing of the Boards of Nursing for all 50 states and U.S. territories, a list of professional nursing associations, books, and websites.

Extras

Because we can all use a little extra help, we've also included some sidebars with useful information to help speed you through your studies:

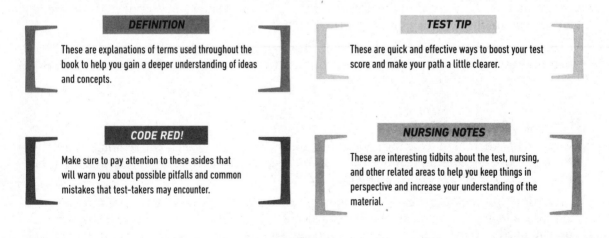

DEFINITION
These are explanations of terms used throughout the book to help you gain a deeper understanding of ideas and concepts.

TEST TIP
These are quick and effective ways to boost your test score and make your path a little clearer.

CODE RED!
Make sure to pay attention to these asides that will warn you about possible pitfalls and common mistakes that test-takers may encounter.

NURSING NOTES
These are interesting tidbits about the test, nursing, and other related areas to help you keep things in perspective and increase your understanding of the material.

Acknowledgments

Maryanne Baudo:

What pleases me most about being an author is the acknowledgement from students who have used the book to gain entrance into the nursing program of their choice. I enjoy hearing from them and thank them for reading it. Robin Kavanagh is very knowledgeable about the process and a pleasure to work with. A thank you to my husband and children for their unending support throughout my career and all undertakings I engage in.

Robin Kavanagh:

Thank you so much Maryanne Baudo, for being the expert in nursing education; Kara LaFrance, for her inspired and always fabulous illustrations; Stephen Butkewitsch, our Technical Editor, for reviewing the math and science chapters for accuracy; my daughter, Jordan Matthews, for being patient as I completed my work on this book; and Marilyn Allen, the best agent in the world. And of course, thank you to our team of editors.

Trademarks

Decision Diagnosis

Deciding to become a nurse is not as easy a decision as many people think. There are many types of nurses and many ways to become a nurse. And for every career and program out there, you'll find a different set of rules and requirements, not the least of which is some kind of entrance exam.

In this part, we introduce you to the different types of nursing careers there are, what your educational options are, and how your certification and career path will affect which entrance exams you'll take. Then we walk you through some of the most commonly used exams and break them down for you, in addition to providing some test-specific tips. Finally, we discuss general test-taking strategies that will help you get through just about any standardized exam.

So, You Want to Be a Nurse?

Some of us are born leaders. Others are born analysts or artists. These types of natural skill sets can make us perfect for some jobs and completely wrong for others. For example, someone who has difficulty understanding basic math concepts, such as percentages or fractions, is not likely to pursue a career as a math professor. Likewise, a person without a sense of tone or rhythm is not likely to become a musician.

Working in the nursing profession requires certain skills, some that you can learn and others that come naturally. Aptitude in math and science are an important part of any job related to nursing, as are communication and analytical skills.

This chapter introduces you to the different types of jobs that fall within the nursing profession and what kinds of education and certifications are needed for them. You'll be able to use this information to decide which career is right for you, to set goals, and to choose which path you want to take to reach them.

The Many Faces of Nursing

The word *nurse* evokes lots of images, depending on your experience with the profession. For example, if you had some kind of surgery or ever needed to go to the emergency room, you may associate nursing with the people who took care of you in the hospital. If you've cared for an elderly relative, you may think of those nurses who work in adult care facilities or come directly to the house.

Although these images of the work a nurse does are accurate, they describe very different types of nursing practices. There are several different career paths you can take within the nursing profession. Choosing which one fits your personal strengths, lifestyle, and preferences will determine what kind of education and certification you should pursue—and ultimately the type of entrance exam you'll need to take.

Here is a look at the two main types of nursing certification programs you're most likely to pursue if you've bought this book.

Registered Nurse

As of the writing of this book, registered nurses (RNs) are the largest group of health-care professionals in the country. About 60 percent of registered nursing jobs are found in hospitals, where RNs are the life-blood of patient care and safety.

RNs perform a variety of functions within the scope of their practice, *assessing* a patient's condition, making decisions on immediate needs, developing a plan of care, executing the plan, and carrying out doctors' orders.

> **DEFINITION**
>
> In nursing, **assessment** refers to asking questions and performing examinations to determine a patient's needs. This leads to taking the proper course of action. Assessment is the main differentiator between RNs and LPNs or LVNs (discussed later in the chapter). RNs are charged with assessing patients as part of their day-to-day responsibilities. LPNs and LVNs usually are not.

RNs also care for patients and their families in ways that doctors often cannot, because doctors specialize in diagnosis and treatment. RNs focus on the following tasks:

▸ Administering treatment plans

▸ Assessing patient needs and reaction to treatment

▸ Informing a patient and family about what is going on and what they need to do

▸ Following up with patients about aftercare or progress of health

▸ Educating the patient and the public about general health issues

Because of this increased interaction with patients, families, and the community at large, RNs are trained in more advanced medical practices and interpersonal communication.

To become an RN, you must be licensed. You can attain this by getting an RN diploma, an Associate's degree, or a Bachelor's degree, and passing the licensure requirements for whichever state in which you are looking to work. These routes are discussed in detail later in this chapter.

Registered nurses can specialize in a variety of areas of medical treatment in four main categories:

▸ Type of setting or treatment, such as emergency or maternity

▸ Type of health issue, such as oncology or rehabilitation

▸ Type of bodily system, such as cardio-vascular or orthopedic

▸ Type of patient, such as pediatric or geriatric

> **TEST TIP**
>
> For an expanded listing of nursing specialties, visit nursing.jnj.com/specialty.

Licensed Practical Nurse/ Licensed Vocational Nurse

Licensed practical nurses (LPNs), also known as *licensed vocational nurses* (LVNs) in some states, have fewer responsibilities than RNs and often work under the supervision of an RN or an advanced practice nurse (APN). Their work is less assessment based and more centered on caring for patients and making sure they have what they need. LPNs focus primarily on the following tasks:

- ▶ Monitoring patients
- ▶ Filling out paperwork and completing other administrative duties
- ▶ Recording vital signs and other readings
- ▶ Collecting lab samples
- ▶ Providing other routine bedside care for patients, including maintaining hygiene, changing bedsheets, and helping them stand or walk

Most LPNs work in facilities that provide basic or long-term health care. These include clinics, hospitals, and college or university health-care centers. Many LPNs also work in doctors' offices, home health-care agencies, and nursing homes, each of which has different demands specific to the type of patients it services.

For example, an LPN in a nursing home may have more of an assessment role than one who works in a hospital, or be allowed to administer medications. LPNs in nursing homes are often charged with developing care plans for patients and overseeing the nurses' aides who administer those plans.

NURSING NOTES

After you are licensed as an LPN, you can opt to gain additional training in various specialties, such as pharmacology or hospice care.

Unlike an RN, an LPN usually completes only a year-long program that focuses on nursing skills related to patient needs and some theory. These programs are usually found in technical schools, community colleges, and hospitals and encompass both classroom and clinical instruction.

Clinical instruction includes patient care and some types of procedures, such as applying dressings, irrigating wounds, and conducting special feedings. An LPN is assessed on those skills. Upon obtaining passing marks from the instructors, the LPN is then assigned to a facility to gain some practical experience under supervision.

When a student has completed his program, he must pass a licensing exam to work as an LPN in a particular state. LPN programs vary from school to school and are sometimes administered through a specific hospital, but most require an entrance exam, such as those discussed in this book.

Advanced Practice Nurses

If your goal is to work as a nurse-midwife or a nurse practitioner, you need to become an advanced practice nurse (APN)—and getting your RN license is just the first step. The RN license can come from a diploma program, an Associate's degree program, or a Bachelor of Science in nursing (BSN) program. You need to complete a BSN in order to apply to a Master's program for nursing (MSN). MSN programs usually require 500 to 700 hours of supervised practice to earn the degree.

As of 2015, APN certification has been incorporated into the Doctor of Nursing Practice degree (DNP). DNP programs require an internship and writing a thesis. A DNP graduate can then sit for the certification exam. Every five years, an APN has to log at least 1,000 hours of clinical practice for recertification.

But after all of that hard work, the payoff can be very rewarding, both personally and financially. APNs use their advanced education in pharmacology and assessment, and expertise in a specialized area, in many different ways that are not open to RNs. They also command higher salaries.

NURSING NOTES

The U.S. Bureau of Labor Statistics estimates that job growth for APNs will be around 31 percent from 2016 to 2026—much higher than the 7 percent projection for all occupations. This is due to increased emphasis of preventative care and need for health-care services among aging populations. Increasingly, APNs are also being viewed as a source for primary health care.

The term *APN* applies to the job titles covered in the following sections.

Nurse Practitioners

Nurse practitioners (more generally called *APNs*) have greater clinical responsibilities than RNs. They have the necessary skills to manage adult and elderly patients with acute and chronic illnesses, order and interpret diagnostic tests, provide counseling and education, and can also perform a wider array of medical procedures. They can diagnose and treat patient illnesses, prescribe medications, perform complete examinations, and follow up with patients, much like a doctor.

You will find nurse practitioners in hospitals, clinics, doctors' practices, home care settings, public health clinics, schools, and other medical facilities, often working side by side with doctors treating patients.

Clinical Nurse Specialists

A clinical nurse specialist (CNS) usually has an area of specialized expertise and works in a hospital or a specialized facility, such as a mental health or a rehabilitation center. They primarily act as a collaborating member of a team that focuses on specific patients with specialized health issues. As a collaborator, they can act in various roles, such as a consultant or a researcher, to improve the quality of care given to the patient.

Nurse-Midwives

Nurse-midwives specialize in gynecological care. As with nurse practitioners, they can assess, diagnose, and treat patients much like a doctor. They can also prescribe medications, such as birth control. Nurse-midwives care for women, both pregnant and not, and help them manage their reproductive health. You'll find nurse-midwives in OB/GYN practices, on-staff in hospitals, and at birthing or family planning centers, as well as in homes conducting home births.

Nurse Anesthetists

Nurse anesthetists specialize in managing anesthesia in patients before, during, and after surgery. They are trained to administer pre-op anesthesia, to monitor its usage and effects during surgery, to bring a patient down from anesthesia, and to manage post-op recovery. Nurse anesthetists work in hospitals and surgical centers under the guidance of an anesthesiologist.

Pediatric Nurse Practitioners

Pediatric nurse practitioners specialize in caring for newborn babies, children of all ages, as well as adolescents up to 18 years old. They monitor growth and development, immunizations, and management of common childhood acute and chronic illnesses. They also provide well-child care to children from birth through young adulthood.

Nurse Educator

After earning an advanced degree in nursing, you can also become a nurse educator. These are APNs who have experience in clinical practice and work in schools of nursing, institutions, and agencies that have staff development departments and education departments. They are a vital part of nursing education—responsible for teaching courses to student nurses and training nursing staff about new procedures or changes taking place.

Nurse educators also work with new employees and recently certified nurses to help them gain their bearings and learn their new jobs. They need to keep current with practices and trends within the health-care field and can also specialize in certain areas, such as diabetes education or wound care.

Education Options

Now that you're familiar with some of the different types of jobs in the nursing field, let's talk about the education you'll need to become one of these highly skilled professionals. Your career goal will determine what type of certification program you'll need to complete. Here is a more detailed look into degree and certificate programs, how they work, and the pros and cons of each.

BSN

The Bachelor of Science in nursing (BSN) degree is a four-year program through which you will gain the kind of education and clinical experience you need to become a licensed RN. But you will also be able to get a lot more out of the time and money you spend on this route to RN certification than you would with a shorter program.

First, your education is broader. BSN programs require more general education courses (usually in liberal arts) than an Associate's degree program. So you can expect that you'll be taking philosophy, arts, and political science courses, in addition to math and English.

Second, your core nursing classes are also significantly different from those found in an Associate's program. In addition to completing several clinical rotations in various specialties (emergency, pediatrics, etc.) at an area hospital, BSN students are required to complete courses in nursing theories, community health, research methodologies, and more. BSN curricula also usually have a thesis seminar that produces a significant body of researched work.

RNs with a BSN are generally considered higher up on the clinical ladder than those with an Associate's degree. Why? One reason is the extra time spent in school. The general education courses, additional theoretical and research studies, and electives in nursing specialties required of Bachelor's degree candidates result in a more mature and experienced RN. They are also considered more educationally rounded.

NURSING NOTES

During the next 10 years, there will be more job opportunities for RNs who have a minimum of a BSN degree than for those who have an ADN or AAS.

ADN/AAS

An Associate's degree in nursing (ADN) or an Associate's degree in applied science in nursing (AAS) can be earned through a technical school or community college. These programs run about two to three years and result in an Associate's degree that can transfer to a Bachelor's program (usually called an RN to BSN program). There may be additional testing that you would have to take before being accepted into a BSN program through this route, but many programs are making it easier for Associate's degree RNs to earn a BSN.

Required courses encompass general education (math, English, humanities, etc.), sciences, health, nursing, medicine, and clinical work at a local hospital, where you apply the skills you've learned. After you've completed all your requirements, you'll need to pass the licensure exam to finish the program. Once this final hurdle is cleared, you will be an RN. The RN licensure exam is the same for the graduate from a diploma program, a BSN program, or an ADN program.

This is a great option for someone who wants to work as a nurse while pursuing a higher degree in nursing, whether for the experience or for the money. It's also a great way to explore the profession before committing to any one specialty or job.

For example, if you're working as an RN with an Associate's degree, you might find a specific area of nursing that you like more than the others. When you pursue a higher degree, you can then get more clinical experience in that specific area. Though most BSN programs have set clinical courses, students can request to be assigned to a certain area for at least one rotation.

Diploma

Some hospitals offer diploma programs for RN licensure. They usually run from two-and-a-half to three years in length and are administered directly through a hospital. Though this path to education and certification is seen less and less these days, it is still a viable option for someone looking to become an RN. It's worth checking out the hospitals in your area to see what programs are offered.

Though you will not have a degree when you take your licensure exam at the end of your program, you should be able to transfer at least some of your classes and experience to an ADN/AAS or BSN program. You will be an RN once you pass the licensure test.

You will, however, need to follow the same admissions process as everyone else—including taking an entrance exam, depending on the program. If the school you're applying to has an accelerated program, you may not have to take the entrance exam. Throughout the program, you will be tested on clinical skills and have to receive passing marks on each in order to continue.

Admissions

After you choose a program to pursue, your next step is applying—a process that is often easier said than done. Nursing programs are very popular and competitive. This is because of the increasing need for qualified professionals in the field, as well as job diversity, salary, and stability that other professions do not offer. Unlike liberal arts or humanities degree programs, nursing programs often require that you have minimum grades in specific courses before you can even apply.

Many programs (mostly two-year Associate's degrees) cap the number of students accepted per year. One of the main reasons for this is because every program needs to provide adequate clinical sites to give students the practical experience they need to become qualified nurses. There is also a declining number of qualified nurse educators who work nursing programs. Fewer educators means fewer students who can attend a clinical course. Board of Nursing guidelines state that the maximum ratio of students to teachers in a clinical unit be 10:1.

This is where nursing school entrance exams come into play. These scores act as a numerical qualifier, so that only the candidates with the most potential to finish and become licensed are admitted into the program. That is not to say that scoring is the only or even the most important variable when applying to a nursing program. It's just one component of many that administrators struggle with every semester when it comes to admitting new students.

CODE RED!

Always aim to get as high a score as possible on your entrance exam. Even though minimums are set, that doesn't mean meeting that score will get you in. For example, if a program only allows in 100 new students per semester, the 100 candidates with the highest scores will move on to the next step in the process.

Admissions testing specific to a nursing program varies from school to school. Most Associate's programs require one of the tests discussed in this book in order to be eligible for admission, while many Bachelor's programs require no entrance examinations at all. These programs use the SAT or the ACT as a qualifying exam.

Very often you'll find that both Associate's and Bachelor's programs will require students to complete prerequisite and general education coursework before being allowed to apply for a nursing major. Completing one of the nursing school entrance exams discussed in Chapter 2 is part of that application process.

Others are less restrictive. Many Bachelor's programs accept incoming high school graduates, without having them take a nursing school entrance exam or prerequisites. One of the reasons for this is that with a four-year education, students have the ability to change their minds and apply the classes they've already taken to a new major. They also have much longer to figure out if nursing fits with their personalities.

CODE RED!

Make sure to check with the program you're applying to for the most up-to-date test requirements. Information on the school's website may not reflect current policy and older materials may reference a testing company that has discontinued offering a particular exam.

Even if you have your heart set on one program or school in particular, there's no guarantee you'll be admitted. Make sure to apply to multiple schools when you're looking to begin your nursing education. True, this may mean that you have to take multiple types of entrance exams. But it's worth it if it means that you are able to begin a program that is right for you at the time that's right for you, as well.

No matter what type of program you're applying to, you should always speak directly with an admissions counselor about the following questions:

▸ What are the admissions requirements?

▸ How are students evaluated for admission?

▸ Is there a maximum number of students allowed into the program, and are applications accepted per semester, per year, or on a rolling basis?

▸ How many people usually apply during an admissions period, and how many are accepted?

▸ What entrance exams are required and what are the minimum scores needed on each?

▸ What prerequisites are required and what are the minimum grades needed for each?

Licensure

After you have completed a nursing school program, you will have to pass one final exam to qualify for licensure. The National Council of State Boards of Nursing administers two standardized exams on the national level for obtaining registered and practical nursing licenses. These are the NCLEX-RN and the NCLEX-PN. It's important to note that passing these exams does not qualify you for a national license. Each state has its own board that oversees licensure and policy, and the state board may require additional training for a nurse to be allowed to practice.

When deciding on a nursing education program, you should take into consideration the state in which you intend to work after you are licensed. Knowing this will help you meet all the requirements that state needs fulfilled in order to practice in that specific state.

Many states have reciprocity, meaning that your license in one state will allow you to practice in some neighboring states. You should contact your state board of nursing (see the appendix for a complete listing) to find out exactly what are your state's requirements for licensure, if they offer reciprocity, and if so, for what other states.

The Least You Need to Know

▸ Research different career paths in nursing and set short-term and long-term goals.

▸ Use your goals to decide which educational route is right for you.

▸ Thoroughly investigate all the programs that meet your needs, and evaluate their entrance requirements.

▸ Apply to more than one program at a time.

▸ Be prepared to take multiple types of entrance exams.

Tests You Need to Make the Grade

As the saying goes, "Anything worth having is worth fighting for." Although you won't be fighting for your nursing certification per se, you will have to complete a lot of work in order to reach your goal—starting with passing your entrance exam.

As discussed in Chapter 1, there are lots of different types of nurses and many different paths to becoming one. Knowing what you want to do with your career and what you need to do to get there is a huge step in advancing toward those goals.

This chapter walks you through the different types of entrance exams you can expect to see when applying to various types of nursing programs, what those exams test you on, how you're evaluated, and how knowing what to expect can help you raise your scores.

Many Paths to the Same Career

After you decide what kind of nurse you want to be, your next step is to choose where to get your education. As you know, there is an array of possibilities to choose from. We recommend researching the different programs available in your area and speaking with an admissions counselor to find out what is required for entrance and expected of students. From there, you can decide which one fits best with your needs.

One thing you may find, however, is that more than one program can help you achieve your goal, but that their entrance requirements are different—particularly when it comes to nursing school entrance exams. For example, both Bergen Community College and Essex County College, located in neighboring counties in New Jersey, offer AAS in nursing programs. Bergen Community College requires the Health Education Systems Exam (HESI), while Essex Community College requires the ATI Test of Essential Academic Skills (ATI TEAS) for all prospective RN students.

Someone who lives close to both schools would likely apply for both programs to increase their chances of being accepted into a local school, and therefore take both exams. That's where this book comes in handy.

The remainder of this chapter introduces you to the five most commonly used nursing school entrance exams and the vital stats you need to know before taking them.

National League for Nursing Pre-Admission Exam (NLN PAX)

The National League for Nursing (NLN) is the leading professional association for nursing education and provides a vast array of educational materials used throughout RN and LPN programs. These include a preadmission exam (called the *PAX*), tests in various subject areas for educators to administer during a nursing program, and preparation for the NCLEX certification exams.

There have been some significant changes to the test in recent years. Though there used to be two versions of the NLN PAX exam, there is now only one: NLN PAX. This is a computer-based test with three sections: verbal, math, and science. Rarely, it may be administered as a paper-and-pencil exam.

When you complete a section or run out of time on one, your answers will be scored behind the scenes, and you will click through to the next section. Experimental questions have been eliminated, so all questions will count toward your score. For this test, always complete as many questions as you can, even if you are making an educated guess.

Scores are reported as both an overall composite and percentages of correct answers for each section. However, unlike many types of computer-based exams, your scores will not be generated immediately. Contact the nursing program to which you are applying for information about how to receive your scores.

NLN PAX Sections and Times

Subject	Skills Tested	Number of Questions	Minutes
Verbal	Word knowledge	60	40
	Reading comprehension		
	Critical thinking		
Math	Numbers and operations	40	40
	Fractions		
	Decimals		
	Percents		
	Algebra		

Subject	Skills Tested	Number of Questions	Minutes
	Geometry		
	Measurement conversions		
Science	Biology	60	40
	Anatomy/ Physiology		
	Chemistry		
	Physics		
	Health		
Total		160	120

Scoring

NLN PAX score reports are relatively simple in their assessment of your test performance and come with a guide to interpreting your scores. When you receive your score report, you can expect to see the following items broken down by section (verbal, math, and science):

▶ **Raw score.** Raw scores show the percentage of questions you got right. The highest raw score for each section is 100 percent.

▶ **Composite score.** Your composite score ranges between 0 and 200 and is an overall score for the totality of your exam. This score is a weighted value of the raw scores based on how you did in relation to the average raw scores of a sample group. The average composite score is 100 and most people's scores range between 50 and 150.

▶ **Percentile norms.** This is a series of three scores for each test section that represents the percentage of test-takers in a sample group who earned raw scores lower than yours.

This means if you got an 89 in Verbal Ability, 89 percent of test-takers in the sample group scored lower than you on this section.

NLN PAX Vital Stats

Now that you've got a general idea of what you're facing on this exam, here are some must-know details about the NLN PAX:

▶ Count on taking the computer-based version of the NLN PAX. This format is talked about specifically later in this chapter.

▶ The NLN PAX will cost about $75.

▶ Every program has different requirements concerning NLN PAX minimum scores. Make sure you know what minimum scores you need to achieve for entrance.

▶ You'll be able to access your scores through your online account, which you create when you register for the exam.

Health Education Systems Exam (HESI) A²

The Health Education Systems Exam (HESI) A² (which is specific to nursing program entrance) is administered by Elsevier through its Evolve Learning System, which provides supplemental online and multimedia tools for nursing programs. Because of this, the HESI is only administered electronically through an online version, software that is incorporated into a school's network, or in testing centers nationwide.

The HESI A² consists of 9 total subtests, 7 of which are based on high school–level math, science, and verbal knowledge. Finally, the last 2 subtests determine your preferred learning and personality styles.

> **CODE RED!**
>
> You don't necessarily have to take all nine subtests. Many programs do not require one or more of the science-based tests. Make sure to double check with your admissions contact to verify what to take and what to avoid.

The following table gives an overview of each of the HESI subtests. Note: We are not including a total time allotted for testing or number of questions, as every program has different requirements for which subtests need to be completed. Also, these are suggested times. Actual times are determined by individual programs.

HESI A² Subtests and Times

Subtest	Skills Tested	Number of Questions	Minutes
Math	Numbers and operations	55	50
	Fractions		
	Decimals		
	Percents		
	Ratio/ Proportion		
	General math facts		
	Measurement conversions		

Subtest	Skills Tested	Number of Questions	Minutes
Reading Comprehension	Health-related passages	55	60
	Main idea		
	In-context vocabulary		
	Inferences		
Vocabulary and General Knowledge	Vocabulary geneally used in health care	55	50
Grammar	Parts of speech	55	50
	Terms and their use		
	Common errors		
Chemistry	Chemical equations	30	25
	Matter		
	Reactions		
	Periodic Table		
	Atomic structure		
	Nuclear chemistry		
	Bonding		
Anatomy & Physiology	General terminology	30	25
	General systems and structures		

Subtest	Skills Tested	Number of Questions	Minutes
Biology	Basic concepts	30	25
	Water		
	Biological molecules		
	Metabolism		
	Cells and cellular respiration		
	Photosynthesis		
Learning Style	Most effective ways you learn	14	15
Personality Style	How your personality relates to your learning style	15	15

Five questions in each section (except the Learning Style and Personality Style tests) are considered "pilot" questions and are not scored.

Because the HESI A² is broken down into so many subtests, programs can pick and choose which ones to consider for admission. This can work to your advantage if you are proficient in some of these areas because all of the sections you complete affect your total score.

For example, it might be a good idea to take the anatomy and physiology (A&P) subtest if you just finished an A&P course and are scheduled to take the HESI A² soon—even if the program you're applying to does not require it. Because the knowledge is fresh in your mind, scoring well on this subtest can raise your overall score. However, if you

struggled in that A&P class, you may want to skip it after all.

Scoring

Because the HESI A² is a CBT, your scores are available immediately after completing the exam. Your *proctor* can print a copy of your scores to take with you, and you can access your scores electronically through the school where you take the test or with the program where you assign your scores.

Score reports are broken down into the following sections:

▸ **Percentage scores.** These scores are given for each subtest and indicate the percentage of questions you answered correctly. Each program sets its own score minimums, though Elsevier gives a recommendation of "excellent," "very good," "satisfactory," and "needs improvement" based on the test-taker's performance on the exam. For most RN programs, you need to score a minimum of 75 percent in all required subtests.

Hospital-based and PN programs usually list 70 percent as their cut-off score.

▶ **Subject-area composite scores.** These scores reflect the average for all subtests completed in a subject area. Depending on which subtests you're required to take, you can see composite scores for English Language and Science.

▶ **Composite scores.** This is your average score for all of the subtests you completed.

HESI A² Vital Stats

The HESI A² is one of the more complex nursing school entrance exams required by different programs nationwide. To help you prepare, here are some extra must-know tidbits:

▶ Fees for taking the HESI A² vary from school to school. They can be as low as $40 and as high as $90.

▶ Some schools may have you take an additional critical-thinking subtest. These results, along with those from the Learning Style and Personality Style subtests, do not count toward your overall score.

▶ The results of the Learning Style and Personality Style subtests include tips for improving study habits and approaching your nursing education.

▶ The HESI A² is highly customizable for different nursing program needs, which is why it's so popular. It's your responsibility to know what's required for your entrance application.

ATI Test of Essential Academic Skills (ATI TEAS)

The Test of Essential Academic Skills (ATI TEAS) is administered by ATI, a nursing education company based in Kansas. ATI produces educational materials and assessment tools for nursing programs to use when selecting potential candidates, teaching student nurses, and preparing them for the National Council Licensure Examination (NCLEX).

ATI TEAS tests nursing candidates on their basic skills in subjects that they have encountered throughout high school. The following is a breakdown of the sections and skills you can expect to see on the ATI TEAS.

ATI TEAS Sections and Times

Subject	Skills Tested	Number of Questions	Minutes
Reading	Key ideas and details	53	64
	Craft and structure		
	Integration of knowledge and ideas		
Math	Numbers and operations	36	54
	Algebra		
	Data interpretation		
	Measurement		
Science	Anatomy and physiology	53	63
	Life science		
	Earth science		

Subject	Skills Tested	Number of Questions	Minutes
	Physical science		
	Scientific reasoning		
English and Language Usage	Conventions of standard English	28	28
	Knowledge of language		
	Vocabulary		
Total		170	209

The ATI TEAS includes about 20 pretest questions that are not scored. This brings the total number of questions to 170, but the number of scored questions to 150.

[**CODE RED!**

Learn more about the ATI TEAS test and access study guides and practice tests at ATITesting.com/TEAS.]

Scoring

ATI TEAS score reports are very detailed in their evaluation of your performance on the test. Each section is broken down into total scores for the section as a whole and every type of question that was presented. For example, the English section report has a total score for the section, and scores for Grammar and Vocabulary in Context, Spelling and Punctuation, and Structure content areas. Each of these content area scores are further broken down into the exact number of questions that were present on the test.

On your score report, you'll find several different metrics by which your performance is measured. They are as follows:

▸ **Adjusted Individual Total Score.** This is provided as a total score for the test, each section, and each proficiency tested within each section. It's calculated by dividing the number of correctly answered questions by the total number of questions. The result is then adjusted based on the assigned difficulty of the form in which it was given (paper-based test versus CBT).

▸ **Overall Academic Preparedness.** This is a classification score that evaluates how prepared you are academically to take on a nursing program. Test-takers are scored from high to low as Exemplary, Advanced, Proficient, Basic, and Developmental. The Basic and Developmental categories are the ones that fall below average.

▸ **Mean Ranks.** These scores tell you what the average score was for your exam among all test-takers within a specified sample. These numbers are reported in terms of test-takers nationally and those who took the test to get into the same type of program to which you're applying.

▸ **Percentile Ranks.** This score shows how you did on the test when compared to a specified sample of test-takers who took the same exam. This is presented in terms of percentages that tell how you did in relation to others who took the exam nationally and for your specific program. Your percentile score represents the percent of test-takers who scored the same or lower than you did.

ATI TEAS Vital Stats

Now that you know what to expect on these exams, let's get into some specifics:

- Every question on the tests is weighted equally.

- Unanswered questions are considered incorrect and scored accordingly. Make sure you answer every question, even if you have to randomly fill in bubbles or click answer choices. Leaving them blank guarantees they'll be marked wrong. However, if you choose an answer, even randomly, you have a 25 percent chance of getting it right.

- Registration fees for the ATI TEAS vary from program to program, but usually range between $20 and $60.

Psychological Services Bureau Registered Nursing School Aptitude Exam

This exam is one of several produced by Psychological Services Bureau, Inc. (PSB), which has been creating entry-level exams for health-care professions since 1955. Participants are asked to respond to 360 items in about 105 minutes.

This exam is broken up into five subtests.

- **Part I: Academic Aptitude:** This is your general math and verbal test with a little twist. Within this subtest you'll find three sections.

- **Verbal:** Has 30 vocabulary-based questions; you'll see synonym, antonym, and analogy questions here.

- **Math:** Has 30 arithmetic-based questions at about an eighth-grade level.

- **Nonverbal:** Has 30 questions related to visual intelligence. You'll be asked to mentally picture shapes and objects and answer questions about their spatial relationships.

- **Part II: Spelling:** Has 50 questions that give you three versions of a word. It's up to you to choose the one that's correctly spelled.

- **Part III: Reading Comprehension:** Has 40 questions based on passages, usually relating to health or science.

- **Part IV: Information in Natural Sciences:** Has 90 questions covering general high school–science topics, such as biology, chemistry, physics, and earth science.

- **Part V: Vocational Adjustment Index:** Has 90 personality-based questions designed to estimate what kind of working environment you would do best in. You only have two choices: agree or disagree. There are no wrong answers.

> **NURSING NOTES**
>
> PSB offers a different exam for those entering PN or VN programs. The Aptitude for Practical Nursing Examination follows the same format, but swaps out the reading comprehension section for one called Judgement and Comprehension in Practical Nursing Situations.

Scoring

Score reports are broken down into several sections and represented in two ways. First is the raw score. This indicates how many questions you answered correctly on a particular part of the test. For example, if you got 50 of the 90 questions on the

Information in Natural Sciences test correct, your raw score would be 50.

The second type of score you'll receive is the percentile score. This shows how your performance on each section of these tests rates in comparison to a group of others who took the PSB test as a requirement for applying to nursing programs throughout the United States and Canada.

Going back to the Information in Natural Sciences example, say your raw score of 50 is better than 72 percent of all the other people who took that section in a specified comparison group. This means your percentile score is 72 and that only 28 percent of test-takers did better than you on this section of the test.

For each test, you'll get a raw and a percentile score. For the Academic Aptitude test, you'll get a total score for the test and scores for each of the subtests.

PSB Vital Stats

To help you prepare, here are some extra must-know tidbits:

▸ PSB offers a few tests for nursing program entrance. They include Registered Nursing School Aptitude Examination (RNSAE); Aptitude for Practical Nursing Examination (APNE); and the Health Occupations Aptitude Examination (HOAE).

▸ Make sure you register for the appropriate test your program requires.

▸ PSB provides several resources for preparing for its exams at psbtests.com/test-resources.

Types of Administration

In this day and age, test administration is serious business. There are entire buildings with strict security standards and high-tech computer systems devoted solely to administering standardized tests. On the other hand, many institutions are still giving exams the old-fashioned way, using pencils, papers, and proctors.

Nursing school entrance exams are no exception to this rule. Just as every program has a different exam requirement, how the tests are administered also varies. Generally, you'll only encounter two formats: paper-based and computer-based tests.

Paper-Based Tests (PBTs)

When most people envision taking a standardized exam, they think of a paper-based test (PBT): booklets, answer sheets with rows and rows of tiny bubbles, number 2 pencils, and a proctor to make sure everyone is completing the exam according to the rules.

When you get to the testing site (usually at the school you're applying to, though you may be directed to a specialized testing center), you'll be checked in and given instructions on where to go, what to do, and when. Make sure you bring a picture ID and a few sharpened pencils. Leave the calculator, food, and beverages at home, as most test-taking facilities ban them.

After all of the administrative stuff is out of the way, the proctor will begin reading instructions and test booklets and answer sheets will be handed out. You will be expected to follow these instructions to the letter.

After the test begins, you will only be allowed to complete one section at a time, and the proctor will let you know how long you have to do so. If you're done with a section before time is called, you'll be allowed to make changes to answers in that section only.

After all the sections have been administered, you will hand in your test materials to the proctor and leave. Official results will be distributed to you and the program you are applying to a few weeks after you take the exam.

Pros: Although this may seem restrictive, the PBT format has its advantages. Remember, the name of the game is to get as many points as possible. PBTs allow you to skip around within a section so that you can play to your strengths and get to all the questions you can easily answer first. This will help you set a pace for the section, enable you to rack up easy points up front, and spend your remaining time on the more difficult questions.

TEST TIP

The skipping-around technique can also help battle test-taking anxiety. Knowing that you're quickly conquering questions can boost your confidence and help you navigate the test more easily.

You also have the ability to write in your test booklet, circle answers, cross out choices you think are wrong, and complete your math work right next to the problems, all of which can help you get to the best answer more quickly.

Cons: You have to wait until the time for each section runs out before you can move on to the next section, which means you are going to be taking the test for the maximum amount of time possible. Speaking of waiting, that's exactly what you'll be doing to find out how you did. Official score reports are sent via snail mail, as opposed to the computer-based tests, which generate unofficial results at the end of the test.

Scheduling may also be more restrictive if you have to take a PBT. A proctor must be present to handle all the paperwork and maintain a controlled environment, so there is often a minimum number of test-takers that must be signed up for the exam in order for it to be scheduled. The center or school administering the test may also only offer it on set dates.

There is also a certain margin of error when filling out the answer sheets. Because the answer bubbles are so close together in tight rows, it's easy to skip a line or fill in two choices in one line (which is a no-no). If you notice right away, no big deal; just erase, fix the error, and move on. But if you complete several questions after making this kind of mistake, fixing it can eat up your test time. And then there's always the possibility that you don't notice at all, which can have dire consequences on your score.

Computer-Based Tests (CBTs)

You'll find that more and more test companies are providing nursing programs with a computer-based test (CBT) option. These can be administered on campus, at a specified testing center, or online, depending on the test. CBTs offer test-takers a great alternative to the traditional fill-in-the-bubble paper test, which is why many programs are now choosing this type of administration.

Generally, there are two types of CBTs you'll encounter for entrance exams: computer adaptive (CAT) and *linear*.

DEFINITION

Linear means "in a line." In relation to CBT administration, this means that the questions are given to you in a way similar to a PBT. A paper-test booklet has a set number of questions listed in a set order, usually offering several on one page. Linear CBTs still have those questions in a set order, but you're limited in how many you can see at one time.

With a CAT test, the program draws from a large bank of questions. The test then adapts which questions you are given based on how you perform on previous questions. For example, the first question in every section is at a medium level of difficulty. If you get that one correct, the next question will be a little harder. If you got that first question wrong, the second will be a little easier. As of the time this book was written, the nursing school entrance exams do not use a CAT format; however, this could change in the coming years.

Many standardized tests, such as the GMAT, GRE, MAT, and other academic evaluations, are administered through a CAT system, which is currently not used for nursing entrance exams. It is important to know about this type of exam, however, so that should you learn about CAT strategies from other resources, you know that they don't apply to all CBTs. Also, the NCLEX is given in CAT format, so your experience on your nursing school entrance exam may not help you so much when it comes to approaching the licensing exam.

The entrance exams discussed in this book follow the linear format. This type of test draws from a finite number of questions of various levels of difficulty. The questions usually are not given in any type of order related to their difficulty, so there's no way to gauge how you are doing throughout the test.

You will be presented with one question at a time within a section, along with a timer so you can keep track of your pace. Work through the question, click on your answer, and move on. Unlike with a CAT test, linear CBTs allow you to skip a question and come back to it later. When you have completed all the questions in a section, you submit the whole section to be scored and move on to the next.

TEST TIP

No matter which version of the test you take, always answer every question. Try to narrow down your answer choices and make an educated guess—one based on logic rather than chance.

Pros: Being able to jump around in a section is very helpful because you can quickly answer questions that are easy for you, saving time for the more difficult ones. You can also go back and change your answer if you have second thoughts or if you remember some important information that influences your answer.

Another great thing about CBTs is that they are easier to administer, offer test-takers more flexibility in scheduling, and can deliver scores more quickly. At the end of your CBT, you will get an unofficial account of how you did; official score reports are generated later and sent out via snail mail.

Finally, you can move through the test at your own pace, not a proctor's. With PBTs, you have to wait for a section's time limit to run out before moving on to the next part. With a CBT, you can start the next section the moment you're done with the previous one. That means less overall time spent testing.

Cons: Though the ability to skip around on a linear CBT is a big pro, it also has its drawbacks. First, it increases the chances that you'll forget to answer a question. Say you skip question 2 because you weren't sure how to answer it. You can't see that the line of bubbles on your answer sheet for question 2 is blank, so it's easier to forget that you have to go back and try that one again.

Second, you can't cross out answer choices or complete math work on a computer screen. For more visual or kinesthetic learners (those who learn and work best by seeing or doing), this can be a big drawback. You can use scratch paper to keep track of your thoughts, jot down notes, or work out your math problems. This creates distance, though, between your thought process (on the paper) and where you record your answer (on the screen), which increases your margin of making a mistake.

TEST TIP

Use your scratch paper when you take a CBT to complete your process of elimination. Writing lists of A, B, C, D and then crossing out the ones you want to discard can make it easier for you to get to the right answer. It also is a good back-up if you forget which answer you want to select between looking at your scratch paper and the screen. See Chapter 3 for more format-specific test tips.

How to Use This Info

Knowing how your entrance exam will be administered can really help you in determining your test-taking strategy. Take the information we've given you and use it to evaluate your strengths and weaknesses and to devise a plan-of-action for scheduling and taking your test. For example, if you know that you're not comfortable with computers, but you're scheduled for a CBT version of the

NLN PAX, you can plan to spend some time beforehand becoming familiar with the demo version on the NLN website.

Similarly, if you know that writing things down helps you remember better or figure out questions, you might want to look into registering for a PBT version of your exam if possible. Then you'll be able to write on your test book and cross off answer choices without having to go back and forth between scratch paper and a computer screen.

Do some research into what your options for taking your entrance exam are and then use the information we've given you in this chapter to devise an approach that works best for you.

The Least You Need to Know

▶ There are a variety of different exams used for nursing school entrance criteria.

▶ Each exam has different parameters, requirements, and scoring methodologies.

▶ Every nursing program uses entrance exam scores differently and has different standards.

▶ There are two main types of testing administration: paper-based tests and computer-based tests.

▶ The type of test you take will determine your test-taking strategy.

Positive Test Results— Stat!

At some point, somebody must have told you that you can't study for a standardized test. If that were true, test preparation companies wouldn't be making millions teaching high school and college students how to pass their college or grad school entrance exams—and there wouldn't be books like this one on library shelves.

The truth is test prep works! Unlike an English or a math test you may have taken in high school or college, mastery of the material you're being tested on is only one piece of the puzzle when taking a standardized exam. Knowing how to take the test is as much a part of your score as finding the right answers. This is what most test-preparation courses focus on: teaching you how to take the test. And believe it or not, your scores do go up when you understand how the questions are structured, what to look for, and what to expect at every turn.

This chapter introduces you to some different ways of approaching how you prepare for and take standardized exams. These strategies will help you use the test structure to your advantage, calm your anxieties, and keep you focused on what you need to do to succeed.

Practice Tests and Planning Strategies

Although studying the subject areas you'll find on the test and learning about new strategies for taking this type of exam are extremely helpful tools, practicing is the best way to prepare. But blindly taking practice test after practice test just to get experience doesn't make much sense. It also takes a lot of time that you could be using more wisely. Your best bet is to think strategically about what you need to accomplish when you take your actual nursing school entrance exam and then plan your study approach accordingly.

Aim High

In Chapter 1, we talked about how getting into the nursing program of your choice is dependent on many factors. Probably the most important is the limit on the number of new students accepted at any one time.

A quick way for admissions committees to whittle down the list of candidates is to require minimum test scores. These scores are general guidelines for admission, but attaining that minimum score does not guarantee that you've made it over this particular hurdle. It also depends on how many other candidates scored higher than you, and how they stand up to the rest of the admission requirements.

Admissions committees will often take a list of scores and choose those who have scored highest and then make their way down the list until they've reached their admissions quota. These candidates are moved on to the next round of consideration. Should one not meet the program's requirements during the rest of the admissions process, the next person on the list of scores will be forwarded along. This goes on and on until the quota is filled.

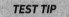

TEST TIP

Applying to multiple programs at the same time will help you increase your chances of being accepted in the semester you want to start your nursing education. Remember, though, that nothing is guaranteed.

Because of this method of candidate evaluation, you want to score as high as possible

on your entrance exam so that you have the best chance of being moved to the next round of consideration.

Play to Your Weaknesses

Ever hear the phrase, "work smart, not hard"? That's good advice for life in general, but especially when it comes to preparing for standardized exams. Because time and energy are usually at a premium when studying for these types of tests, you need to take a strategic approach to how you prepare. A good rule of thumb is to spend more time on the subjects you know have been difficult for you in the past than on subjects you are strong in.

For example, you may have a natural aptitude for science. It has always come easily to you and you genuinely enjoyed taking every science class you've ever had. Because of this, chances are that you will know a good amount of the science-based materials on whichever nursing school entrance exam you take. Refreshing yourself on the topics specific to the test should have you in good shape rather quickly.

However, say you've never been particularly strong in your English courses. Because verbal skill is a core component of every nursing school entrance exam—and some schools may not require that you take certain science sections at all—it makes sense to focus a good amount of your study time on strengthening your verbal skills.

Rethink Your General Approach

If you're like most people, in school you liked multiple-choice tests better than any other kind. Who can blame you? Essay tests were full of writing out ideas and facts that you may or may not know. Same with definitions or fill-in-the-blank tests. But with multiple choice, all of the answers were already there! Even though many people hope for multiple-choice quizzes in the classroom, when it comes to standardized tests, the thought of them can be very nerve racking—even though logically they shouldn't be. The answers are all still there; the main difference is that there are more questions to answer.

We're here to tell you to relax. Most nursing school entrance exams are based on general knowledge you've gained by finishing high school—not on what you will know by the time you're certified. So you're already starting off with a big advantage because you've essentially been studying for the test for at least 12 years. With a little brushing up on the subject matter, you should be in good shape for handling the questions.

Now, let's talk about how to attack those questions. It's your job to choose the answer that will get you the points, which can be more complicated than it sounds. Multiple-choice exams are essentially guessing games. How you would phrase the answer isn't necessarily how the answers you have to choose from are presented.

However, if you adjust the way you approach these questions, you'll be able to get to the correct answers more easily and quickly. The following sections outline some smart steps that should be your general approach to any multiple-choice question on a standardized exam. Although throughout this book you'll see more individualized techniques suggested for specific types of questions, these steps should be your go-to approach when faced with most standardized test questions.

Read Carefully

First, always start by making sure that you read the directions and your question very carefully before deciding what a likely answer is. One of the biggest mistakes test-takers make is to assume they know what they're supposed to do on every question. And because you're under tight time constraints, it's very tempting to do this.

However, this is a surefire way to end up missing crucial information in the question itself that leads to the correct answer. Always take your time and make sure you fully understand what the question is asking.

> **TEST TIP**
>
> Pay close attention to questions that have the word not in them. They ask you to do the reverse of what you normally would on a question. Instead of searching for the one answer choice that the question content supports, you're looking at three answer choices that the question backs up and one that doesn't fit. That one is your answer.

Speak for Yourself

After reading the question, your first instinct may be to go right to the answer choices. But doing this may sway your opinion on the correct answer, which you want to avoid.

Instead, take a minute to jot down your own answer to the question. You can use your test booklet if you're taking a paper-based test (PBT) or scratch paper if you're taking a computer-based test (CBT). This will help ensure that your answer makes sense to you and that you remember it when you look at the answer choices. Believe it or not, it's very easy to forget your original answer when you start evaluating the answers on the test.

Find the "Best" Answer

Now that you have the answer you think is right, it's time to look at the answer choices you have to work with. Most standardized questions don't ask you to choose the right answer; they ask you to find the best answer out of the four choices you're given. Chances are, your answer is a lot better and makes more sense to you than the answer choices. But your task is to find the choice that the test says is the right one.

This is all part of the test design strategy. Those who write these exams want to see that you can not only come up with the correct answer but also recognize it in varying forms.

The test writers also have to be very careful about how their answer choices are worded so that there are very definite reasons why one is better than all the rest. This works to your advantage as a test-taker. Look for specifics in the question or within your realm of knowledge to give logical reasons why the answer you select is correct. If the logic isn't there, chances are the answer is wrong.

Use Process of Elimination— Every Time

Process of elimination is your best friend with multiple-choice exams in general. If you think about it, it makes more sense to look for answers that are wrong simply because there are more of them. Some will be so obviously wrong that you can cross them off quickly. However, others will give you pause. This is where having an answer in mind will help you the most.

Use the answer you came up with on your own to help you narrow possible "best" answers when there is more than one possibility. Consider each choice and eliminate anything that doesn't fit your

original answer. If you can get your odds down from one correct answer out of four to something like one correct answer out of two, your chances of selecting the correct answer go way up.

> **CODE RED!**
>
> Always choose an answer choice that makes a logical connection to the information you're working with—don't just take an instinctual guess.

Go through all the answer choices before making your selection—even if you're 100 percent sure that your answer is right. Often answer choices are arranged to make you think one is correct at first glance. Using process of elimination will slow you down a little, and you'll be able to think your answer through a little more before marking your choice.

It's also important to be flexible when it comes to your answers; the choices you're given may not match what you were thinking. When this happens, try thinking about the question and your answer from a different direction, or go over the way you came up with your answer to make sure you didn't miss something.

For example, if you're working on a vocabulary question and none of the answer choices match the definition you have in your head, ask yourself if there is another definition of the word that the question could be asking you about. Many words have multiple definitions, and it's a common test design strategy to use these lesser-known definitions on the exam.

The Guessing Game

One question most test-takers have is whether they should guess on the test. The answer is yes—and no—for nursing school entrance exams. Some tests will not penalize you for leaving questions blank. Those questions are not scored and your score is calculated based on the number of questions answered. For other tests, particularly the ATI TEAS (see Chapter 2), unanswered questions count the same as incorrect answers, which could affect your score.

Either way, it's in your best interest to complete each question. On tests where you're not penalized for leaving answers blank, you can pick up extra points. On the tests where you are penalized, there's really nothing to lose by guessing at the answers. If you're wrong, your score will be the same as if you just skipped it. But if you're right, you get the points.

So when we talk about guessing, does that mean you should just randomly select answers on questions you're having trouble with? No way. This is a wasted opportunity. If you don't know what the answer to the question is, you can still eliminate answer choices that you know are not correct and then make an *educated guess* based on what's left.

> **DEFINITION**
>
> An **educated guess** is when you choose an answer based on some kind of logic or using information that you have. It's always best to make an educated guess instead of a random one because it increases your chances of getting the question correct.

Eliminating answers that you know are not right is a great way to start making your educated guess. It automatically increases your chances of getting the question right. Think about it. On any given question ...

▸ You have a 25 percent chance of choosing the answer that will get you points.

▸ If you can eliminate one answer, you increase your chance to 33 percent.

▸ If you eliminate two answers, you have a 50 percent chance of choosing the right answer.

Even if you have no idea what the question is asking, you tip the odds in your favor by eliminating at least one of the answers. The beauty of the standardized test format is that you can do this, even if you don't know what the question is asking!

Here are some specific things to look for in answer choices—usually, telltale signs that those choices are not the best answer:

▸ **Extremes or absolutes.** Test writers like to keep things neutral. If an answer choice has words that indicate some type of condition that is too far to one side—good or bad—it's likely this is not what you're looking for. Watch out for words such as *never, always, furious, enraged, overjoyed,* or anything else that hints at an extreme situation.

▸ **Contradictory information.** Many times, particularly in verbal sections, answer choices directly contradict information given in the question, information you're asked to read in a passage, or even another answer choice. If it goes against what's in the question or passage, that's a dead giveaway that the choice is most likely wrong. If it goes against another answer choice, this is a signal that at least one of these answers is wrong—and that one is right. Spend some time here to figure out which one is your best bet.

▸ **Similarities.** When you see two answers that are very close in meaning, it's easy to get stuck trying to figure out whether there's a trap there. Generally when this happens, neither answer is correct, and the only thing you gain is more time passed on the clock. If your instincts are telling you that something's there, see what other answer choices you can eliminate; then come back to these and look for specific reasons you think one might be correct. In most cases, you'll find the correct answer elsewhere.

Test-Specific Strategies

In Chapter 2, we talked about how nursing school entrance exams are administered as PBTs and CBTs—though most are CBTs these days. You'll need to know which type of test you're going to be taking and adjust your test-taking strategies based on this information. Use these test-specific strategies in addition to the general tips we give you throughout this book.

For paper-based tests, follow these tips:

▸ **Take notes.** Make use of the test booklet (which you can write on) or scratch paper you're given during the test to write down your thoughts, take notes, and cross off answer choices you don't need. These can be invaluable ways to work through questions, especially if you learn best by both seeing and doing.

▸ **Watch where you mark.** Filling in the right bubble on the wrong line is common. To prevent this, block out all the lines of answer bubbles for the questions following the one you're answering with your test booklet or scratch paper. Also, always check and double-check that you are filling in the right bubble in the right space. If you make a mistake, make sure you completely erase your mark.

▸ **Skip carefully.** You can move back and forth among questions in a single section. Use this to your advantage by skipping questions that you're having difficulty answering and move on to something else. When you do this, make sure that you continue to mark your answer in the correct spaces on the answer sheet.

▸ **Keep an eye on the clock.** Keep your pace steady by not spending too much time on any one question. This will help you get to each question before time is called.

▸ **Know about penalties.** Some exams treat unanswered questions like ones that are incorrect. Others give no penalty at all. Knowing how your test is scored will help you when it comes to crunch time. If it looks like you're running out of time and your test penalizes for unanswered questions, fill in random answers to complete the section. You have nothing to lose, but you could pick up a few stray points by doing this. If there's no penalty, then answer as many questions as possible.

> **TEST TIP**
>
> One of the best but most-overlooked study strategies is taking timed practice tests. Make sure you study the subject matter for each section. Then practice completing those sections in the time frame you'll face when taking the real thing.

For computer-based tests, follow these tips:

▸ **Skip carefully.** As with PBTs, some CBTs allow you to skip questions and go back to them before submitting the section you're working on for scoring. If your test allows you to do this, skipping difficult questions is a great strategy to use on a CBT—but only if you remember to go back to the question later. First, make absolutely sure that you can go back and forth among questions before choosing to skip anything. Then if you do, make a note for yourself on your scratch paper to remind yourself to return to those questions.

▶ **Watch where you click.** Choosing a different letter than the choice you mean to mark is a common mistake on a CBT. To avoid this, use your scratch paper to write down the answer choices and cross off the ones you want to eliminate. Circle the one that you believe is correct and then check and double-check that the answer you're selecting onscreen matches it. After you make your selection, you'll be prompted to confirm that this is your choice. Take this opportunity to check again. Better safe than sorry.

▶ **Know before you go.** Get as familiar with your exam as possible before test day. Many of the companies that administer CBT nursing school entrance exams have some kind of online or app-based practice version. Go to the company website (see the appendix for a list of URLs) and look to see what's available. When you sit down for the test, spend as much time going through the tutorial as you need so that you're comfortable moving forward.

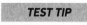

TEST TIP

The time spent on the tutorial is free time, so make the most of it.

Practice Makes Perfect

Planning a path to your future is exciting stuff. Riding the wave of adrenaline at the thoughts of your life to come as a nurse can get you pumped for studying for your entrance exam. So pumped, in fact, you may be tempted to set unrealistic goals for yourself, which can undermine your efforts to prepare.

You can plan to invest quite a bit of time and effort into preparing for your exam—in addition to school, work, family, friends, sports, or whatever else you have going on in your life. But finding a balance is essential to your success. That's why it's important that you get the most out of your study time. Let's look at some often-overlooked yet highly effective ways to make sure your efforts will make the most impact on test day.

Timing Is Everything

A certain amount of anxiety accompanies any timed test and is a major contributor to poor test performance. If you're a slow reader or have marked test-taking anxiety, these issues can become even more pronounced when taking your nursing school entrance exams. The best remedy for this is to practice under the same time constraints you'll face on test day.

The more you practice at home, the better idea you'll have about what pace to set, how much time to spend on your questions, and how to keep yourself on target with the clock. Timing yourself also goes a long way toward making you more comfortable with working against the clock. The calmer you are when you take the test, the better the experience will go.

Study Strategically

It doesn't matter whether you're preparing for every section of your exam or only one or two, breaking down the material you're studying into smaller parts is a great way to manage your study time. This will keep you from feeling too overwhelmed with information in one sitting. Keeping your mind concentrated in one area will also increase your chances of retention.

Additionally, always make sure that no matter what you're studying, you work on a handful of practice questions every time. Reading and memorizing is great, but you'll benefit from it more if you can apply it right away. For example, if you're studying word roots to prepare for a vocabulary section, answer a few practice questions in the book or online, to apply what you learned to actual questions.

TEST TIP

Completing practice questions is a great way to study. You'll learn new information from the ones you got wrong. And because you missed the right answer the first time, you're more likely not to miss it if you see a similar question later.

Study Smart

When you sit down to take your entrance exam for real, you'll want to be as comfortable with it as possible. So it's not very realistic to expect to be ready for the test in a week or even two. To effectively study for this test, you need time. Our advice is to schedule a little time every day over a few weeks to work on your skills, so it doesn't seem like such a huge task. An hour a day is all you need. This will spread out the work and keep your stress level down.

Some tips for doing this include the following:

▶ Give yourself enough time to realistically prepare for the test. Take the time you need to study now so you can do your best the first time around.

▶ Look at your schedule for the next six to eight weeks and pencil in some study time every day. Then stick to it.

▶ Choose a place where you're comfortable and where you'll be undisturbed, preferably someplace without a phone or computer.

▶ Leave the rest of your hectic life behind. Your study time is yours. Don't let any other worries or concerns about other aspects of your life take precedence.

▶ Have everything you need close at hand. Having to go from one room to another wastes a lot of time.

▶ Don't beat yourself up for missing a study session or two. Life can be unpredictable. Try to adjust your routine if you need to, or sneak in some extra study time later.

Final Preparations

After weeks of preparing and thinking about the worlds of possibilities riding on your results, your blood pressure may be sky-high the week you're scheduled to take your entrance exam. Putting everything in perspective now is more important than ever.

Taking a nursing school entrance exam is not rocket science, nor is it your one-and-only shot at a prosperous future. It's a test, plain and simple. It's made of paper and ink (or, in the case of the CBTs, software coding). Spill your water on it, and it goes back to just being man-made material that sits on your desk.

Now that you've got your head in the game, here are some other things you can do to make sure you're in the best shape possible—and they have nothing to do with studying.

The Week of the Test

Your first instinct the week leading up to your exam date may be to cram as much study time in as possible. This can actually be counterproductive. Some better choices would be to ...

▸ **Take some time off.** A day or so before the test, ease back on the preparation. Better yet, stop altogether. This will give your brain a chance to rest so that it's in top shape on test day. Instead, schedule in some leisure time with friends, family, or your favorite Xbox game.

▸ **Get some sleep.** Try to get as much sleep as you can the week of the test. One night's rest is not enough if you want to be as rested and relaxed as possible for the test.

▸ **Pack what you need the night before.** Make sure you have everything you need for the exam with you and ready to go. A photo ID is a must. If you have to borrow or sharpen pencils in the middle of the test, you'll lose precious time. Bring at least five sharp no. 2 pencils for the PBT. Find out from your test administrator other specifics you'll need, and what you can't bring to the site.

The Day of the Test

There are a few things that you'll need on test day to help get you through the hours ahead:

▸ **Eat something.** Have a little something with protein the morning of the test. This will help keep your blood sugar up and hunger at bay. The last thing you want is a grumbling stomach while you're trying to concentrate. You also don't want to be overly full, so keep it light. Protein bars are a good (and tasty!) idea.

▸ **Arrive early.** Arrive at least 15 minutes before the test begins, to take care of any administrative business and ensure you get the seat you want. Traffic and unforeseen events are not excuses for being late to the test, so allow yourself ample time.

▸ **Come up with a plan B.** If you're not feeling well, have a fever, or have recently gone through a stressful or emotional event (good or bad), your test scores may not accurately reflect your abilities. Don't be afraid to reschedule the test. Talk to the test administration company or your admissions contact about options if your personal circumstances are not optimal on test day or the days leading up to it.

After the Test

Whether you think you did great on your test, bombed it, or simply aren't sure about your performance, now is the time to chill. The worst is over; take some time to …

- **Celebrate!** Congratulations! You made it through. Make sure you do something nice for yourself as a reward. Now is not the time to worry about how well you did or worry about whether or not you're going to make the admissions cut. You've worked hard to get through your test and that is worth celebrating.

- **Keep things in perspective.** Waiting for the final word on your scores can be daunting in the weeks following your exam. Try to focus on other things in your life so that the waiting game doesn't get to you.

The Least You Need to Know

▸ Rethinking your general approach to taking a standardized test can help you score better.

▸ Use the multiple-choice format of the test to your advantage by eliminating incorrect answers.

▸ When in doubt, take an educated guess on a question you're not sure about to increase the chances of choosing the correct answer.

▸ You can use different strategies to approach the PBT and CBT versions of various nursing school entrance exams, so know which one you're taking and study accordingly.

▸ Make the most of your study time by taking a strategic approach, timing yourself, and practicing good study habits.

▸ Preparations for what to do before, during, and after the test can help take some of the stress off of you.

PART 2

Say It Right: Verbal Review

For nurses, being able to read, write, and use vocabulary is a necessity. Whether it's for building relationships with colleagues and patients or for accurately carrying out orders, nurses need strong verbal skills to do their jobs effectively and safely.

In this part, you'll learn about the different kinds of verbal sections you'll encounter on most nursing school entrance exams. These include grammar, vocabulary, and reading comprehension. You'll also get some good practice for the types of questions you'll likely face on test day. Plus, you'll get lots of tips for improving your vocabulary, breaking down questions, and translating those pesky paragraphs into real English.

Ⓐ Ⓑ Ⓒ Ⓓ

Ⓐ Ⓑ Ⓒ Ⓓ

Ⓐ Ⓑ Ⓒ Ⓓ

Ⓐ Ⓑ Ⓒ Ⓓ

Ⓐ Ⓑ Ⓒ Ⓓ

Ⓐ Ⓑ Ⓒ Ⓓ

Grammar: It's How You Say It

Ah, grammar. It's the glue that holds our sentences together, enabling us to understand each other through a shared knowledge of how ideas are communicated through language. But so many rules about proper grammatical structure and usage make it difficult and frustrating for many people to get a clear understanding of how grammar works.

What's more, most primary school curricula spend years teaching you all about grammar, but taper off in this area of education in high school. Many who are preparing for a nursing school entrance exam haven't studied grammar since the eighth grade! Yet five out of the six main exams have some kind of grammar component included in their verbal assessments, which means it's time to bone up on your skills.

That's where this chapter comes in. It takes you through the basic grammatical concepts that you'll likely encounter on the test and gives you an idea of what these questions are going to look like. You'll also get some review in spelling, punctuation, and commonly misused words that will help you get through those verbal sections that aren't quite about grammar, but are close enough.

What to Expect

If you are taking the HESI A², ATI TEAS, or PSB, you can expect to see some kind of grammar, punctuation, or spelling component on your exam. This may sound like a scary prospect, but the fact that you're taking a multiple-choice test works to your advantage here.

In Chapter 3, we talked about how this format makes taking a test much easier because all the answers are there, you just have to figure out which one is the right one. When we're talking about grammar, this also means that you don't need to recite rules and define terms, you just have to be able to identify when these rules and terms are applied correctly—and when they're not.

In many cases, this is as easy as spotting the sentence or answer choice that doesn't "look" or "sound" right. When this happens, look for telltale signs of one of the common errors we discuss in this chapter. Chances are, you'll find one and know how to answer the question.

> **CODE RED!**
>
> Be careful here. When something doesn't sound right, you should pay extra attention to that issue, but don't automatically assume it's wrong. There is a big difference between proper grammar and the grammar used in everyday language. How you say something doesn't mean that it's grammatically correct.

Another great thing about the format these exams have is that they're standardized, which means that the types of questions you'll get are pretty predictable. Here is what you can expect to see:

▸ **Grammar:** Choose the answer that shows the version of a sentence is grammatically correct or incorrect; answer choice or type of word will make the sentence grammatically correct; answer choice is an example of a certain part of speech or structure in a sentence; word in the sentence is not used correctly; and word should be used to replace a specific word in a sentence.

▸ **Common errors:** Choose the answer that defines or identifies various structures, such as subject, predicate, independent clause, subordinate clause, etc.; identifies and/or corrects the type of structural error shown in a sentence, such as a misplaced modifier, preposition at the end of a sentence, incorrect subject/verb agreement, etc.; identifies/corrects run-on sentences and fragments; uses the correct tense, spelling, or case of a word; and defines sentence structures.

▸ **Punctuation:** Choose the answer that shows which punctuation mark is missing from the sentence; which sentence is correctly punctuated; and where the punctuation should go to make the sentence correct.

▸ **Spelling:** Choose the answer choice that is spelled correctly or presents the correct spelling of a word within the context of a sentence.

Not too bad, right? To make it even easier to get to the right answers on these questions, you'll want to follow the general approach described in Chapter 3, with a little twist:

1. Read the question carefully and identify what kind of issue you're being asked to address (use the preceding information as a guide).

2. Identify what kind of answer you're looking for or the rule that's being tested. Write down what you think the answer should be or should look like.

3. Use process of elimination to get rid of the answer choices that do not match your answer.

Now it's time to jump into a review of the basic parts of speech, sentence structures, and punctuation. Then we'll move on to common errors to look out for and misspelled/misused words you'll want to memorize.

Parts of Speech

It's probably been a long time since you were introduced to parts of speech, the building blocks of our language. You were probably in first or second grade when you moved from being able to read to learning the mechanics of how those sentences worked. It's here that you first heard about nouns, verbs, adjectives, and adverbs—and then addressed them in every language arts or English class until you got to high school.

Well, not much has changed since then—except for the fact that knowing what these types of words do and how they relate to each other is essential to passing your nursing school entrance exam. To help you out, here is a quick overview of the main parts of speech you'll need to be familiar with for the test.

Nouns

These are words that name people, places, things, or ideas. *Cat, boy, shoe, communism,* and *park* are all nouns and generally fall into one of two cases: singular (meaning one) or plural (meaning more than one).

Here are a couple types of nouns you should be aware of:

Common nouns: These are your general nouns, like the ones mentioned here. These can be either singular or plural: one cat, two cats; one boy, two boys.

Proper nouns: These identify specific people, places, things, or ideas. For example, *Fluffy* is the proper noun for a specific cat who is named Fluffy. *George* is the proper noun for a boy with that name. Proper nouns are always capitalized and are often singular, but can also be plural.

Possessive nouns: These are nouns that show ownership of something. For example, the phrase "the cat's toy" is broken down into a definite article ("the"), a possessive noun ("cat's"), and a common noun ("toy"). Possessive nouns are differentiated from plural nouns with an apostrophe. With a singular possessive noun, the apostrophe is placed between the end of the word and the "s"; the plural possessive noun has the apostrophe after the "s":

▸ Singular possessive noun: "cat's toy" means one toy belonging to one cat

▸ Plural possessive noun: "cats' toy" refers to one toy belonging to more than one cat

> **TEST TIP**
>
> A good trick for quickly distinguishing between a simple plural case and a possessive case is to look for an apostrophe. If it's there, you're dealing with possessive. If not, you're dealing with plural.

Collective nouns: These nouns are used to name a group and are generally treated as singular, even though they refer to many people or things. For example, a nursing class is made up of many students. *Class* is a collective noun because it names the group of students. When you refer to the class as a whole, you treat it as a singular noun and give it a singular verb:

> The class *is* taking a field trip tomorrow.

However, should you use the plural form of a collective noun, your verb will still be plural:

> The classes *are* taking a field trip tomorrow.

Some common collective nouns are: band, troupe, troop, clan, gaggle, battery, deck, class, den, belt, armada, army, herd, convoy, fleet, athletics, physics, and economics. The rule of thumb is that it's a collective noun if the term is used to identify one entire category, group, association, or school of thought.

Proper names of countries are also considered collective nouns and should take the singular case:

> Indonesia *is* recovering from a recent earthquake.

However, if you're talking about the specific people of a country, you are then looking at a plural case, because you are no longer focusing on the country itself, but its people:

> The people of Indonesia *are* recovering from a recent earthquake.

These last few examples will come into play when we discuss subject/verb agreement later in the chapter, because this is a common grammatical bugaboo on these types of tests.

Pronouns

These are words that stand in the place of nouns. *He, she, it, they,* and *we* are all pronouns. It's important to note that pronouns fall into several categories, and many are subject to singular and plural cases.

The following table explains the different types of pronouns, what they do in a sentence, as well as their singular and plural forms. This is a good table to memorize if you're not comfortable with how pronouns are used.

Types of Pronouns

Type	Function	Singular	Plural/ Example
Personal	Replaces person or thing	he, she, it, me, you, him, her, I	we, us, they, you, them
Possessive	Shows possession, ownership	his, hers, its mine, yours, my, your	our, ours, their, theirs, your, yours
Relative	Begins a clause that modifies the antecedent	who, whom, whose, which, that	Ex: The man *who* bought the necklace was kind.

Verbs

These are words that show action or some state of being. A sentence needs to have a verb to be considered a sentence. Although verbs are a necessary part of our language, they can also be very tricky.

Verbs in their base form are called *infinitives* and are preceded by the word *to.* Changing a verb from its base form into some other form is called *conjugation*. These are good terms to know for your exam.

There are several types of verbs and *tenses* in which they are used. Most verb issues you'll see on your entrance exam will have to do with subject/verb agreement, which is discussed later in this chapter. (You can find a more detailed explanation of verb tenses on the Word Power website: www. wordpower.ws/grammar/gramtoc.html.)

> **DEFINITION**
>
> Grammatically speaking, **tense** refers to how a verb indicates time. Past, present, and future are your basic tenses, though there are others that indicate more specific points in time.

Verbs that you're likely to see on your entrance exams include the following:

Regular verbs: These are the types of verbs you're most familiar with: *to walk, to play, to sing,* and *to dance* are all verbs because each shows action. Regular verbs don't change all that much when you change their tense. It's usually just a matter of adding an –ed or an –s to the end of the word, or including *will* before the verb. For example:

- Present tense: I fast
- Past tense: I fasted
- Future tense: I will fast

Irregular verbs: These are verbs that change completely when you go from tense to tense. The verb *to be* is a classic example. Depending on the subject of the sentence, its present tense can be *am, are,* or *is,* which are very different from the base form. When you conjugate the verb "to be," things get really interesting:

- Present tense: I am
- Past tense: I was
- Future tense: I will be

There are hundreds of irregular verbs in the English language—and they're usually the ones that you have to think twice about how to use correctly in a sentence. *Do, go, know, swim, break, dig, cast, get, have, hear, bear, mistake, prove, sell, sing, wake,* and *sling* are just a few. Georgia State University has a great list of irregular verbs and their conjugations at success.students. gsu.edu/download/irregular-verbs/ ?wpdmdl=931&ind=0.

Adjectives

Nouns, pronouns, and verbs tell you who is doing what in a sentence; adjectives tell you when and/or how it's done. These words are used to describe or modify a noun or pronoun. They provide context for you, the reader, and add color to language.

For example, which of the following sentences is more descriptive?

> I walked down the driveway.
>
> I walked down the slick, wet driveway.

The second sentence tells you much more about what's going on because of the two adjectives (*slick* and *wet*); they modify our understanding of the state of the driveway, which is why adjectives are often called modifiers.

Pay attention to whom or what the adjective in a sentence is referring when you're tackling a grammar question on your exam. The adjective usually comes before the noun or pronoun it modifies, but not always, and that's where errors happen. When you see an adjective, ask yourself what it's describing and look to see if its placement in the sentence is conveying that relationship.

Adverbs

Adverbs work just like adjectives. But where adjectives only apply to nouns and pronouns, adverbs modify just about everything else: verbs, adjectives, and other adverbs.

> **TEST TIP**
>
> Many adverbs end with –ly, as in evenly, quietly, and hungrily. If you're asked to identify an adverb, look for these kinds of words first.

To figure out if a word is an adjective or an adverb, identify what word within the sentence it's modifying. If it's a noun or a pronoun, then you definitely have an adjective. If it's anything else, it's an adverb.

Prepositions

The last part of speech we're going to talk about is the preposition. Like the verb, this can be a rather tricky part of a sentence to deal with in terms of proper grammar. Prepositions link nouns, pronouns, and phrases to other words in a sentence by describing some kind of relationship (location, time, logic, etc.).

Look at the following sentence:

> I left my groceries in the trunk of the car.

What are the prepositions? If you said *in* and *of*, you're right, because these words begin a phrase that defines a specific relationship— a prepositional phrase to be precise.

You would have enough for a complete sentence with just "I left my groceries" (subject, predicate, and direct object). It's the prepositional phrase (defined in the next section) that describes where the groceries were left. There are two prepositional phrases here, and they build on each other to give the reader a more precise description of where the groceries were left than one would alone: "in the trunk" and "of the car."

There are about 150 prepositions in the English language, which unfortunately you just have to memorize in order to recognize. Some include *about, above, across, after, before, beneath, down, for, in, instead of, on, off, since, through,* and *with.*

> **NURSING NOTES**
>
> Daily Grammar (www.dailygrammar.com) is a great website for building up your grammar skills and getting in some extra practice. You can also go there for more in-depth information about additional parts of speech. They even have a Daily Grammar Lessons blog to which you can subscribe.

Common Errors

Now that you're refreshed on the building blocks of our language and up to speed with definitions and concepts you'll need to identify examples of each, it's time to move on to the types of grammatical errors that are often seen on nursing school entrance exams. We're also going to further build up your understanding of parts of speech within this section. But first, let's look at some basic terms and examples of sentence structures. You can find a more detailed look at these structures at http://grammar.ccc.commnet.edu/grammar.

Parts of a Sentence

Type	Function	Example
Subject	Shows what's performing the action in the sentence. Can be simple (just the subject with no modifiers) or compound (more than one subject for one verb).	**Simple:** _High school seniors_ wrote letters to pen pals. **Compound:** _Bill and Amy_ wrote letters to pen pals.
Predicate	Shows the action the subject is performing. Can be simple (just the verb or verb string) or compound (more than one verb for one subject).	**Simple:** High school seniors _wrote_ letters to pen pals. **Compound:** Bill and Amy _wrote_ letters to pen pals and _sent_ them out.
Direct object	Shows who or what receives the action in the sentence.	High school seniors wrote _letters_ to pen pals.
Indirect object	Shows to whom or for what the action is performed.	High school seniors wrote letters to _pen pals_.
Clause	A group of words that has a subject and a verb. Can be independent (can stand alone as a sentence) or dependent (can't stand alone; depends on the rest of the sentence for meaning).	**Independent:** _High school seniors wrote letters_ to pen pals. **Dependent:** High school seniors were writing letters _when the bell rang_.

Type	Function	Example
Phrase	A group of words that doesn't have a subject and a verb but acts as a unit.	_While in English class_, high school seniors wrote letters to pen pals.
Prepositional phrase	Phrase that has a preposition, a noun/pronoun as the direct object, and sometimes a modifier.	Bill and Amy mailed their letters _before going to lunch_.
Comma	Punctuation that separates sentence structures to make them more manageable to read. Some rules for commas: to introduce a sentence, to indicate a pause in reading, to separate two independent clauses joined by a coordinating conjunction, or to separate items in a list (like this one).	**Introduce a sentence:** Come, take a look. **Separate independent clauses:** Bill and Amy mailed their letters, and they went to lunch.

(continues)

Parts of a Sentence (continued)

Type	Function	Example
Semicolon	Use a semicolon when you need to connect two related independent clauses or separate items in a list that contains commas.	**Two related independent clauses:** Bill and Amy mailed their letters; they went together. **List with commas:** They took with them a package, which was handmade; a card; and stamps.
Colon	A colon is used when joining two independent clauses and you want to emphasize the second of the two. Also use after an independent clause to indicate to your reader that you are starting a list, a quotation, an example, or another related idea.	**Emphasize second clause:** Bill and Amy mailed the letters: they went together in his car. **Starting a list:** They took with them: a card, a package, stamps, and scissors.

Subject/Verb Agreement

Let's start this discussion with two basic concepts:

1. Sentences can be written from three perspectives:

   ▶ **First person:** The speaker of the sentence is the subject: I walked the dog. I see the light.

   ▶ **Second person:** The speaker is addressing someone specific (you): You walked the dog. You see the light.

   ▶ **Third person:** The speaker is detached from the subject (he/she/it): He walked the dog. He sees the light.

2. Subjects and verbs can also be singular or plural, as discussed earlier in this chapter.

The most important thing to remember is that subjects and verbs *must* always agree in number and person. This is an extremely common error you'll see on grammar sections of nursing school entrance exams and is also very easy to spot. More often than not, these sentences will not "sound" right to you. Although some of the examples you'll see are rather obvious, others are not. Look out for these three following errors:

1. **Distance between your subject and verb:** When there are a lot of words between your subject and verb, it's very easy to get confused as to whether or not they agree.

   Example: The king, after a long and drawn-out speech, finally named his successor.

TEST TIP

Sometimes you'll find that your subject and verb are reversed in a sentence. It doesn't matter where they're placed, they still have to agree.

Quick fix: Cross out all the words in between so that your verb directly follows your subject. Then check if they agree. If you get rid of everything between the subject and verb in the previous example, you'll find that they do, in fact, agree: The king named his successor.

2. **Compound subjects:** With more than one component in a subject, it's hard to figure out if it's singular or plural sometimes. The rules are pretty simple, though:

   ▸ If the nouns in the subject are connected with *and*, treat them like they're plural in most cases: The bathroom door and the garage *are* closed.

   ▸ If they're connected with an *or* or a *nor*, the verb agrees with the last noun's case: Either the bathroom door or the <u>garages *are*</u> next on the list.

   Quick fix: Ask yourself if you could replace the compound subject with the pronoun *they*. If you can, then your subject is plural. If you can't, your subject is singular.

3. **Collective nouns:** We discussed these earlier in the chapter, but it's worth revisiting when discussing subject/ verb agreement. Collective nouns are generally singular and take singular verbs.

   Quick fix: When you're facing a collective noun that looks like it's plural, stop to think about what it's really referring to. For example: *Mechanics is a specialization within physical science.* This sentence might sound strange, but it's correct because *mechanics* is referring to a field of science and not the plural form of *mechanic*.

Ambiguous Pronoun

Just as with subjects and verbs, pronouns need to agree with their antecedent. You can't have a singular noun in the subject and its plural pronoun later in the sentence. But very often there will be a lot of distance between antecedent and pronoun, making it seem like the pronoun agrees, when it really doesn't.

Example: The fire crackled throughout the evening, and *it* was very pleasant.

Quick fix: If there is a pronoun in the latter part of the sentence, match it up with its antecedent. More often than not, you'll find that something doesn't match up or that it's not clear which noun the pronoun is replacing. Look at the previous example; what does "it" refer to? It's hard to tell, isn't it? When you see things like this on the test, look for answer choices that fix this error.

Misplaced Modifier

These can be kind of funny little mistakes in grammar that we often overlook in our own writing. When this happens, a modifier within a sentence is not placed where it needs to be to modify its intended word or phrase.

Example: The tree was struck by lightning from the grove.

In the previous sentence, the prepositional phrase "from the grove" is meant to modify "the tree." But its place in the sentence makes it seem like it is modifying "lightning" instead, which doesn't make sense.

Another example of a misplaced modifier is known as the *dangling modifier*. This happens when a sentence begins with a phrase that ends in a comma, and the noun that follows is not what the phrase is modifying.

Example: In the gorgeous velvet gown, he felt like a king watching his queen enter the room.

Unless the man in this sentence was wearing that gorgeous velvet gown while he felt like a king, that opening phrase is not modifying the correct noun. Chances are it was the woman entering the room in that gown that made him feel like a king.

Quick fix: Look for answer choices that reword the opening phrase, change what's being modified, or move the modifier to a position in the sentence where it is clear what it is modifying.

Commas in Compound Sentences

You already know all about simple sentences: subject + verb = complete thought. You've been dealing with them all of your life. But there are other kinds of sentences out there, and you're going to have to deal with them on your exam. One in particular is the compound sentence, which is a sentence made up of two independent clauses that are joined with a *coordinating conjunction*.

> **DEFINITION**
>
> A **conjunction** is a word that connects two structures in a sentence. A **coordinating conjunction** links grammatically similar parts of a sentence, like two independent clauses. You are very familiar with these words: and, but, or, nor, for, yet, and so.

Example: Tori went to her interview, and Casey dropped off the baby.

Quick fix: If your sentence has two complete ideas that can stand by themselves, look to see how they are separated. There should be a comma at the end of the first independent clause and before the coordinating conjunction.

Run-On Sentences

Run-on sentences are usually suffering from a lack of proper punctuation. When you have a sentence that has two or more independent clauses that are not joined with an appropriate conjunction or punctuation, it's a run-on.

Example: The rain washed away all of the chalk on the ground and that made the kids really upset they broke all the chalk.

Quick fix: If your sentence is long and complicated, look to see if it could be a run-on. In this sentence, you have three independent clauses that need separating: a comma between "ground" and "and" and a semicolon between "upset" and "they."

> **TEST TIP**
>
> When a compound sentence does not have a coordinating conjunction, you need to place a semicolon or colon (if appropriate) between the two independent clauses.

Fragments

Sentence fragments are just the opposite of run-ons. Instead of having too much information or too many words, these beauties don't have enough. A fragment is basically a dependent clause that stands alone.

Example: Broke into the hotel room.

Quick fix: Look to see if your sentence has a subject and a verb. If one is missing (like the subject is here), it's a fragment. To fix it, add the missing structure.

Preposition Placement

According to the rules of grammar, you should not end a sentence with a preposition. When writing informally, however, you do this all the time because it's commonly accepted and understood. If you notice, we write this way throughout this book. The reason? Our tone and purpose is to communicate with you as if we were having a conversation. Nursing school entrance exams don't care about this, though. They want to know that you know what the rules are and that you can correct these formal errors.

Example: That's the person I want to rehearse with.

Quick fix: Here is where knowing what a preposition is will help you get through a question pretty quickly. If you see a grammar question that has a sentence with a preposition as the last word, you will probably have to reword the sentence to change this. In this example, "with" is a preposition and should not be at the end of the sentence. Correct by rewording: That's the person with whom I want to rehearse.

Spelling

When it comes to spelling, there's not much more you can do to prepare for your exam except memorize some basic rules, recognize correct spellings, and practice using them. The following chart gives you an overview of some important rules to learn and remember during your exam.

Basic Spelling Rules

Rule	Example/Exceptions
I comes before *e* in a word, except after *c*, or if together they make the ay sound.	receive, weigh, believe, relief, deign, freight **Exceptions:** neither, either, height, seize, weird
When a word ends in *y*, change *y* to *i* and then add the suffix. Exception: When the suffix is *-ing*, or when a vowel comes before the *y*.	marry>married supply>supplied **Exceptions:** marry>marrying convey>conveyed
Drop the silent *e* at the end of a word when adding a suffix that begins with a vowel. Exception: If the word ends in *-ce* or *-ge* and the suffix begins with an *a*, *o*, or *u*, or when a vowel comes before the silent *e*.	advise>advising care>caring **Exceptions:** advantage> advantageous see>seeing
You don't change anything in the base word when you add a suffix that begins with a consonant.	advise>advisement father>fatherhood
Double the consonant when you add a vowel suffix to a word that ends in an accented short vowel sound or a modified vowel sound.	**Accented short vowel:** forbid>forbidding **Modified vowel sound:** Flip>flipped

Commonly Confused Words

Here is a sampling of words that are commonly confused, which leads to misuse and misspelling in writing. But don't worry—we also give you some tricks to help you keep them straight. Weber State University has a more comprehensive list at https://bit.ly/2PspPYA.

Accept/Except: To *accept* means to receive something. To *except* means to exclude something. To remember the difference, think of the *ex* as the differentiator: Your ex is excluded from your life.

Affect/Effect: The difference between these two words is their parts of speech. *Affect* is a verb that means to have an effect on something or to stir up emotion. *Effect* is a noun that refers to a result, force, impact, or appearance. Good association: *The movie's special effects did not affect the audience.* In the sentence, *affect* is the verb.

CODE RED!

Effect can sometimes be used as a verb, meaning to cause or produce. Even though you will most likely encounter the noun form on the test, you should be aware of this lesser-used definition. It just might show up!

Allude/Elude: *Allude* means to reference something. *Elude* means to try to avoid or get away. To tell the difference, think "to elude is to evade."

Alright/All Right: *Alright* is the more modern, informal version of all right—most likely used to shorten the intent of the phrase in writing. Language tests like the ones you'll be taking soon, however, are looking for formal use of language and grammar. For the purposes of the exam, go long, not short, and stick with *all right*.

Complement/Compliment: *Complement* means to go with something, like colors that complement each other or a specific wine that complements the flavors in your meal. Compliment is when you say something nice to someone.

Elicit/Illicit: *Elicit* is a verb that means to cause or generate. *Illicit* is an adjective that describes something illegal. Use that "ill" as your association: illicit = illegal.

Farther/Further: *Farther* is used when discussing distance. Remember this by looking at the smaller word far, which implies distance. *Further* means to progress.

Imply/Infer: When you *imply*, you communicate information without stating it outright. When you *infer*, you are taking in information and drawing a conclusion based on it. The difference is with *imply* you communicate outward, and with *infer* you communicate inward.

Insure/Ensure: *Insure* means to place insurance on something. *Ensure* means to make sure or make certain. Remember: insure = insurance.

Its/It's: *Its* is an exception to the possessive pronoun rule. The reason for this is because *it's* is a contraction that combines *it* and *is*. Therefore, *its* is the possessive form of *it*. Think of *it* like *his* and *hers*, which are also possessive pronouns that don't get apostrophes.

TEST TIP

Contractions combine two words into a shorter word that has an apostrophe. When reading a sentence, look at the words with apostrophes to determine if they're being used to show possession or if they're contractions.

Less/Fewer: Use *less* when you're referring to something that can't be measured in quantity: less friction. Use *fewer* when you're referring to something that can be measured in quantity: fewer doughnuts.

Than/Then: *Than* indicates some kind of comparison (greater than). *Then* indicates time.

There/Their/They're: *There* refers to a place (*here* is a smaller word within it to remind you). *Their* is a possessive pronoun. *They're* is a contraction of *they* and *are*.

Wary/Weary: *Wary* means to be alert to what's going on around you. *Weary* means tired.

Who/That: *Who* indicates a person or animal. *That* refers to a thing or group.

Your/You're: *Your* is a possessive pronoun. *You're* is a contraction that combines *you* and *are*.

Practice Questions

For each of the following questions, choose the best answer from the choices provided.

1. What is the adverb in the following sentence?

   I was barely three years old when I broke my wrist.

   (A) I
   (B) broke
   (C) barely
   (D) wrist

2. Choose the word that is spelled incorrectly:

   (A) calendar
   (B) begger
   (C) boundaries
   (D) despair

3. What is the subject of the following sentence?

   Eliza's death was tragic.

   (A) Eliza
   (B) Eliza's death
   (C) death
   (D) tragic

4. What punctuation is needed to correct this sentence?

   Where can I put my bag

   (A) question mark
   (B) comma
   (C) semicolon
   (D) colon

5. Which word will make the following sentence grammatically correct?

   Mark and Jim played cards and talked about going to the gym; then _____ got into the car and left.

   (A) him
   (B) them
   (C) his
   (D) they

6. Which verb tense is shown in the following sentence?

   George brought a sandwich to work today for lunch.

   (A) past
   (B) present
   (C) future
   (D) present perfect

7. Which word in the following sentence is used incorrectly?

   There was no one in the warehouse accept Louis and me.

   (A) one
   (B) in
   (C) was
   (D) accept

8. Which is the correct pronoun to stand in for South Korea in the latter part of the following sentence?

South Korea hosted the Summer Olympic Games in 1988, and _____ has bid for the chance to host again several times since then.

(A) they
(B) it
(C) we
(D) our

9. Which of the answer choices is grammatically correct?

(A) Offending the queen, the general removed the foul-mouthed protester from the meeting room.
(B) Because he offended the queen, the general removed the foul-mouthed protester from the room.
(C) Because he offended the queen, the foul-mouthed protester was removed from the room.
(D) Because the general offended the queen, the foul-mouthed protester was removed from the room.

10. Which word pair would make the following sentence grammatically correct?

After deciding to get some air, the pair of friends ran into a group of teenagers swimming _____ pool.

(A) in the
(B) in their
(C) on the
(D) under the

11. What kind of error is present in the following sentence?

Like the sands of time.

(A) run-on sentence
(B) sentence fragment
(C) subject/verb agreement
(D) ambiguous pronoun

12. What punctuation is needed to correct this sentence?

Adrienne melted the chocolate first then she added the cream to the pot.

(A) a comma between "Adrienne" and "melted"
(B) a semicolon between "first" and "then"
(C) a comma between "first" and "then"v
(D) a comma after "then"

13. Choose the word that is spelled correctly:

(A) tempermental
(B) synonomous
(C) yield
(D) resevoir

14. Which form of the verb *to be* would make this sentence grammatically correct?

Either Jack or Wilson _____ coming to the picnic.

(A) are
(B) am
(C) be
(D) is

15. Choose the word that is spelled incorrectly:

    (A) tyrany
    (B) separation
    (C) irresistible
    (D) acclaim

Answers and Explanations

1. **C.** When looking for adverbs, look for words that end in *ly* first. *Barely* modifies the verb *was*, which makes it the adverb. Answers A and D are nouns. Answer B is a verb.

2. **B.** This choice should be spelled *beggar*.

3. **B.** It might be tempting to choose A or D as your answer, but the subject isn't talking about Eliza or death alone; it's talking about Eliza's death, which makes it the subject.

4. **A.** *Where* is an interrogative pronoun. If you associate the word *interrogate* with TV crime shows where the cops question witnesses, you already know what this means. Interrogative pronouns indicate a question. Therefore, a question mark is the appropriate punctuation.

5. **D.** "Mark and Jim" is your subject. In fact, it's a compound subject connected by *and*, which makes it plural. Thus, it takes a plural pronoun.

6. **A.** *Brought* is the past form of *bring*.

7. **D.** You want *except* here. *Accept* is a verb, so it doesn't make sense where it's placed in the sentence. Plus, except means to exclude, which is what the sentence is trying to convey: Louis and me are the only ones left in the warehouse and are thus excluded from whoever already left.

8. **B.** This is a collective noun issue. Your subject is South Korea, which as a country has bid to host the Olympics. Your pronoun needs to be singular, and *it* is the only one that is.

9. **C.** This is a misplaced modifier issue. Who offended the queen? The protester. This needs to come directly after the introductory phrase, which eliminates Answers A and B. Answer D is wrong because it doesn't make sense and this construction changes the meaning of the sentence.

10. **A.** If you chose Answer B, you're putting an ambiguous pronoun in the sentence. Does the pool belong to the pair of friends or to the teenagers? You don't know if you add in *their* as a pronoun here, which makes it not a good choice. The other two choices don't make sense.

11. **B.** There is no verb in this sentence, which makes it a fragment.

12. **B.** You have two independent clauses here and no coordinating conjunction. This calls for a semicolon.

13. **C.** *Temperamental, synonymous,* and *reservoir* are the correct spellings for the other options.

14. **D.** You have *either* as an indefinite pronoun. Because of this, you know that a verb is needed that agrees with the part of the subject closest to the verb.

15. **A.** It is spelled *tyranny*.

Mark Your Words

Ⓐ Ⓑ Ⓒ Ⓓ

Ⓐ Ⓑ Ⓒ Ⓓ

Ⓐ Ⓑ Ⓒ Ⓓ

Ⓐ Ⓑ Ⓒ Ⓓ

Ⓐ Ⓑ Ⓒ Ⓓ

Ⓐ Ⓑ Ⓒ Ⓓ

Just about every teacher you had in school probably stressed the importance of building your vocabulary. Back then, you needed it to pass tests and write papers that made you sound like the greatest living expert on whatever your topic was. Today, you need it to pass the verbal sections of every nursing school entrance exam.

Most verbal components of these exams are focused heavily on vocabulary, making them really not much more than big vocabulary tests, only better. If you remember back to high school, your vocabulary tests were probably nothing more than a list of words you had to define. On your entrance exam, you get four answers to choose from and, a lot of the time, context clues to help you make the right choice.

This chapter gives you the tools you need to ace this section. You'll see what types of questions are most often found on nursing school entrance exams, essential strategies for approaching them, and ways to build up your vocabulary skills so that you can figure out the correct answer, even when you don't know what a word means.

What to Expect

Your vocabulary says a lot about you as a person. Right or wrong, you are judged based on the words you use. Although this may or may not have much of an impact on your day-to-day interactions with people, how you communicate and how you're perceived is extremely important in nursing.

Nurses need to be able to put people at ease and form at least short-term relationships with their patients. They also need to be able to accurately communicate with their patients, their colleagues, and others within the health-care environment. And when the health of people is at stake, miscommunications can have extremely negative consequences.

That's why all of the nursing school entrance exams test vocabulary knowledge. It enables them to get a read on your communication abilities, as well as your ability to recognize and manipulate written language.

There are four types of questions you can expect to see on nursing school entrance exam verbal sections:

▸ **Synonyms:** Synonyms refer to two words with similar meanings. With this type of question, you'll be given a word (either on its own or used within a sentence), and then you'll have to choose the answer choice that means nearly the same thing.

▸ **Antonyms:** Antonyms are literally the opposite of synonyms; instead of having to find the answer choice that means nearly the same thing as the word you're given, you need to find the answer that means the opposite. These can get tricky, as they're sometimes mixed in with many different types of verbal questions.

▸ **Sentence completion:** These questions give you a sentence with a missing word. Your job is to determine which of the answer choices fits best in the sentence.

▸ **Analogies:** These questions show a relationship between two "stem" words. Your job is to figure out which pair of stem words in the answer choices has the same relationship as the original stem pair.

When faced with vocabulary questions, following the general strategies for multiple-choice questions outlined in Chapter 3

should be your first response. But for this to work, you have to know or figure out what all the words in the question mean. Let's look at some additional strategies for addressing these specific types of questions.

NURSING NOTES

The vocabulary you encounter on your entrance exam will include general SAT-level words, but may also focus on terms used in health care. EnglishClub.com has a nice list of common terms at www.englishclub.com/english-for-work/medical-vocabulary.htm.

Synonym and Antonym Questions

The first type of question to look at is the most straightforward: simple definitions for synonyms and antonyms. You're given a word, and your job is to choose the answer choice that is closest to the meaning of that word, or the opposite in the case of an antonym question:

Joyous most nearly means

(A) happy.
(B) drab.
(C) original.
(D) different.

Seems simple enough, right? Sure, if you know what everything means. If you don't, you still have lots of ways to narrow your answer choices and get to a word's meaning.

Get to the Root of the Problem

Just about every word in the English language is made up of smaller parts. If you've ever wondered why the word *contradict* is used to describe saying something that goes against something else, just look at the word's roots:

- The prefix *contra* means "against" or "opposite."
- The root *dict* means "speak."

Now put these meanings together and you can see a clear definition: to speak against or oppose.

Many of the words commonly used on standardized tests like the nursing school entrance exams use words that have Greek and Latin word roots, prefixes, and suffixes. Don't forget that you're looking for the answer that *most nearly* matches or opposes the word you're given, not the definition that is exactly the same or opposite. This is one way that roots can be a powerful tool for eliminating answer choices.

You can make this work for you by memorizing a handful of these roots (more on this in "Learn Your Roots," later in this chapter). Then when you see them in a word, you can get a good idea of what the word generally means. Based on this information, you can then eliminate answer choices that do not match up with this idea.

Try it with the following example:

Enamored most nearly means

    (A) hated.
    (B) melodious.
    (C) infatuated.
    (D) angelic.

Look at the root word in the middle, *amor*. Pretty much everyone knows that *amor* means "love," thanks to American pop culture. So the correct answer choice will have something to do with love.

Now look at your answer choices. "Hated" just isn't going to do it. If you don't know what *melodious* means, see if you can pick out a familiar word within the main roots. Look closely, and you'll pick out *melody*, which doesn't mean love. Try the same strategy with "angelic," and you have *angel*. Although angels often are associated with love, they are defined as heavenly beings. Love is not used to define what an angel is. That means this answer choice is likely wrong.

Even if you didn't know that *infatuated* means "possessed of an unreasoning passion or love," you've eliminated all of the other answer choices as being unsuitable for "most nearly" meaning the same as the word in the question.

Now how should you approach this question if you were asked to choose the antonym of *enamored*? Do the same things, but tweak your process of elimination. You'll need to figure out the meaning of the word you're given before you can do anything else. When you go to the answer choices, eliminate answers that are similar to that definition or have nothing to do with it at all. Your best answer will be the complete opposite of the given word. In this case, your answer would be A, because *hated* is the polar opposite of *enamored*.

What's the Connotation?

If you're not sure what the definition of a word is, ask yourself if it has a positive or negative *connotation*.

> **DEFINITION**
>
> **Connotation** is the implied meaning or the feeling associated with a word. You may choose to say "car accident" instead of "wreck" or "crash" because "accident" doesn't imply as much violence as the other words. Don't confuse *connotation* with its opposite, *denotation*, which is the literal or dictionary definition.

When looking for synonyms, a correct answer choice will have the same connotation as the word in the question (and vice versa for antonyms), so depending on what word you're struggling with, you can use this technique to help you eliminate answer choices:

1. If you know that the word in the question is a positive, you can eliminate any negative answer choices right away.

2. If you're not sure what one of the answer choices means, see if you can determine whether it is positive or negative using word roots. Then compare it to the question word's connotation.

3. If the word you're given in the question is neither positive nor negative, the correct answer must also be neutral. Eliminate any obviously positive or negative answer choices.

To determine the connotation of a word, think about how you've heard it used before and in what context. Say you don't know what the word *malicious* means, but there it is in a practice question. Ask yourself where

you've heard that word before and in what situations. What can you connect to it?

Chances are the context in which you've heard this word used have been negative, because *malicious* describes something as being intentionally harmful. This means you can be pretty confident that its connotation is negative, too.

Prefixes and suffixes can also give you a good idea of whether the word you're looking at is a positive or a negative. Again, memorizing word roots will be a big help here. Here are some to get you started:

▶ Prefixes that connote positive meanings: *am/ami/amor, ben/bene, gen, grat, pac*

▶ Prefixes that connote negative meanings: *ant/anti, bel, dys, mal, mis, mor/mort, neg, pug*

> **TEST TIP**
>
> You're not limited to using only one strategy at a time when approaching questions. Combine those that make the most sense and you will get to the correct answer fastest.

Determine Part of Speech

The correct answer choice will be the same part of speech as the word in the question. If you know that the word you're given is a noun, you can eliminate any answer choice that is not a noun. For a review of parts of speech, flip back to Chapter 4.

Looking at parts of speech can work both for and against you. It can work against you because some words have multiple definitions and are multiple parts of speech; it can work for you because looking at the part of speech of other words in the question can help you determine which definition of the word is being used in this instance.

Look at the following example:

<u>Cow</u> most nearly means

    (A) energize.
    (B) levitate.
    (C) aggravate.
    (D) intimidate.

Your first instinct is likely to define *cow* as a noun, an adult female bovine, whale, elephant, manatee, or other animal. But if you look at the answer choices, you'll see that they're all verbs: to energize, to levitate, to aggravate, to intimidate. This means that the definition of *cow* you need to concentrate on is the verb form, which means "to frighten or threaten."

Words in Context and Sentence Completion

Another type of question you'll see on vocabulary sections of nursing school entrance exams gives you sentences with a single underlined word or a place to insert a word to complete the sentence. Your job is to choose the answer choice that gives the meaning of how the word is used in the sentence or makes the most sense in completing the sentence:

When her money ran out for the third time that month, the girl <u>entreated</u> her parents to send some more for her basic expenses.

    (A) annoyed
    (B) begged
    (C) smiled
    (D) soothed

The sentence isn't there just to make the test question longer. It actually gives you more information that will help lead you to the correct answer. The strategies discussed

earlier for simple definition questions can still be used with these questions. However, two additional techniques work specifically for these types of questions.

Look for Clues

Look for context clues within the sentence that hint at the meaning of the word. Some are very obvious, like specific words that modify or apply to the underlined word. Others require a little logic on your part to draw conclusions about what's going on in the sentence and how it relates to the underlined word.

In the previous example, the word you need to define is *entreated*. You know that the word is being used as a verb, because it's the action the subject is taking (the girl entreated). Based on the context of the sentence, you can infer that she's asking her parents for money, because she doesn't have any more.

What else does the sentence tell you? This is the third time she's run out of money. You also know that her parents are supporting her because the sentence says "to send her *more* money," which implies that they have done so before.

Now look at the answer choices:

    (A) annoyed
    (B) begged
    (C) smiled
    (D) soothed

Based on what you've learned about what's going on in the sentence, *annoyed* would not fit; the girl would most likely not get very far in her attempts to get money from her parents if she annoyed them, so Answer A is out. Answer B could fit, because there seems to be a note of desperation in the connotation of the sentence. Plus, you're looking for an answer choice that means something close to *ask*, and begging fits the bill. But let's look at the other answer choices before committing to this one. Yup, Answers C and D don't really make sense for this question. Your best answer (though not a great word to replace *entreat*, which means to ask) is B.

Swap It Out

The second approach is to simply replace the underlined word with the answer choices. This works well with sentence completion questions or with words-in-context questions when you know the definitions of the answer choices but are not sure about what the underlined word means. If the answer choice makes sense in the sentence without changing the meaning, chances are that answer is a keeper.

Read the following example:

> Mark was such a(n) _____ guy, it was no wonder that his many friends voted him the most popular boy in his class.
>
> (A) lackluster
> (B) unusual
> (C) affable
> (D) original

Your task is to find which answer choice best completes the sentence. First, let's get an idea of what kind of word you're looking for. The sentence tells you that Mark is a pretty good guy: he has lots of friends and was voted most popular. You're looking for a word that has a positive connotation and communicates these qualities.

Based on this info, plug each of the answer choices into the sentence, and see what works best:

> (A) Mark was such a lackluster guy, it was no wonder that his many friends voted him the most popular boy in his class.
> (B) Mark was such an unusual guy, it was no wonder that his many friends voted him the most popular boy in his class.
> (C) Mark was such an affable guy, it was no wonder that his many friends voted him the most popular boy in his class.
> (D) Mark was such an original guy, it was no wonder that his many friends voted him the most popular boy in his class.

If you don't know what *lackluster* means, you can use one of our previous strategies to get a clue to its meaning: look for smaller words in this complex one that are familiar. The word *luster*, when it stands alone, means "shiny." *Lack* suggests that something is missing—in this case, shine, because that's part of the word. A good guess would be that *lackluster* means "dull" (which it does).

Now that you're familiar with all of the words, what fits? Would a dull or unusual guy have lots of friends and be voted Mr. Popularity? Probably not. How about an original guy? *Original* is a neutral word, suggesting neither positive nor negative connotations. The sentence, however, leans more to the positive than anything else, so *original* is likely not your answer.

This leaves us with *affable*. Even if you don't know what this word means, it's a better choice than *lackluster* if only based on the loose definition formed by looking at the smaller words that make up the whole. It so happens that *affable* means "likable," which makes the most sense out of the answers you're given.

Analogies

The last type of question you're likely to see on some nursing school entrance exams is the analogy. Analogy questions are all formatted the same way and look like this:

> hedonist : pleasure ::
>
> (A) jurist : conviction
> (B) doctor : prescription
> (C) musician : improvement
> (D) addict : drugs

When you first encounter analogies in school, you're taught to read them like this: "hedonist is to pleasure, as what is to what?" This construction is really vague and tends to be confusing. But like we said earlier in the chapter, these questions are really identifying relationships between words.

Some common relationships you'll see:

▶ Type: banana : fruit—a banana is a type of fruit.

▶ Synonym: braid : plait—braid is another word for plait.

▶ Antonym: smile : frown—smile is the opposite of frown.

▶ Degree: pneumonia : cold—pneumonia is a more severe infection than a cold.

▶ Cause and effect: cancellation : opening—a cancellation can cause an opening in a schedule.

▶ Part of a whole: goose : gaggle—a goose is part of a gaggle.

▶ Definition: hedonist : pleasure—a hedonist is a person who is devoted to indulging in pleasure.

When you approach an analogy question:

1. Define the relationship in a clear, specific sentence like the ones used previously.

2. After you define your relationship in a sentence, substitute the answer choice pairs for the original stem pair.

3. Use process of elimination.

Let's try it out with *hedonist* and *pleasure:*

Relationship sentence:

> A *hedonist* is a person who is devoted to indulging in *pleasure.*

Plug-in answers:

> A *jurist* is a person who is devoted to indulging in *conviction.*
>
> A *doctor* is a person who is devoted to indulging in *prescription.*
>
> A *musician* is a person who is devoted to indulging in *improvement.*
>
> An *addict* is a person who is devoted to indulging in *drugs.*

The only answer choice that makes sense here is the last one, which makes it your best bet.

Build Your Vocabulary

Probably the best thing that you can do to raise your score on the verbal section of your nursing school entrance exam is to simply increase your vocabulary. The more words you know or are familiar with going into the test, the faster and more efficient you'll be on this subtest.

The key to bulking up your vocabulary is to do it slowly and steadily. A little work on this each day can pay off big time in terms of words you know walking into the exam. The following are easy and even entertaining ways to get started.

Word of the Day

You can subscribe to a word-of-the-day website that will email you a new vocabulary word and definition every day. Just click open your message and use that word sometime during the day for maximum retention. You can also download a word-of-the-day app or follow Merriam-Webster on Twitter. A quick online search nets several services that you can subscribe to.

Hit the Books

Simply reading will help you increase your vocabulary. It doesn't matter much what you read, as just about anything you pick up will likely introduce at least one new word to you. Yes, that romance novel, mystery, issue of *Sports Illustrated,* or even daily newspaper can help you pick up new words. The increased interaction with language will seep into your mindset and familiarize you with more words than you could ever imagine—and it happens automatically. Also, underline words you don't know the definitions of and look them up later.

You can also head to your local library in search of vocabulary guides. Use one of these books to make a list of words you want to learn, and work on learning them a few at a time over a couple weeks. Making up your own flashcards is an excellent way to do this.

Memorize in Clusters

So many of the words you'll likely encounter on standardized exams have similar meanings. For example, *florid, embellish, bombastic, ornate, overblown, flowery,* and *elaborate* all have similar meanings: excessively decorated, spoken, or written. Use a good thesaurus and make a list of synonyms for any vocabulary word on your list. This is a great way to get the most out of your study time.

Learn Your Roots

We talked earlier about being able to recognize prefixes, suffixes, and word roots. This is really an invaluable tool for improving your vocabulary because it gives you the tools for understanding how words are built—which, in turn, clues you in to their meaning. The following table identifies some common roots, prefixes, and suffixes.

Common Roots, Prefixes, and Suffixes

Root	Meaning	Example
acer/acri	sour, sharp, bitter	acid
beli/bel/pug	fight, war	pugnacious
bene	good	benefit
chron	time	chronological
circ	around	circuit
dic/dict/dit	speak, talk	dictate
loqu/locut/log	speak, talk	dialogue
luc/lum/lun/lus	light	illuminate
mal	bad	malaise
omni	all, ever	omnipresent
path	feel	sympathy
phot/photo	light	photograph

Root	Meaning	Example
pop	people	population
simil/simul	same	simultaneous
spec/spic	see	conspicuous
sym/syn	together	synchronize
terr/terra	earth	terrain
ver	true	verify
vid/vis	see	visual
viv/vita/vivi	life	vitality

Prefix	Meaning	Example
a/ab/an	away from, without	abdicate
ante	before	antechamber
anti/de	against, opposite	antihero
com/con	with, fully, together	congregation
contra/counter	against, opposite	counteract
inter	between	interoffice
intra	within	intramural
post	after	posthumous
super/supra	above or over	supersede

Suffix	Meaning	Example
able	worth or ability, suggests adjective	capable
acy/cy	state of, suggests noun	accuracy
ant/ent	noun that does something	defendant
ary	relating to, suggests adjective	reactionary

Root	Meaning	Example
ation/ness	action or condition, suggests noun	intimidation
ed	past, suggests verb	walked
ful	having/giving, suggests noun/adjective	bountiful
fy/ify	to cause or form, suggests verb/adjective	justify
ise/ize	cut off, suggests verb	excise
ism	belief, suggests noun	feudalism
ist	person, suggests noun	nudist
ly	in the manner of, suggests adverb	normally

Let's get in some practice figuring out the meanings of words based on looking at their roots. For each of the following, list as many roots as you can in the first column. Then write what you think the word means in the second column. Look them up in a dictionary to check.

Word	Roots	Meaning
Interoffice	_____	_____
Acerbic	_____	_____
Luminous	_____	_____
Circumvent	_____	_____
Omnipotent	_____	_____
Antebellum	_____	_____
Pugilistic	_____	_____

Malodorous	_____	_____
Anachronistic	_____	_____
Sympathetic	_____	_____

TEST TIP

PrefixSuffix.com (www.prefixsuffix.com) has an extensive list of word roots that you can access for free.

Make Associations

One of the easiest and most lasting ways to learn new words is to associate their meanings with something that makes sense to you. You can do this in a few ways. The first is to come up with a little rhyme or word association that reminds you of the meaning. These are called *mnemonic devices*, and as long as they make sense to you, they can consist of just about anything. Here are a few to get you started:

▸ Pretentious: Pretends to be all that

▸ Nullify: Make nada or nothing

▸ Miser: Scrooge was a miserable miser

▸ Levity: Levitates or lifts your mood

▸ Concrete: Hard evidence

▸ Intrepid: Bold, gutsy, like the famous aircraft carrier

You can also make associations with words based on where you heard them (a conversation, a book, a movie, a song, and so on), what you were doing when you heard them, the context of what was going on, how you were feeling, and more. A few that work for us include these:

▸ *Curious:* Mr. Olivander, the wand-maker in *Harry Potter and the Sorcerer's Stone,* used *curious* when Harry's wand had the same core as Voldemort's.

▸ *Indubitably:* Burt, in *Mary Poppins,* would say *indubitably* when agreeing with Mary.

▸ *Vapid:* In the movie *10 Things I Hate About You,* a character used *vapid* to describe the boring and unoriginal student population.

With a little time and practice, you will be in excellent shape to take on any vocabulary-based question on your nursing school entrance exam. And all your hard work will pay off—not only on the test, but for the rest of your life as well. A great vocabulary is an asset that can give you an advantage when applying for future jobs and help you make a good impression on new people you meet.

Practice Questions

For each of the following questions, choose the best answer out of the choices given.

1. <u>Perverse</u> most nearly means

    (A) able.
    (B) wicked.
    (C) appreciative.
    (D) wired.

2. Jade's friends loved how friendly and _____ she got when they went out on Friday nights.

    (A) reticent
    (B) reserved
    (C) sociable
    (D) suspicious

3. The <u>spare</u> room had only a cot and a pillow in it.

    The underlined word in the previous sentence most nearly means

    (A) small.
    (B) unadorned.
    (C) ornate.
    (D) spacious.

4. <u>Hasten</u> most nearly means the opposite of

    (A) accelerate.
    (B) pause.
    (C) cry.
    (D) drop.

5. florid : embellished ::

    (A) arid : wet
    (B) evil : condescending
    (C) quiet : loud
    (D) talkative : chatty

6. <u>Raze</u> most nearly means the opposite of

    (A) demolish.
    (B) uplift.
    (C) create.
    (D) fasten.

7. With the help of the increased winds and dry weather, the smoking leaves where the cigarette had been dropped had quickly turned into a <u>conflagration</u> that endangered whole neighborhoods.

    The underlined word in the previous sentence most nearly means

    (A) inference.
    (B) blaze.
    (C) creation.
    (D) beast.

8. <u>Invigorate</u> most nearly means

    (A) appreciate.
    (B) value.
    (C) refresh.
    (D) concentrate.

9. vapid : creative ::

    (A) engaged : distracted
    (B) committed : enamored
    (C) credible : believable
    (D) wealthy : generous

10. The damage the illness did to my immune system leaves me _____ to all sorts of common infections.

    (A) vulnerable

    (B) over-the-top

    (C) brilliant

    (D) aged

11. Astronomical most nearly means the opposite of

    (A) valid.

    (B) ordinary.

    (C) negligible.

    (D) huge.

12. displeasure : rage ::

    (A) tower : building

    (B) interest : obsession

    (C) boxcar : train

    (D) pallet : colors

13. Vogue most nearly means

    (A) search.

    (B) fad.

    (C) model.

    (D) belief.

14. Though she smiled when she said she was delighted to be part of the committee, her resentful tone proved her words to be _____.

    (A) serious

    (B) believable

    (C) angry

    (D) disingenuous

15. Sacred most nearly means the opposite of

    (A) reviled.

    (B) exceptional.

    (C) belated.

    (D) perfect.

Answers and Explanations

1. **B.** Perverse can mean "stubborn" or "wicked." None of the other answer choices make sense with this definition.

2. **C.** Using the context clues, you can tell Jade is friendly and active with her friends. Answers A and B mean "quiet" and "keeping to oneself." Answer D means "doubtful." Answer C makes the most sense.

3. **B.** Don't be fooled here into thinking "spare room" automatically means "extra room." If you look at the context clues in the sentence, you'll see that it's talking about how the room is decorated. There is very little in the room and no indication of its size. Answer B is the best choice.

4. **B.** The base word here is *haste,* which means "speed" or "hurry." Remember, we're looking for the opposite of this word in the answer choices. Answer A is a synonym—a common trap for antonym questions. Answers C and D have nothing to do with speeding or hurrying. However, when you pause, you are doing the opposite of this, which makes B your best choice.

5. **D.** Define the relationship: florid is another word for embellished. Plug your answer choices into this sentence and the only one that makes sense is D. Answers A and C show opposite relationships. Answer B shows no relationship.

6. **C.** A good connection to make is "raze one building to make room for another," as this is often the context in which you hear *raze* being used. However, it does not mean to build; it means to destroy or demolish.

Because you're looking for the opposite meaning here, the correct answer is C.

7. **B.** The sentence talks about a small flame that grows large. The only answer that makes sense is Answer B.

8. **C.** Invigorate means "to add life to" or "to refresh." None of the other answer choices come anywhere close to this definition.

9. **A.** If you are vapid, you are not creative. Plug your answer choices into this sentence: If you are engaged, you are not .... Answer A fits best because when you are engaged, you are not distracted.

10. **A.** You may want to use Swap It Out for this question. When you do, you'll find that Answers B and C don't fit. This leaves A and D for you to consider. The sentence talks about how an illness damaged the speaker's immune system, which implies that some harm has made it exposed. Age is not necessary to define this, so Answer A is the best choice.

11. **C.** A good association to make with *astronomical* is to think of it in terms of space. Space, the universe, and everything associated with them are so large that you can't even conceive of it all. This fits with Answer D, but we're looking for the opposite. *Negligible* means so small it's insignificant, which fits for this question.

12. **B.** Displeasure is a milder degree of rage. Interest is a milder degree of obsession. Answers A and C show "type of" relationships. Answer D shows a "is made up of" relationship.

13. **B.** An easy association with the word *vogue* is to think about the fashion magazine with the same name. Fashion is all about what's the best now, and those perceptions are fleeting, just like fads are. Answers A and D have nothing to do with this, and though you might be tempted to choose Answer C because of the link between "fashion" and "model," "fad" is the choice that most nearly means "vogue."

14. **D.** The sentence tells us that the woman is being false with her words. *Disingenuous* means "insincere."

15. **A.** Something that is revered is holy or sacred. Reviled is the opposite of this. The smaller word here to give you an inkling of the definition is *vile*, meaning awful. Something that is reviled is loathed, not sacred. *Exceptional* means "special"; *belated* means "late"; and *perfect* means "without flaws."

Read, Comprehend, Conquer

Believe it or not, as a nurse, you will be doing quite a bit of reading. Whether it's reading a patient's chart, brushing up on procedures and protocol, or studying to expand your skills, your ability to understand and analyze the information that you read needs to be strong. Mistakes due to misinterpretation or misunderstanding written information can result in serious consequences for patients.

That's why every nursing school entrance exam has a reading comprehension section, which is about way more than just reading little passages and answering questions. This section is about how you think and communicate. How you do on this portion of the test will tell the program's admissions people if you have a basic level of ability to complete the program.

This chapter introduces you to what you can expect to see on this section of most nursing school entrance exams, how to approach each type of question, and how to make getting through this section of the exam as painless as possible. If reading comprehension has never been a strong subject for you, this chapter will definitely help you out.

What to Expect

As we said earlier, reading comprehension gives insight into your communication skills. So how does reading boring little paragraphs and answering questions tell anyone how you communicate? It's all about analysis. Reading comprehension tests gauge your ability to effectively take in information, process it, and make decisions based on what you've read. When you get the correct answer, you show that you can do this effectively.

On most tests, you can expect to see a series of unrelated short passages ranging from one to eight paragraphs. After each passage, you'll find questions that are based on the information in the preceding passage. The tasks that these questions ask you to do usually fall into a handful of categories (covered in detail later in this chapter). These include identifying the main idea, making inferences based on information given, predicting what comes next, defining a word based on context, and identifying/analyzing specific details.

While the majority of nursing school entrance exams take the same general approach to reading comprehension, the ATI TEAS likes to mix it up a little. On this exam you may encounter passages that give you a set of instructions to draw something. Using your scratch paper, you'll follow the directions and then choose the answer choice that most closely resembles what you drew. This tests you on your ability to accurately follow directions and visualize what needs to be done in your head.

Another type of question you may find on the ATI TEAS reading comprehension section involves deriving information from a table, a chart, or an image. The question asks you to identify certain information based on the item they give you to examine. This tests your analytical and reasoning skills as much as your ability to follow directions. (We cover charts in Chapter 7.)

Be prepared to see a variety of types of writing on the test—anything from journal entries and personal letters to dialogue between two or more people, maps and figures, advertisements, and more.

Because the majority of the reading comprehension questions on these exams center on the more traditional model of passage/question/answer, these are the tips focused on in this chapter. For the other types of

questions, there's not much more you can do to prepare than simply practice.

So let's get down to it. When you're approaching a reading comprehension test, some simple tweaks to your general approach will save you time and brainpower:

1. **Read the question first, not the passage.** There are several different types of questions, which we'll detail later in this chapter. If you know what type of question you're dealing with, you'll know what to look for in the passage—which can save you a bunch of time. For example, if you have a question that asks you what a word means in a particular sentence, you only have to read enough to figure out how it's used in that one instance. Also, make sure you read through the answer choices and understand what they mean.

2. **Read as little of the passage as possible.** Contrary to what you may have been taught about reading comprehension tests, you don't have to read the whole passage (which is often designed to be dry and boring, making it harder to get through) to get the right answers.

   The type of question you need to answer will determine how much of the passage you need to read. For main idea questions, you will likely have to read the whole passage. However, for a specific detail question, you can scan quickly for key words that can lead you to where the answer is in the passage. Analyze the information and answer the question in your own words.

3. **Answer and eliminate.** Once you have an answer in your head, eliminate answer choices that don't match

up with your original thought. When you read through the answer choices, they may be wordy or complicated. Look for answers that are backed up directly with information from the passage. Get rid of answer choices that are not supported by a specific phrase or sentence in the passage.

> **TEST TIP**
>
> Check reality at the door when you approach a reading comprehension question. The only information that matters is what's in the passage. Make your inferences based on your own logic and specific statements from the passage—not what you know to be true in real life.

Now, let's take a look at some of the types of questions you'll see on a reading comprehension test.

Main Idea

Very often you'll be asked to identify the overall point of a passage. There really isn't a shortcut with this type of question, other than skimming through the passage to get a sense of what it's about. But we don't suggest doing that because very often, paragraphs in this section talk about one thing at the beginning and then transition into something else by the end. Skimming can lead you to a false conclusion about the passage's purpose.

Should you choose to skim, watch out for transitional words, like *but* or *however* in the middle of a passage. If you see them there, it's a good bet that the content of what's being said is about to change, and what follows may be the point the author's trying to make.

Treatment plan:

1. Your best bet with main idea questions is simply to read carefully, make notes about what you're reading if you can, and use the format to your advantage. Most passages have a predictable format, and somewhere there's some kind of topic sentence that states or implies the point of the passage. The rest of the sentences give details or support for that point. Your job is to find that sentence.

2. Look for sentences that explain what the passage is about, rather than how or why something is what it is. These can appear anywhere in the passage. They often are the first or last sentence but can also come in toward the middle.

> **TEST TIP**
>
> Main idea questions may not come right out and ask you to identify the point. When you see questions that ask you to choose the best title or what the passage is primarily about, think main idea.

Purpose

This is a variation on the main idea question. You're not looking for what the passage is about, but what the speaker hopes to accomplish. Some purposes of a passage can be to ...

▸ Inform the reader about something.

▸ Show or explain a process.

▸ Educate or instruct.

▸ Persuade.

▸ State an opinion or position.

▸ Reason something out.

▸ Tell a story.

Treatment plan:

1. Figure out what the main idea of the passage is.

2. Ask yourself why the speaker would try to communicate this message. What is he or she hoping to accomplish?

3. Eliminate answer choices that don't match your idea.

Tone

As discussed in Chapter 5, words can have more to their meaning than what's written in the dictionary. They also can evoke a feeling in the person communicating them and the person receiving the message.

On reading comprehension tests, sometimes you'll be asked to figure out what feelings the speaker in a passage is trying to communicate through their words. This is called *tone*. When you have a tone question, pay close attention to the language in the passage and the impression you get based on what's said.

> **NURSING NOTES**
>
> When we say speaker, we're talking about the narrator of a passage, not the author. Narrators give accounts of events, stories, etc., and may or may not be involved in what's being told. Every piece of writing has a speaker. When you read the following example, ask yourself who the speaker is. If you think it's a college freshman, you're right!

Read the following passage:

> College is so not what I thought it would be. I figured living away from home, away from my parents' restrictions would mean more freedom and lots of time to party. But living in the dorms is tough. My roommate is up all night on his computer and his radio blasting the whole time. I never get any sleep and am always late to my 8 A.M. classes. When I'm there, I start to doze and miss half of the lecture, which makes doing the homework so much harder. I'm spending all of my free time in the library trying to catch up, while my roommate is the one who's partying and having a good time. Who knew being on my own would be so much work?

What kind of vibe do you get from reading this paragraph? Frustrated, shocked, annoyed, and exasperated are all good answers. The fact that the speaker is complaining in every sentence and everything he's saying is negative gives us a clue to what he's feeling.

Treatment plan:

1. Look at the language that's being used, punctuation, and context clues in the passage.

2. Determine if the speaker in the passage is excited, somber, apprehensive, happy, etc.

3. Eliminate answer choices that don't match.

Try it out here:

> The tone of this passage can best be described as
>
> (A) reminiscent.
> (B) argumentative.
> (C) mysterious.
> (D) exasperated.

"Reminiscent" means that you're remembering something fondly, which doesn't really apply here because the passage takes place in present tense—and there is no fondness anywhere. "Argumentative" doesn't work because there isn't a point being made; he may be complaining about his circumstances, but there's no argument being made. "Mysterious" just doesn't make sense for this passage. This leaves "exasperated," which means to be frustrated or at your wits' end. Answer D fits best.

Unfortunately, like main idea questions, you'll have to read the whole passage for tone questions, too. Vocabulary will also play a key role with this type of question, because many of the answer choices may be more sophisticated than what you'd use every day. Be sure to check out our vocabulary-building tips in Chapter 5.

Specific Details

As the name suggests, this type of question asks you to find a specific piece of information in the passage. The beauty of this type of question is that the answers are right in the passage, and often, language similar to what's written in the passage *will* be used in the question. Knowing this will save you time if you use the general approach outlined earlier in this chapter.

Treatment plan:

1. Read and determine what information the question is asking you to find.

2. Skim the passage to determine where the information you need is located. Read just enough to answer the question in your own words.

3. Eliminate answer choices that don't match your answer.

Give it a try:

> A census provides comprehensive data about
>
> (A) job rates.
> (B) electoral votes.
> (C) the population.
> (D) market trends.

The question is asking you to look for a word that has something to do with "comprehensive data." Now skim the passage for those words and see what you find:

> The U.S. Constitution mandates that the federal government take a national census every ten years. The data is used to calculate how many congressional seats need to be appointed per state, the number of electoral votes each state gets, and determine state and municipal funding. Census data also gives comprehensive demographic information about the population.

The second sentence discusses data, but no mention of how in-depth it is. The last sentence, however, talks about "comprehensive demographic information" which means comprehensive data. So what is this information in regard to? Population. Answer C is correct.

It may be tempting to choose Answer B because "electoral votes" are mentioned and in the same sentence as "data." But the content of the sentence talks about what census data is used to calculate, not the information it provides, which is what your question is asking for.

CODE RED!

Beware of questions that ask you to determine what's not in a passage or can't be inferred from what's written. This runs counter to what you're used to (finding the correct answer), and is a huge time drain. In this case, you should compare each answer choice to the information stated in the passage. The one that doesn't fit is your answer.

Vocab in Context

These questions are probably the easiest on the test, because you will likely have already encountered them on a vocabulary or word knowledge section. This means you can use the same strategies here as well; the Swap It Out technique discussed in Chapter 5 works well for this type of question.

Your job is to figure out how the underlined word is being used in a specific sentence. The great thing about this type of question is that you usually only have to read one sentence!

Treatment plan:

1. Go back to the passage and read the sentence that contains the word in the question.

2. Use context clues to determine how the word is being used and what it's intended to mean.

3. Eliminate answer choices that don't match your definition.

Use the previous passage that discusses the census to answer the following question:

> In the passage, <u>mandates</u> most nearly means

(A) enlists.
(B) believes.
(C) requires.
(D) restricts.

The sentence reads: "The U.S. Constitution mandates that the federal government take a national census every ten years." Use your Swap It Out method here and see what works best:

(A) The U.S. Constitution enlists that the federal government take a national census every ten years.

(B) The U.S. Constitution believes that the federal government take a national census every ten years.

(C) The U.S. Constitution requires that the federal government take a national census every ten years.

(D) The U.S. Constitution restricts that the federal government take a national census every ten years.

The only answer choice that makes sense within the context of the sentence is C. "Enlist" means to sign up, which doesn't fit; "believes" isn't possible because the Constitution can't believe because it's not an entity, but a document; and "restricts" means to limit, which also doesn't fit with the content of the sentence.

Inference Questions

Many people consider inference questions to be difficult or tricky because they ask you to think for yourself. They don't give you the answers, as in specific detail or Vocab in Context questions. It's up to you to draw conclusions (or infer) based on information in the passage. You may also be asked to predict what happens next.

These questions are a good way to measure your critical thinking skills. Just like every other question in this section, you'll be presented with a passage of information and a question or prompt such as the following:

▸ The author is most likely to agree with which of the following statements?

▸ Based on the passage, it can be inferred that …

▸ According to the passage, it can be assumed that …

Then you'll get four statements to consider. They can ask you about what happens next, thoughts the speaker might have, where the story takes place, or other conclusions that could be based on the passage.

Now, you may be asking how you're supposed to know what happens next or what the speaker is thinking. That's where critical thinking comes in. It's your job to compare the answer choices to information in the passage. Correct answers will always be supported by specific details in the passage.

Treatment plan:

1. Read the question first.

2. Read the passage.

3. Go to each answer choice and ask yourself, "What in the passage tells me this would likely happen or be true?"

Let's try this out:

> According to the passage, it can be assumed that …

The setup of the question tells us it's a straightforward inference question. Next, read the passage:

> Owning a pet can result in several health benefits. Studies have shown that cat and dog owners tend to suffer fewer cardiovascular ailments, such as high blood pressure or cholesterol. Interacting with pets can also result in increased brain activity and have a calming effect on the body.

Now look at the answer choices, and go through them one by one to see what's supported by information in the passage and what's not:

(A) Pet owners live longer.
(B) Cats and dogs are inappropriate pets for children.
(C) The health benefits of owning a dog are greater than those of owning a cat.
(D) A cat would be a good gift for someone who has anxiety issues.

The passage doesn't mention anything about pets affecting length of life or children.

Answers A and B can be eliminated. Although the passage does talk about different health benefits for dogs and cats, it does not provide a judgment on which is better. This eliminates Answer C. Because the passage says that interacting with a pet can have a calming effect on the body, and a cat is a pet, it can be reasonably assumed that Answer D is correct.

Fact or Opinion

Sometimes you'll get a question that asks you to look at the answer choices and determine which one is a *fact* or *opinion*. This is one of the easiest types of questions you'll find on a reading comprehension test, because all you have to do is figure out what can be proven and what can't.

Treatment plan:

1. Read the question first and figure out what you're looking for: fact or opinion.

2. Compare each answer choice to the information given in the passage. For each, ask yourself, "Can this be proven with information in the passage?" If the answer is yes, it's a fact. If the answer is no, it's an opinion.

3. Use process of elimination to get rid of unlikely answer choices.

If you're really stuck on this type of question, look at the answer choices. Opinion answers will have some telltale signs that you're dealing with a perspective or preference. Look for words such as *good, better, best, prettiest, strongest, fastest, thought, think, believe, feel, love, hate, bad, worse,* and *worst.* Anything that implies an emotion or thought, not verifiable information, is a big red flag that you're most likely dealing with an opinion.

Paragraph Breakdown

Now that you know all about the types of questions you'll see on the test, let's get some practice in getting the information you need out of the passages. Write out the main idea, purpose, tone, and major details for each of the following paragraphs. They might not be as long as a whole passage you'll see on the test, but they'll give you good practice in sifting through sentences to get the info you need.

The idea of the public being able to access information about its government goes back to the days of ancient Rome. During this time, the Roman government published *acta*, official texts that were often openly accessible to the public. However, acta that detailed the goings on within the Senate were not made public until Julius Caesar, in his position as consul, ordered that accounts of such proceedings be open to the people. Though these acta were later censored by the government, their publication shows that our modern democratic ideas that center on the public accessibility of government records have very deep, historical roots.

Main idea: _____

_____

Purpose: _____

_____

Tone: _____

_____

Main details: _____

_____

The centuries of trial and error with the simple process of fermentation have led to the creation of a vast variety of beverages that are consumed every day. For example, wine is produced as a result of fermenting specific types of grapes or other fruits whose chemical compositions are conducive to creating alcohol. Grapes grown specifically for producing wine are first crushed and strained before the skins are discarded. Then yeast is added to the mixture. As the yeast consumes the natural sugars in the grape juice, alcohol is produced. This concoction is kept in climate-controlled containers, such as vats or barrels, to give the yeast time to develop the flavor of the wine. Beer is also produced through a similar process, but grains and hops are used in place of grapes.

Main idea: _____

_____

Purpose: _____

_____

Tone: _____

_____

Main details: _____

_____

Laws regarding car seats vary from state to state. It is important for parents to know what their local regulations are, not only for the safety of their children, but also to comply with the law. Car dealerships, community groups, and health-care agencies often hold free clinics to check that your car seat is installed properly and to give out informational material about child age, height, and weight requirements for different car seats. Every parent can benefit from attending these clinics.

Main idea: _____

_____

Purpose: _____

_____

Tone: _____

_____

Main details: _____

_____

When you fall asleep, your brain literally slows down. The brain waves you create when you're awake take a break and different, slower waves—theta and delta waves—are produced. As you descend deeper into sleep, your theta and delta wave patterns become slower. Your body temperature and respiration also decrease, while your brain's need for oxygen increases. You are more likely to experience longer periods of this type of sleep when you are younger. Children and young adults most often fall into a slow-wave sleep not long after going to bed for the night. As people get older, these periods become fewer, and by the time they are elderly, may not even occur at all.

Main idea: _____

_____

Purpose: _____

_____

Tone: _____

_____

Main details: _____

_____

Practice Questions

Select the answer choice that best answers each question.

Use the following passage to answer questions 1 through 5:

Will listening to loud music make my child go deaf? This question is on the minds of many parents given the increased popularity and use of personal electronics with headphones among children.

The answer, however, is not as simple as the question. Kids who often listen to loud music or are frequently exposed to lawn mowers or motorcycles are at risk of hearing loss. But that risk is dependent on how loud the sounds are and how long the child is exposed.

"Using a personal music player with headphones at a reasonable level is fine, but cranking it up above 90 decibels will, over time, cause irreversible hearing loss in some children," says Lynn Leuthke, PhD, director of the hearing program for the National Institute on Deafness and Other Communication Disorders, in Rockville, Maryland.

A good rule of thumb to follow is that if you can hear what your child is listening to just by standing near her, it's too loud. Also, when buying a personal music player, look for a model that enables you to limit the volume output to no more than 90 decibels.

1. A good title for this passage would be
    - (A) Your Child's Hearing Is in Danger!
    - (B) Why Headphones Should Be Banned from Schools
    - (C) The Dangers of Listening to Music
    - (D) What Parents Should Know about Exposure to Loud Sounds

2. The highest level of sound that does not pose a risk of damaging one's hearing is
    - (A) 120 decibels.
    - (B) 100 decibels.
    - (C) 90 decibels.
    - (D) 80 decibels.

3. The tone of this passage is
    - (A) helpful.
    - (B) alarming.
    - (C) condescending.
    - (D) punishing.

4. According to this passage, a parent should
    - (A) not buy their child a personal music player.
    - (B) have their child's hearing tested regularly.
    - (C) look for personal music products that limit volume.
    - (D) let their child listen to music as loud as they like.

5. The narrator of this passage would most likely agree that

   (A) regular exposure to sounds above 90 decibels pose as much risk to a child's hearing as music.

   (B) hearing tests can't accurately measure hearing loss.

   (C) irreversible hearing loss is an epidemic.

   (D) new studies should be conducted to evaluate hearing loss in children.

Use the following passage to answer questions 6 through 10:

Coffee beans are not actually beans, but rather roasted seeds of coffee berries. After the seeds are separated from the berries, they're fermented, cleaned, and air dried. Now called green coffee beans, they must be roasted before they are consumed. The internal temperature must be raised to at least 205 degrees Celsius to produce caffeol oil, which produces the flavor commonly associated with coffee.

Even so, there are two main types of coffee "beans" that are consumed around the world. The first is arabica and is the more expensive of the two; it is also more popular due to its richer, more developed flavor. Arabica coffee plants need to be grown within certain conditions: at an elevation between 4,000 feet and a mile, and in a climate that has a consistent temperature around 70 degrees.

Robusta is the other type of "bean" that is used to make coffee. Robusta coffee is less expensive than its arabica counterpart, primarily because of the plants that produce the beans; they can be grown at lower, more accessible altitudes, produce more beans per acre grown, and do not have to be handpicked to make it to the roasting process. However, robusta beans do not have as much flavor as arabica beans, which is why you'll most often find them used in coffee blends or instant coffee.

6. What is produced when the internal temperature of a coffee bean reaches at least 205 degrees Celsius?

   (A) caffeine

   (B) caffeol oil

   (C) dark coloring

   (D) extra flavor

7. According to the passage

   (A) Coffee beans can be eaten directly from the plant.

   (B) Coffee beans taste like berries.

   (C) Coffee beans must be cleaned before they are fermented.

   (D) Coffee beans are seeds.

8. Which of the following statements is an opinion?

   (A) Arabica coffee plants need to be grown at least 4,000 feet.
   (B) Arabica coffee is better than robusta coffee.
   (C) There are two main types of coffee beans.
   (D) Coffee beans are not really beans.

9. The purpose of this passage is to

   (A) inform.
   (B) persuade.
   (C) incite.
   (D) evaluate.

10. Robusta beans are often used to make

   (A) cappuccino.
   (B) instant coffee.
   (C) espresso.
   (D) coffee-flavored ice cream.

Use the following passage to answer questions 11 through 15:

Have you ever given any thought to why superstitions still have power in today's modern society? With all of the technology and access to knowledge at the tips of our fingers, most people still place at least some stock in superstitions whose origins they don't really know or don't even make logical sense. For example, how did the number 13 become feared and reviled in our society? The answer is far from simple.

Strikingly similar instances of the demonization of the number can be seen in folklore and religion throughout history. For example, Christian tradition says that Judas, the apostle who betrayed Jesus to the Romans, was the thirteenth member to arrive at the Last Supper. In Norse mythology, it's said that the god Loki tricked the god of winter into killing Balder the Good, the son of the king and queen of the gods, during a feast of 12 gods in Valhalla. As in the Christian story, the arrival of the thirteenth person to the dinner brings horrible consequences.

Historical instances of bad things happening on Friday the thirteenth have also helped further connections between evil or bad luck and the number 13. The wildly popular novel *The DaVinci Code* introduced the idea to millions that the beginning of France's persecution, torture, and execution of the Order of the Knights Templar began on Friday the thirteenth. The tragic crash of Uruguayan Air Force Flight 571, which stranded survivors of the flight in the Andes Mountains for two months without food or water, took place on Friday, October 13, 1972. And the Apollo 13 mission, the United States' third trip to the moon in the infancy of the space program, suffered a devastating blow when an explosion on Friday, April 13, 1970, caused severe damage to the craft.

The most logical explanation, though, is that these cultural assignments that have been developed and attached to this number are simply our way as humans to make sense out of the unexplainable. Mythology, religion, and even historical connections do not provide concrete proof that the number 13 in and of itself has any power in the real world.

Yet, this belief has trickled down from generation to generation through the centuries without any real thought as to the hows or whys of it. Given this history, it is more than likely that this pattern will continue so long as we continue to give such power to beliefs without logically examining their validity in the modern world.

11. In the first paragraph, the word <u>stock</u> most nearly means

   (A) broth.
   (B) commodity.
   (C) value.
   (D) to hunt.

12. The main idea of this passage is

   (A) the number 13 has innate power to cause harm in the world.
   (B) people turn to superstition to explain the unexplainable.
   (C) superstitions are based more on science than mythology.
   (D) even though it makes no logical sense, people still believe in superstitions because they are handed-down beliefs.

13. According to the passage, the crash of Uruguayan Air Force Flight 571

   (A) took place on Friday the thirteenth.
   (B) happened because the flight took place on the thirteenth day of the month.
   (C) occurred in Uruguay.
   (D) caused the survivors to turn into cannibals.

14. Based on information from the passage, it can be inferred that in the future

   (A) science will disprove all superstitions and they will no longer hold power over human behavior.
   (B) superstitions will continue to play a role in human culture.
   (C) new superstitions will be formed.
   (D) science will prove the validity of many superstitions.

15. According to the passage, the most likely reason the number 13 has a negative stigma attached to it is because

   (A) it is written in a holy book that the number is evil.
   (B) a powerful political leader declared the number taboo.
   (C) people throughout history have assigned ideas of evil to the number as a way of explaining the inexplicable.
   (D) history definitively shows bad things happen when associated with the number.

Answers and Explanations

1. **D.** Answers A and B are too extreme and don't accurately reflect what's being discussed in the passage. Answer C is tempting, but it's not only music that's being discussed. This answer is vague enough to be wrong on a standardized exam. The final answer choice is both neutral and detailed enough to convey the main idea of the passage.

2. **C.** This is a specific detail question that asks you to infer just a little. Scan the passage for a number like those in the answer choices. You'll find that 90 is the only one mentioned. If you look further, you'll see the line: "cranking it up above 90 decibels will, over time, cause irreversible hearing loss in some children." Based on this information, you can deduce that 90 decibels is the limit you're looking for.

3. **A.** This is an informative, advisory type of passage. It is generally neutral to positive in connotation. Answer B connotes there is a sense of extreme urgency, which is neither present in the passage nor implied. Answers C and D connote negative tones, which are not present at all in the passage. No one is being talked down to (condescending) or censured, which makes A the best choice.

4. **C.** Another specific detail question here. The only choice directly supported by the passage is C, specifically the last line: "Also, when buying a personal music player, look for a model that enables you to limit the volume output to no more than 90 decibels."

5. **A.** This is an inference question. Based on the information in the passage, which of the statements do you think the narrator would likely agree with? This is just a matter of taking the information in each answer choice and comparing it to information in the passage, which makes no mention of hearing tests, measuring hearing loss, epidemics, or studies. What the passage does address is other types of sound exposure posing a risk to hearing. The following sentence makes A the best answer: "Kids who often listen to loud music or are frequently exposed to lawn mowers or motorcycles are at risk of hearing loss."

6. **B.** This is a specific detail question and the answer is found in the last sentence: "The internal temperature must be raised to at least 205 degrees Celsius to produce caffeol oil ...". Caffeine and coloring aren't mentioned in the passage—flavor is—but it says that caffeol oil produces the flavor you associate with coffee. It does not mention extra flavor anywhere.

7. **D.** This is an inference question. You need to use information in the passage to prove each answer true or false. The passage says that green coffee beans must be roasted before they can be consumed. This eliminates Answer A. The passage says that coffee beans come from berries, but nothing about them tasting like berries. It also says that coffee beans must be fermented before they're

cleaned. These two details eliminate Answers B and C. The first sentence clearly states that coffee beans are "roasted seeds of coffee berries," which makes Answer D the best choice.

8. **B.** All of the other answer choices are backed up by facts in the passage. They are all statements that can be proven. However, even though the passage says that arabica coffee is the most popular, this does not mean that it is better, because better is not something that can be proven one way or another. It's an opinion.

9. **A.** The passage gives information about coffee beans. No opinion or conclusion is stated, so "persuade" and "evaluate" aren't possible answers. The information is very neutral and does not ask the reader to take any action, which eliminates "incite" as an answer. A is the best answer.

10. **B.** None of the other answer choices are mentioned or implied in the passage.

11. **C.** Answers A and B both define "stock," but not in the way it's being used in the sentence from the passage. Answer D is a definition of *stalk*, which sounds like *stock*, but is not the same. Plus, if you use your Swap It Out method, Answer C is the only one that makes sense.

12. **D.** This is a tricky passage because the main idea is presented at the beginning and the end of the passage, but there's a lot of detail in between where you can get lost. Process of elimination is a good way to approach this question. Answer A is directly refuted in the passage: "Mythology, religion, and even historical connections do not provide concrete proof that the number 13 in and of itself has any power in the real world." Answer B is backed up by the passage, but is not the main idea being communicated, it's a detail. Answer C is not supported by the passage at all. That leaves Answer D. This idea is established in the first paragraph and strengthened in the final paragraph.

13. **A.** You have three events here mentioned in the third paragraph of the passage—you know, the one where they talk about events that happened on Friday the thirteenth. The Last Supper, mentioned in the second paragraph, did not.

14. **B.** The passage provides no direct statements to support any other answer choice. Answer B is backed up by the following: "Given this history, it is more than likely that this pattern will continue so long as we continue to give such power to beliefs without logically examining their validity in the modern world."

15. **C.** Holy books and taboos are not mentioned in the passage at all, making Answers A and B unlikely choices. And even though the passage recounts lots of times that the number has been associated with bad things, this is not definitive. Answer D is not a good choice. However, Answer C is directly supported by the following, making it the strongest answer: "The most logical explanation, though, is that these cultural assignments we've developed and attached to this number are simply our way as humans to make sense out of the unexplainable."

Math Matters

There's no getting around it; nurses use math every single day. They have to fill in and analyze data in charts. They measure medications and calculate percentages and proportions. And they do a lot of problem solving. The good news is that to qualify for nursing school, you don't have to be a math genius. You just need high school–level skills in arithmetic, algebra, geometry, and reasoning.

This part will refresh your memory and skills in areas of math that you likely haven't thought about since grammar school, such as adding fractions with different denominators. It also takes you through more complex types of math that you may not have understood all that well the first time you touched on them in high school—but you sure will this time, with a little practice.

Basic Arithmetic

Math—especially basic math—is a skill that you will use every day as a nurse. Working with decimals, calculating percentages, analyzing charts, converting metric units, and more are all part of a day's work. And often it's the accuracy of those calculations that greatly affect a patient's health.

Without a firm grasp of basic math skills, completing any nursing education program is going to be a challenge. It can also become a potential hazard, as most nursing programs require students to take part in clinical instruction. This is why most nursing school entrance exams require some kind of a math assessment as a yardstick for measuring candidate eligibility.

This chapter walks you through the main types of math question formats you may see on your test, in addition to a review of basic concepts you'll likely encounter. We'll also show you how to break these questions down, strategies for getting the right answer, and lots of practice putting it all together.

What to Expect

Though the material on each type of exam will vary, you will generally find a few main types of questions on any given math section. They are straight computation problems (1 + 1 =), word problems, and quantitative comparison. You've been doing straight computation problems since the first grade, so we're not really going to spend much time on those, other than to say to follow the general approach discussed in Chapter 3.

So that leaves us with quantitative comparisons (discussed in Chapter 8) and word problems. Assessment is the key to effectively completing word problems, which makes them a good indicator of your thinking and reasoning skills. Your goal is to determine mathematical objectives out of a short description of circumstances by analyzing the word problem and decide what's important to your task and what's not.

Because you're starting to get into the mindset you'll need to have when working as a nurse, think about word problems as if you were working with a new patient: assess the situation, diagnose the issue, create a treatment plan that will solve the issue, implement that plan, and follow up to make sure it's working.

1. **Assess:** Read the question from beginning to end, and try to figure out what it's asking you to do.

2. **Diagnose:** After you've read the question and assessed what it's asking you to do, you need to translate this into what this means in terms of math. This will give you a better understanding of what the question is asking you to do and a simpler focus moving forward.

3. **Create a treatment plan:** Write out the steps and equations you'll need to solve the problem. Seeing them on your scratch paper will help you keep track of your work as you go along and make sure you're taking a logical approach to solving the problem.

4. **Implement:** Complete all steps needed to formulate the answer. Check and double check your math to make sure that it's accurate and that it makes sense.

5. **Follow up:** In real life, this would be when you check with your patient to assess the effects of your treatment plan. On your exam, this means eliminating answer choices that don't match the one you've come up with.

Let's try this out with the following question:

> The owner of Artie's Furniture Emporium is planning a holiday sale. A five-piece dining room set is one of the main items he wants to feature. He bought the set wholesale for $1,000 and set the retail price at $2,000. If he wants to make at least a 25 percent profit by selling the set, what's the lowest amount that he can set the sale price?

1. **Assess:** The question seems to have a lot of parts that you need to understand:

    ‣ Dining set wholesales for $1,000; Artie marked up to $2,000.

    ‣ Artie wants to feature the set as part of a sale and needs to figure out how much he can mark the price down and still make a 25 percent profit.

2. **Diagnose:** In math terms, the question is asking you to figure out how to make this 25 percent profit. Profit refers to money that is made after expenses are recouped. In this case, Artie paid $1,000 for the set, which means that to make a profit he will have to sell it for more than this amount. Now you have to figure out how much is 25 percent more than $1,000.

3. **Create a treatment plan:** How do you figure this out? To calculate percentage, you multiply the decimal form of the percentage amount by the number you're trying to find the percentage of. (We discuss decimals and percentages later in this chapter.)

$$.25 \times 1,000 = x$$

But you're not done. You now need to add that answer to $1,000 to find out the total price Artie can set to make his 25 percent profit:

$$x + 1,000 = \text{ANSWER}$$

4. **Implement:** Now, let's solve the expressions you've written and find out what answer choice you need to look for:

$$.25 \times 1,000 = 250$$

$$250 + 1,000 = 1,250$$

5. **Follow up:** If this were a question on your exam, you'd now eliminate answer choices that are not $1,250.

Arithmetic Review

Now that you're feeling more comfortable with word problems, it's time to review some of the math you'll be using. To start, take a look at some basic terms and symbols. Some may be familiar, while others may be new.

Arithmetic Vocab

Term	Definition
Natural numbers	Counting numbers, such as 1, 2, 3. Natural numbers are always positive, and 0 is not a natural number. When a set of numbers includes 0 (0, 1, 2, 3), you're dealing with whole numbers.

Term	Definition
Integer	Any whole number or its opposite. (The opposite of 3 is –3; the opposite of –5 is 5.) –2, –1, 0, 1, and 2 are all integers; 3.1 or –2.5 are not.
Prime number	A natural number that can only be divided by 1 and itself. 2, 3, 5, 7, 11, 13, and 17 are prime numbers. 1 is not a prime number because 1 is its only factor.
Factor	A natural number that can be evenly divided into a number. Factors of 12 are 1, 2, 3, 4, 6, and 12. They all divide into 12 evenly.
Multiple	The product of two natural numbers: 36 is a multiple of 9 because $9 \times 4 = 36$. 14 is a multiple of 7 because $7 \times 2 = 14$.
Term	A single number, variable, or combinations thereof. Examples: $8x$, x, xy^2, 15.
Product	Answer to a multiplication problem. This and words such as *times*, *double*, and *of* in a word problem can indicate the need for multiplication.
Quotient	Answer to a division problem. This and words such as *per*, *out of*, and *into* in a word problem can indicate the need for division.
Sum	Answer to an addition problem. This and words such as *total* and *combined* in a word problem can indicate the need for addition.
Difference	Answer to a subtraction problem. This and words such as *minus*, *decrease*, and *fall* in a word problem can indicate the need for subtraction.

Now let's look at some specific types of arithmetic you can expect to see on your exam.

Order of Operations

You may remember the "Please Excuse My Dear Aunt Sally" or PE(MD)(AS) rule from grade school. This mnemonic applies to order of *operations,* or the order in which you perform mathematical processes in an expression with more than one type of the following symbols: +, × (or), ÷, and –.

> **DEFINITION**
>
> In math, an **operation** refers to one of four mathematical processes: addition, subtraction, multiplication, and division.

You need to follow a specific order to solve these problems correctly. First, look for any expressions that are separated into parentheses and solve these by applying any exponents (discussed in Chapter 8) that may be present.

Next, move on to multiplication and division and solve these parts of the expression moving left to right. Finally, perform the addition and subtraction operations, moving left to right. When the expression in the parentheses has been reduced to a number, repeat the order of operations on the entire expression.

Try this with the following expression: $2 \times (2 \times 3)^3 + 7 - 10$.

- ▸ **Parentheses:** Solve the expression in parentheses: $2 \times 3 = 6$.

- ▸ **Exponent:** Apply the exponent to the 6 in the parentheses. (For more about exponents, see Chapter 8.) This is the same as saying $6 \times 6 \times 6$. The product is 216.

- ▸ **Multiplication:** The new expression is $2 \times 216 + 7 - 10$. Multiply 2 by 216 to get 432.

- ▸ **Addition and Subtraction:** Now the expression is $432 + 7 - 10$. Solve left to right to finish: $432 + 7 = 439$, and $439 - 10 = 429$.

Always keep order of operations in mind when you have a mixed expression like this. Solving in a different order can lead you to a wrong answer.

Positive and Negative Integers

If you think of numbers in terms of a line, you'll be able to understand positives and negatives. At the center of the line is 0. All numbers to the right of 0 are positive, and all numbers to the left are negative. (0 is a neutral number.)

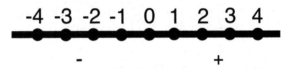

Easy enough, right? The tricky part with positives and negatives comes when you start moving up and down that line through addition and subtraction.

Look at the following expression: $2 - 1$. Your first instinct might be to read this as 2 minus 1, but really, what you're seeing in terms of the number line is $+2 + (-1)$. This expression is telling you to start at the +2 position on the number line and move one step to the left, or –1. The result is that you end up at +1 on the number line. Try it out on the previous diagram.

This is the basic idea of how we deal with adding and subtracting positives and negatives in math. Use the previous number line to illustrate the following:

- Positive + positive = Move up the number line: 3 + 1 = 4

- Positive + negative = Move down the number line: 2 + (− 3) = −1

- Negative + positive = Move up the number line: −1 + 4 = 3

- Negative + negative = Move down the number line: −2 + (−2) = −4

- Negative − negative = When you have two negative symbols, they cancel each other out and make a positive. For example, −1 − (−3) is the same as −1 + 3, and you would move up the number line when you solve. The answer is 2.

- Positive − negative = With this type of problem, you have two negatives, as well: 3 − (−1). The negatives become a positive, so you need to move up the number line: 3 − (−1) = 3 + 1 = 4.

Multiplication and division problems are a little different:

1. Multiply or divide the numbers in the problem like you normally would.

2. Then figure out whether it's positive or negative. Only the negatives affect the sign of the answer:

- An odd number of negatives will result in a *negative* answer: −12 ÷ 3 = −4 (one negative); (−4)(−2)(−6) = −48 (three negatives).

- An even number of negatives will result in a *positive* answer: −24 ÷ −3 = 8 (two negatives); (−2)(−6)(−5)(−1) = 60 (four negatives).

Multiples and Factors

When you need to factor a number, what you're doing is figuring out the pairs of natural numbers that can be multiplied to get the number you're factoring. For example, what numbers can you multiply to get 10? There are only two sets: 1 × 10 and 2 × 5. Guess what? You just calculated the factors of 10! The numbers 1, 2, 5, and 10 are all factors of 10.

Up next are the three things you need to know when calculating multiples and factors.

Prime Factorization

This action breaks down a number into the product of its prime factors. To factor a number into primes you should ...

1. Divide by a prime number again and again until you have 1 as an answer.

2. List all the primes you used and multiply.

Let's try this with the number 36:

$$3 \underline{|36}$$
$$3 \underline{|36}$$
$$2 \underline{|4}$$
$$2 \underline{|2}$$
$$1$$

Now list out the prime numbers you've used on the outside (3, 3, 2, and 2) and then multiply: 3 × 3 × 2 × 2 = 36.

A good place to start dividing with prime factorization is 2 if you have an even number; 3 if the sum of the digits is a multiple of 3 (ex. 3,654; $3 + 6 + 5 + 4 = 18$, which is a multiple of 3); and 5 for numbers ending in 0 and 5.

Greatest Common Factor (GCF)

The general idea here is to multiply all the common prime factors of two numbers. The product is the highest factor they have in common.

To find the GCF of two numbers:

1. Use prime factorization.

2. Multiply the common factors.

Try it out with 24 and 28:

$$3 | 24 \qquad 7 | 28$$
$$2 | 8 \qquad 2 | 4$$
$$2 | 4 \qquad 2 | 2$$
$$2 | 2 \qquad 1$$
$$1$$

$$3 \times 2 \times [2 \times 2] = 24$$

$$7 \times [2 \times 2] = 28$$

As you can see, the only shared factor here is 2×2, or 2^2, which, when multiplied, gives you a highest common factor of 4. (See Chapter 8 for more about exponents.) If there had been more than one shared factor, you would multiply them all, and the product would be your GCF.

Least Common Multiple (LCM)

This is the smallest number that can be divided by two specific numbers. To figure out LCM:

1. Use prime factorization.

2. Use each individual digit as a factor the greatest number of times it appears in any one factorization.

Take a look at the following example, where you need to find the LCM of 20 and 30:

$$20 = 2 \times 2 \times 5$$

$$30 = 2 \times 3 \times 5$$

The factors are 2, 3, and 5. The greatest number of times you see 5 in one factorization is once; 3 is once; and 2 is twice. Combine each of these occurrences in the expression $2 \times 2 \times 3 \times 5$ and find that 60 is the smallest number that 20 and 30 can both divide into evenly.

Fractions

Fractions represent a part of a whole, which means that every number can be expressed as a fraction. They follow a specific format: The bottom number (denominator) tells us how many pieces make up the whole. The top number (numerator) tells us how many parts of that whole we are dealing with.

Basic concepts in regard to fractions that you should know include the following:

▶ When the numerator is less than the denominator, you have a proper fraction: $\frac{9}{11}$

▶ When the numerator and denominator are the same number, the fraction equals 1: $\frac{5}{5} = 1$

▶ When the numerator is either equal to or greater than the denominator, you have an improper fraction, which represents something that is either more than or equal to one: $\frac{16}{5}$

▶ When you simplify an improper fraction, you break it down into a mixed number (a whole number and a fraction together in one term). To do this, divide the bottom number into the top (that result is your whole number) and use the remainder as the numerator of a new fraction with the denominator remaining the same: $\frac{16}{5} = 3\frac{1}{5}$

For the most part, you'll be working with proper fractions on your exam and should be familiar with the following concepts.

Simplification

This means to reduce a fraction to its simplest form. To do this:

1. Break down both the numerator and denominator into prime factors.

2. Get rid of any factors each side has in common. What's left is the simplified fraction.

Take a look: $\frac{4}{16} = \frac{2\times2}{2\times2\times2\times2} = \frac{\cancel{2\times2}}{\cancel{2\times2}\times2\times2} = \frac{1}{4}$

Addition

When you have to add two fractions, add only the numerators when the denominators are the same. If your fractions have different denominators, you have to get them to match. To do this, multiply each fraction by the other fraction's denominator over itself in a new fraction.

Let's try it with: $\frac{3}{5} + \frac{7}{8}$

1. Multiply the first fraction by the opposite denominator (which is 8) over itself in a new fraction: $\frac{3}{5} \times \frac{8}{8} = \frac{24}{40}$

2. Now do the same with the second fraction: $\frac{7}{8} \times \frac{5}{5} = \frac{35}{40}$

3. Finally, add the two new fractions you created and reduce to simplest terms: $\frac{24}{40} + \frac{35}{40} = \frac{59}{40} = 1\frac{19}{40}$

So, what do you do if you have to add mixed fractions? Add the fractions first and then add the whole numbers, including any whole numbers that result from adding the fractions.

Let's try it with $4\frac{1}{3} + 6\frac{4}{5}$:

1. Add fractions first: $\frac{1}{3} \times \frac{5}{5} = \frac{5}{15}$ $\frac{4}{5} \times \frac{3}{3} = \frac{12}{15}$ $\frac{5}{15} + \frac{12}{15} = \frac{17}{15} = 1\frac{2}{15}$

2. Now add the wholes. This would include the 4 and 6 from the original expression and the 1 that was created by adding the fractions: $4 + 6 + 1 = 11$

3. Your final answer is $11\frac{2}{15}$.

Subtraction

The same rules you apply for addition, you use for subtraction, except for when you're dealing with mixed numbers that have different denominators. When this happens, you should do the following:

1. Turn each mixed number into an improper fraction before doing anything. To do this, multiply the whole number by the denominator. Then add the product to the numerator. Your denominator stays the same.

2. After all of your fractions are converted, follow the steps to make two fractions with matching denominators.

3. Subtract your fractions and simplify the answer back to a mixed fraction.

Let's see how this works with $5\frac{2}{3} - 1\frac{2}{4}$:

1. Turn each fraction into a mixed number: $5\frac{2}{3} = \frac{17}{3}$ $1\frac{2}{4} = \frac{6}{4}$

2. Make two fractions with matching denominators: $\frac{17}{3} \times \frac{4}{4} = \frac{68}{12}$ $\frac{6}{4} \times \frac{3}{3} = \frac{18}{12}$

3. Subtract your fractions and simplify: $\frac{68}{12} - \frac{18}{12} = \frac{50}{12} = 4\frac{2}{12} = 4\frac{1}{6}$

Multiplication

Multiply the numerators and denominators straight across. Then simplify the resulting fraction: $\frac{4}{5} \times \frac{6}{7} = \frac{24}{35}$

If you have to multiply mixed numbers, turn them into improper fractions and follow the same previous steps. When you simplify the answer, turn it back into a mixed number.

Division

Set up your problem as if you were multiplying. Then flip the numbers of the second fraction. (The result is called a *reciprocal*.) Multiply across and simplify: $\frac{7}{10} \div \frac{1}{2} = \frac{7}{10} \times \frac{2}{1} = \frac{14}{10} = 1\frac{4}{10} = 1\frac{2}{5}$

When dividing mixed fractions, turn them into improper fractions and proceed as you would with any other division problem.

Decimals

Just as every whole number is a fraction, every whole number is a decimal. The decimal place is directly behind the whole number: 4 = 4.0. Everything after the decimal point is a portion of a whole.

Every number has a place that is named in relation to its distance from the decimal point. Below is a listing of these places; the 5 indicates the position of the place from the decimal:

Thousands:	5,000.0
Hundreds:	500.0
Tens:	50.0
Ones:	5.0
Tenths:	0.5
Hundredths:	0.05
Thousandths:	0.005

As you can see, each place represents a place to the left or right of the decimal point. These places continue into infinity on either side.

Now let's look at how we apply operations to decimals.

Addition and Subtraction

Perform these operations like you would with any other problem. Line up your decimal points before you attempt to solve these problems. This ensures that you keep your numbers in line and that your answer has the decimal in the right place:

$$\begin{array}{r} 12.3 \\ + 1.2 \\ \hline 13.5 \end{array}$$

Multiplication

Multiply the problem as you normally would. Then count up the *total* number of decimal places in *each* factor of the original expression, and put the decimal point that many places to the left of the last number in your product. Try it with 5.4×2.3:

1. Multiply like normal:

$$\begin{array}{r} 54 \\ \times 23 \\ \hline 162 \\ +1080 \\ \hline 1242 \end{array}$$

2. Because there are two decimal places (one number after the decimal in each of the factors) in the original expression, place the decimal in the answer two places from the right: 12.42

Division

The trick to dividing decimals is working with a whole number divisor. Turning decimals into whole numbers is as simple as moving the decimal point in the right direction. Here's how you'd approach $1.729 \overline{)215.35}$:

1. The outside number is the divisor. Move the decimal point three places to the right so that you have a whole number: $1729 \overline{)215.65}$

2. Now move the decimal point of the dividend (the inside number) three places to the right. Because the decimal point is only two places in, add in as many 0s as needed to make up three places: $1729 \overline{)215650}$

3. Divide like normal and get 124725. Because the decimal point in the dividend is after the 0, just move it straight up into the quotient:

$$1729 \overline{)215650.00} \quad \frac{124.73}{}$$

Converting Decimals to Fractions

To convert a decimal to a fraction, make the decimal the numerator and 1 the denominator. Then move the decimal point to the right until you have a whole number.

For each place you move the decimal to the right, add a zero to the denominator. Finally, simplify the fraction: $.75 = \frac{75}{1} = \frac{75}{100} = \frac{3}{4}$

To turn a fraction into a decimal, simply divide the
numerator by the denominator:

$\frac{3}{4} = 3 \div 4 = .75$

Rounding

Rounding refers to making a number easier to work with by estimating its value to the nearest decimal place. For example, if a question asks you to round 10.36 to the nearest tenth, you'll have to decide if the 3 (which is in the tenths place) should stay a 3 or become a 4.

The rules for rounding are pretty straightforward:

1. Determine to what place you're being asked to round the number.

2. Look to the number to the right of the place you're being asked to round to. If the number is 1, 2, 3, or 4, drop that digit and leave the digit to be rounded alone. If it is 5, 6, 7, 8, or 9, drop that digit, but round the previous one up to the next number.

In the previous example, you would round 10.36 up to 10.4 because the number to the right of the tenths place is 6.

Percent

Percents represent a part of 100. Whenever you have a question that involves percent,

you're dealing with either decimals or fractions (whichever works best for you).

In decimals, 100 percent is the same as 1. Anything less than 100 percent is shown to the right of the decimal place: 4% = .04; 50% = .50.

In fractions, 100 percent is $\frac{100}{100}$ or any fraction where the numerator and denominator are equal. When you want to turn a whole number into a percent expressed as a fraction, simply make the number the numerator and use 100 as the denominator:

2%= $\frac{2}{100}$. Then, if possible, reduce: $\frac{2}{100} = \frac{1}{50}$.

A common type of percent problem on your entrance exam involves finding a certain percentage of another number, like we did with the furniture store sale example earlier in this chapter. When asked to do this, divide the smaller number by the larger to find the percentage.

Try it here:

What is 52% of 326?

To solve, multiply .52 by 326:

$$
\begin{array}{r}
326 \\
\times\ .52 \\
\hline
652 \\
+16300 \\
\hline
169.52
\end{array}
$$

The answer is 169.52.

Ratios

Ratios compare two values and are expressed in three main ways: with fractions, with a colon (:), or using the word *to*. Ratios in general usually express some sort of group relationship. The easiest way to work with ratios is to turn them into fractions and reduce:

An outpatient clinic sees 25 men and 45 women on Tuesday. What's the male-to-female ratio of patients for that day?

Here, you're being asked to write a mathematical statement that shows the relationship of men to women. Write the fraction the way you read it. That means the value for men is the numerator and the value for women is the denominator: $\frac{25}{45} = \frac{5}{9}$.

Proportions

Proportions compare two amounts or quantities. Like with ratios, it's easiest to treat these as fractions. Two must-knows for your exam:

Test for equality: Sometimes you'll be given two ratios and be asked if they are equal. To figure this out, cross-multiply the fractions. If the products are the same, your proportions are equal.

Try it out: Does $\frac{5}{8} = \frac{3}{4}$? If $8 \times 3 = 4 \times 5$, then it does.

In this case, the values on either side of the equals sign are not the same ($8 \times 3 = 24$ and $4 \times 5 = 20$), so these two fractions are not proportional.

Solve for an unknown quantity: Cross-multiply the two proportions in fraction format and use a variable (see Chapter 8) for the unknown value.

Try it out with the following: $\frac{2}{8} = \frac{x}{12}$

Start by cross-multiplying: $12 \times 2 = 24$ and so $8 \times x = 24$

To find the value of x, divide both sides of the second equation by 8:

$$\frac{8x}{8} = \frac{24}{8}$$

$$\frac{8x}{8} = \frac{24}{8}$$

$$x = 3$$

This gives you a final answer of $x = 3$.

Rates

Rates are special ratios that compare two different measurements. Examples include unit price $\left(\frac{\text{Price}}{\text{Number of items}}\right)$; speed $\left(\frac{\text{Distance}}{\text{Time}}\right)$; distance(rate × time); simple interest (amount borrowed × interest rate × time of loan); time $\left(\frac{\text{Distance}}{\text{Rate}}\right)$.

When you encounter a rate question on your exam, figure out what kind of rate you're being asked to calculate and then plug your values into the appropriate equation. Solve for the missing value.

Averages, Median, and Mode

Calculating averages (also known as *mean*) is simple math. When asked for an average of something, add up all of the terms that are given and then divide by the number of terms. For example, the average of 3, 4, 6, and $7 = \frac{3+4+6+7}{4} = \frac{20}{4} = 5$.

When you're asked to find the median of a set of numbers, you're looking for the one in the middle. Reorder the numbers from least to greatest. If you have an odd number of values in a set, the middle is easy to find: 2, 3, 4, 5, 6. If you have an even number of values, add the two values in the middle and divide by 2 to find the median: 2, 3, 4, 5, 6, 7; 4 + 5 = 9; 9 ÷ 2 = 4.5.

Mode simply refers to the value that occurs most often in a number set. In the following set, the mode is 4: 2, 3, 8, *4*, 9, *4*.

U.S. and Metric Measurements

Measuring dosages and converting one kind of measure to another are skills that nurses use every day when treating patients. It's no wonder that nursing schools want to gauge your ability in this area before admitting you into their program.

You will likely see some kind of conversion type of question on your entrance exam. Usually, all you have to do is plug the values into a proportion and solve for the missing quantity. But you also have to know what measures you're dealing with, too.

Here are some of the basic measures you'll find in the U.S. and metric measurement systems. Memorize them. You will need to know them.

Metric measures of length:

Millimeter (mm) = .1 centimeter

Centimeter (cm) = 10 millimeters

Meter (m) = 100 centimeters

Kilometer (km) = 1,000 meters

Metric measures of weight:

Milligram (mg) = .001 grams

Gram (g) = 1,000 milligrams

Kilogram (kg) = 1,000 grams

Metric ton = 1,000 kilograms

Metric measures of fluid:

Milliliter (mL) = .001 liter

Centiliter (cL) = .01 liter

Deciliter (dL) = .1 liter

Liter (L) = 1,000 milliliters

Kiloliter (kL) = 1,000 liters

U.S. measures of length:

12 inches (in.) = 1 foot (ft.)

3 feet = 1 yard (yd.)

5,280 feet = 1 mile

U.S. measures of weight:

16 ounces (oz.) = 1 pound (lb.)

2,000 pounds = 1 ton

U.S. measures of fluid:

8 fluid ounces = 1 cup (c.)

2 cups = 1 pint (pt.)

2 pints = 1 quart (qt.)

4 quarts = 1 gallon (gal.)

Approximate U.S. to metric conversions:

1 ounce = 28.35 grams

2.21 pounds = 1 kilogram

1 inch = 2.54 centimeters

3.28 feet = 1 meter

1 mile = 1.61 kilometers

1 fluid ounce = 29.57 milliliters

1.06 quarts = 1 liter

1 gallon = 3.79 liters

Graphs, Charts, and Tables

Math questions involving graphs, charts, and tables are nothing more than graphic presentations of data. These questions test you on your ability to evaluate the information given in graphic form and use it to answer the question. Chances are you're already pretty familiar with graphs, charts, and tables. You've already seen a table at the beginning of this chapter. (In case you missed it, it's where we define basic math terms.) Here are some examples of different kinds of graphs and charts.

Bar Graph

Bar graphs present information in terms of filled-in columns that are placed on an *x/y* axis, which is just a mathematical way of saying that the information is presented between two perpendicular lines that represent different values:

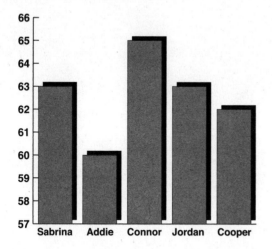

In this graph, the values on the left are represented by numbers. The values on the bottom are represented by names. When you compare the two, you find that each column measures up to a number on the left, which tells you the value of the column.

Here, Sabrina = 63; Addie = 60; Connor = 65; Jordan = 63; and Cooper = 62. Depending on the question associated with this graph, you can use this information to answer it.

One of the great things about graphs and charts is that you can quickly get a visual sense of quantity. A quick look at this bar graph tells you that one person has more than the others and three people have around the same amount. Information like this can help you get to your answer very quickly.

Line Graphs

This is another type of graph that enables you to make comparisons. But instead of columns, you have lines that mark certain points on the chart to show data:

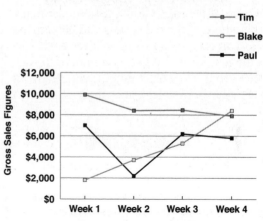

You can see that this chart represents the sales performance of three men during the month of March. They all stayed within the $2,000 to $10,000 range, but their sales numbers per week vary greatly. What a graph like this shows, which the bar graph did not, is how this information played out over time. Line graphs are most often used to present and analyze this type of data.

Pie Chart

As the name suggests, a pie chart presents data as portions of a circle:

Class of 2015

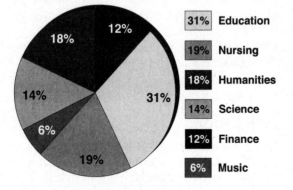

31%	Education
19%	Nursing
18%	Humanities
14%	Science
12%	Finance
6%	Music

The title of this chart tells us that we're looking at some kind of distribution of the Class of 2015. It is broken down into percentages (the whole of the pie equals 100 percent), and you can see how much space each percentage takes up. When you match up the colors to the key on the right, you see what each slice of the pie represents.

CODE RED!

Though overall, graphs, charts, and tables are pretty easy to get information out of, you always want to make sure that you understand the information that's being presented to you. Make sure you always read the title, values, and other notations so that you fully understand the context of the data.

Practice Questions

For each of the following questions, choose the best answer:

1. Place the following numbers in order from least to greatest: 2.5780, 2.725, 2.5782, 2.469, 2.5728, 2.697

    (A) 2.469, 2.5780, 2.5728, 2.5782, 2.697, 2.725

    (B) 2.469, 2.5728, 2.578, 2.5782, 2.697, 2.725

    (C) 2.469, 2.5782, 2.5780, 2.5728, 2.697, 2.725

    (D) 2.469, 2.5782, 2.5780, 2.5728, 2.725, 2.697

2. What is $\frac{17}{24}$ as a decimal rounded to the nearest hundredth?

    (A) .69

    (B) .70

    (C) .71

    (D) .72

3. .48 equals what fraction in its simplest form?

    (A) $\frac{24}{50}$

    (B) $\frac{48}{50}$

    (C) $\frac{6}{9}$

    (D) $\frac{12}{25}$

4. $4.75 + 3.2 + 2.87 + 1.1 =$

    (A) 8.05

    (B) 10.33

    (C) 11.92

    (D) 12.67

5. $2.73\overline{)16.425}$

    (A) 2.265

    (B) 6.016

    (C) 60.16

    (D) 601.6

6. A waitress makes $215.67 in tips during a night of work. She must give 10% to the bartender and 5% to the bus boy. After she does this, how much money in tips will she have to take home for the night?

    (A) $32.35

    (B) $76.67

    (C) $183.32

    (D) $215.52

7. $\frac{4}{5} \div \frac{6}{8} =$

    (A) $\frac{3}{4}$

    (B) $\frac{30}{32}$

    (C) $1\frac{4}{5}$

    (D) $1\frac{1}{15}$

8. What is negative four plus positive eight?

    (A) −4

    (B) 4

    (C) −12

    (D) 12

9. Find the LCM of 16 and 12:

   (A) 48
   (B) 62
   (C) 86
   (D) 120

10. The pediatric wing of a hospital has a total of 120 patients. Of these, 30% are critical care patients, 20% are long-term patients, and the rest are short-term patients. What is the ratio of long-term patients to critical care patients?

    (A) 3:2
    (B) 2:3
    (C) 2:5
    (D) 3:5

11. There are about 33.81 fluid ounces in a liter. How many full liters would you have if you filled a bucket with 275 ounces of water?

    (A) 6
    (B) 7
    (C) 8
    (D) 9

12. You check a patient's heart rate four times an hour for two hours. Your readings are 89, 86, 82, 95, 100, 98, 92, and 95. What is the patient's average heart rate during this time?

    (A) 90
    (B) 92
    (C) 93
    (D) 94

13. Two runners leave the same starting point at the same time. Runner A moves at a pace of 4.2 miles per hour. Runner B moves at a pace of 3.6 miles per hour. After 2.25 hours, how much farther has Runner A gone?

    (A) 1.35 miles
    (B) 1.58 miles
    (C) 2.34 miles
    (D) 8.31 miles

14. Fourteen is what fraction of 21?

    (A) $\frac{2}{3}$
    (B) $\frac{7}{8}$
    (C) $\frac{2}{21}$
    (D) $\frac{14}{3}$

15. If it takes 4 cups of sugar to make one batch of brownies that yields 24 pieces, how many cups of sugar would you need to make 132 brownies?

    (A) 22
    (B) 23
    (C) 25
    (D) 28

Answers and Explanations

1. **B.** Because each of these numbers begins with 2 in the ones place, you need to start with the tenths place. That puts 2.469 first. In determining the second number in the sequence, there are three numbers with 5 in the tenths place, so you need to compare the digit in the hundredths place with those numbers. Continue this pattern until you sort out all three of the 2.5 numbers and then tack the 2.6 and the 2.7 numbers on to the end of the list.

2. **C.** Divide 17 by 24 to get .7083. You now have to figure out if your 0 should stay a 0 or round up to become a 1. The number in the place to the right is an 8, so that means you round up. Your answer is .71.

3. **D.** Start by turning .48 into a fraction: $\frac{48}{100}$. Then reduce by dividing both numerator and denominator by 4: $\frac{12}{25}$. This fraction can't be simplified any more.

4. **C.** Straight addition here; make sure you keep your decimals straight. You could also estimate the answer quickly by just adding up the numbers to the left of the decimal point: $4 + 3 + 2 + 1 = 10$. That would help you eliminate Answers A and B right away.

5. **B.** Straight decimal division here. The key is figuring out where the decimal goes. You move it to the right two places in both your dividend and divisor. The smallest number 273 goes into is 1642, which means the decimal in the answer comes after the first 6.

6. **C.** You're being asked to calculate 15% of 215.67, and then subtract that amount from 215.67:

   $.15 \times 215.67 = 32.3505$

   $215.67 - 32.3505 = 183.3195$

   The closest answer is C.

7. **D.** Remember to flip the second fraction and multiply across:

   $\frac{4}{5} \div \frac{6}{8} = \frac{4}{5} \times \frac{8}{6} = \frac{32}{30} = 1\frac{2}{30} = 1\frac{1}{15}$

8. **B.** Write this as an expression: $-4 + 8$. You start on the negative side of the number line and move eight steps to the right. When you stop, you're at $+4$.

9. **A.** Use prime factorization on both numbers:

   $16 = 2 \times 2 \times 2 \times 2$

   $12 = 2 \times 2 \times 3$

   The factors are 2 and 3. The most times that 2 appears in one factorization is four, while 3 only appears once. Multiply $2 \times 2 \times 2 \times 2 \times 3 = 48$ to find that 48 is the lowest number that both 16 and 12 can divide into evenly.

10. **B.** You're looking for the ratio of long-term to critical care patients. First you have to figure out how many patients there are of each type:

    Long-term patients: $.20 \times 120 = 24$

    Critical care patients: $.30 \times 120 = 36$

    Now plug the values into a ratio and reduce: $24:36 = 2:3$.

    Alternatively, you could compare the given percentages, since they are percentages of the same total number of patients. Long-term is 20%. Critical care is 30%. The ratio is, thus, 20:30 or 2:3.

11. **C.** Divide 275 by 33.81 to get 8.133. Because this question is asking how many full liters you would have, you have to round down and say 8.

12. **B.** To calculate average, add all the numbers together: $89 + 86 + 82 + 95 + 100 + 98 + 92 + 95 = 737$. Now divide by the total number of readings (8) to get 92.125. Here, round down to get 92.

13. **A.** Calculate the distance per rate each runner goes using the Distance = Rate × Time formula: Runner A: $D = 4.2 \times 2.25 = 9.45$; Runner B: $D = 3.6 \times 2.25 = 8.1$. Now subtract Runner A's distance from Runner B's to get 1.35 miles.

14. **A.** Start by dividing 14 by 21 to get the percent: .6667. You could then convert this to a fraction, by placing 66 over 100 and reducing. However, .66 is a common decimal and percent that is roughly equal to $\frac{2}{3}$. This is good to memorize.

15. **A.** A quick way to solve this is to turn it into a proportion:

$$\frac{4 \text{ cups}}{24 \text{ brownies}} = \frac{x \text{ cups}}{132 \text{ brownies}}$$

To solve for x, multiply 4 by 132 to get 528. Now divide 528 by 24 to get the value of x: $\frac{528}{24} = 22$

Algebra and Geometry

Believe it or not, algebra and geometry are not all they seem on the surface. Yes, they are required math courses you had to take in high school and likely in college, but what you learn in these classes goes far beyond simple classroom application and academic requirements.

When you're learning about the properties of a triangle or how to factor a quadratic expression, you're gaining a greater understanding of how the world around you works. You're also strengthening your critical thinking skills and ability to solve problems by taking multiple steps.

Beyond looking to test your reasoning abilities, nursing schools look to your performance on these more advanced mathematic abilities to gauge how you may do in the many science courses you'll need to complete during your program. Physics, chemistry, and anatomy and physiology courses all have a heavy dose of algebra and geometry integrated into them.

Because each of the nursing school entrance exams differs in terms of skills tested within any subject, this chapter goes over some general concepts of algebra and geometry, strategies for working out these types of questions, and lots of practice.

What to Expect

As we've said, every exam for nursing school entrance tests you on different concepts within any given subject. For example, the NLN PAX-RN/PN usually tests your knowledge of numbers, operations, fractions, decimals, percents, algebra, geometry, and measurement conversions.

The HESI A² tests all of that, plus other things, like dosage calculations, measurements/conversions, and data interpretation. The ATI TEAS exam tests you on numbers, operations, algebra, data interpretation, and measurements. Your best bet for preparing for your test is to look at the tables in Chapter 2 to determine what concepts you need to know and then concentrate your study efforts on those specific areas.

The good news is that although algebraic and geometric concepts are more advanced than those discussed in the previous chapter, the types of questions you'll encounter here are very straightforward. Expect to apply these concepts through solving equations and the occasional short word problem.

Keep in mind that many questions will require you to take several steps to come up with the correct answer, so be prepared to look beyond the surface before attempting to solve any of these questions.

TEST TIP

Complete all your math practice without using a calculator. Most tests don't allow you to use one, so it's best to not get used to it.

Steps for Panic-Free Success

Now that you have a general picture of what to expect, let's talk about how to get through this section of your test without getting flustered or letting second-guesses get the upper hand. Here are a few tricks to take some of the guesswork out of working on these kinds of questions:

▶ **Translate the question.** Standardized math tests are notorious for asking you to complete complex questions with many steps. Take some time to really read and understand the

question before diving in. Put it in your own words, if you can. You may find that it's asking you to do something other than what you thought at first glance.

▶ **Estimate the answer.** After reading the question, try to come up with a general idea of what the correct answer should be. Eliminate anything that doesn't fit these criteria. This is a quick way to narrow your choices and help you decide whether the answer you've calculated is reasonable. In some cases, it can even lead you to the right answer without having to do much math at all.

▶ **Substitute.** If the question you're dealing with asks you to solve for a variable, try to plug the answer choices into the equation you're working with. This means you don't have to deal with unknowns and you can do simple math with real numbers. The right answer is the one that works in the equation. This will save you a lot of time and effort.

▶ **Eliminate.** Again, we can't stress enough how important it is to eliminate answer choices you know are wrong.

CODE RED!

Always be sure to double check your math. Simple errors are the reason for more wrong answers than you can imagine.

Now let's look at some algebraic concepts that will help you on a number of questions you may find on your nursing school entrance exam.

Algebra Review

The language of mathematics is complex. If you're not familiar with the words used to describe numbers, parts of equations, and actions you're supposed to take in a problem, you'll be confused throughout our discussion about the types of math you need to know. So before diving into the basic concepts of algebra, familiarize yourself with the terms in the following table.

Algebra Vocab

Term	Definition
Expression	Mathematical statement that combines terms and operations, such as $4 + 2$, 12×3, or $6 \times 4 + 8 \times 2 - 5$.
Operation	Action you need to take with a value: addition, subtraction, division, or multiplication. See Chapter 7 for more on this.
Equation	A mathematical statement that shows two equal expressions: $2 + 3 = 5$ or $12x = 48$.
Variable	Letter in an equation or expression that stands in place of an unknown quantity; in $12x = 48$, x is the variable.
Coefficient	Number that multiplies a variable; in $12x = 48$, 12 is the coefficient and means $12 \times x$.
Term	A single number, variable, or combinations thereof. Examples: $12x$, x, x^2y^2, 3.
Constant	A number that stands by itself in an expression or equation; in $2x + 3$, 3 is the constant.

Equations

Working with equations is one of the most basic tasks in algebra. If you remember the definition of *equation* discussed earlier, you're dealing with two amounts that equal each other. Your job is to either solve the equation or solve for one term in the equation. To do this, you'll have to move terms around and make sure what you do to one side of the equation, you do to the other.

Let's say that you're asked to solve for a variable. You do this by isolating the variable to one side of the equation and the numbers to the other.

How do you do that? Get rid of the numbers on one side of the equation by canceling them out with a reverse operation (subtraction is the reverse of addition, and division is the reverse of multiplication, and vice versa). Then do the same to the other side. Try it out on this example:

Solve for a: $a - 10 = -2$

The first thing you need to do is get rid of the -10 so that the a is alone on the left side of the equation. Because the 10 is negative, you add a positive 10 to cancel it out, and then you do the same to the expression on the other side of the equals sign.

$$a - 10 + 10 = -2 + 10$$

$$a \; \cancel{- 10 + 10} = -2 + 10$$

$$a = -2 + 10$$

The rest is simple arithmetic. According to order of operations, you solve the expression from left to right, which means you're adding 10 to -2.

If you remember from Chapter 7, when you add a positive to a negative, you go up the number line. Because you're starting with -2, you would go 10 steps to the right, which brings you to 8. Your final answer is $a = 8$.

Unfortunately, not every problem will have such a nice and neat answer. More often, you're going to have to solve for a variable equaling an expression. Your answers can look more like $x = y + 2$ instead of a simple $x = 2$. If the question asks you to solve for one variable "in terms of" another, here's what to do:

1. Isolate the variable you're asked to solve for on one side of the equation, the same as you would with a number. The only difference is that you're moving around terms, not just numbers. For example, if you're asked to solve for a in terms of y if $8a - 2y = 6a + 10y + 2$, your goal is to solve until you have a by itself on one side of the equal sign.

   Start by adding $2y$ to both sides:

   $8a - \cancel{2y} + \cancel{2y} = 6a + 10y + 2 + 2y$

2. Now combine *like terms:*

   $8a = 6a + 12y + 2$

3. Next, add $-6a$ to both sides:

   $8a + -6a = \cancel{6a} + \cancel{-6a} + 12y + 2$

4. Now combine like terms again:

   $2a = 12y + 2$

5. Finally, divide every term on both sides of the equation by 2:

   $\frac{2a}{2} = \frac{12y}{2} + \frac{2}{2} \rightarrow a = 6y + 1$

DEFINITION

Like terms refers to terms that have the same variables and exponent. For example, with $8 \times 2 + 10x + x - x^2$, the only terms you can add are $10x$ and x to make $11x$ because they share the same variable and exponent. (In this case, the exponent is 1, which is implied. See our explanation of exponents later in the chapter.)

Some equation problems will give you the values of the variables. When you see this, just plug in the numbers and solve according to order of operations.

Inequalities

When you see something that looks like an equation but has a $>$, $\geq$, $<$, $\leq$, or $\neq$ sign, you're dealing with an inequality. Here's what these symbols mean:

▸ **Greater than symbol ($>$).** The value to the left is greater than the value to the right.

▸ **Greater than or equal to symbol ($\geq$).** The value to the left is greater than or equal to the value to the right.

▸ **Less than symbol ($<$).** The value to the left is less than the value to the right.

▸ **Less than or equal to symbol ($\leq$).** The value to the left is less than or equal to the value to the right.

▸ **Not equal symbol ($\neq$).** The values are unequal.

TEST TIP

A good way to remember your inequality symbols is to look at their shape. The smaller end of the symbol points to the smaller value. The larger end of the symbol points to the larger value.

Your job with inequalities is not to find one answer, but to find a range of answers (which you don't have to write out). To do this, work an inequality through like you would any other equation:

$12 + b < 32$

$\cancel{12} - \cancel{12} + b < 32 - 12$

$b < 20$

Here, your answer is saying that the value of b is some number less than 20.

Simple, right? It is when you're dealing with addition and subtraction. Multiplication and division, however, are a little different. When you multiply or divide an inequality by a negative number, you have to flip the inequality symbol. Take a look:

$$36 > -12a$$

This says 36 is greater than $-12a$. To solve for a in this inequality, you have to divide both sides by -12:

$$\frac{36}{-12} > \frac{-12a}{-12} \rightarrow -3 < a$$

The -12s on the right cancel each other out, leaving only the a. Divide 36 by -12 and flip the symbol, and you're done: $-3 < a$.

Exponents

When you see a term like x^2, you may automatically think *exponent*. However, this is actually a *power*. The main number or variable in the term is called the base, while the raised number is the exponent. For example, in 4^3, 4 is the base, ^{3} is the exponent, and all together it's read 4 to the third power (or 4 cubed).

No matter how you say it, though, exponents tell you one thing: how many times to multiply the base times itself. All 4^3 means is $4 \times 4 \times 4$.

Some rules to remember with exponents:

▶ A base to the first power (x^1) is just the base shown. A base to the zero power (x^0) equals 1.

▶ When you multiply like variables, you get an exponent: $y \times y = y^2$.

▶ When multiplying two like variables with exponents, keep the variable the same and add the exponents: $x^2 \times x^4 = x^6$.

▶ When you apply an exponent to terms in parentheses that have powers, you multiply exponents to simplify the expression: $(x^3)^3 = x^{3 \times 3} = x^9$.

▶ When you multiply separate powers, you multiply the coefficients and then add the exponents: $3x^2 \times 2x^2 \times 2x^2 = 12x^6$.

▶ When you divide powers, subtract the exponents: $x^3 \div x^2 = x^{3-2} = x$. You can also treat it like a fraction and reduce. Write out the base the number of times indicated in the exponent and cancel out like terms:

$$x^3 \div x^2 = \frac{x^3}{x^2} = \frac{x \times x \times x}{x \times x} = \frac{\cancel{x \times x} \times x}{\cancel{x \times x}} = \frac{x}{1} = x$$

▶ When you multiply unlike variables with exponents, combine them into one term: $x^2 \times y^2 = x^2 y^2$.

▶ A negative exponent, such as 8^{-2}, doesn't tell you the number of times to multiply the base by itself. Instead, it tells you how many times to divide the number itself from 1: Take a look at how this works with 8^{-2}:

1. Calculate the value of 8^2: $8 \times 8 = 64$.

2. Write the answer as a fraction: $\frac{64}{1}$.

3. Flip the fraction: $\frac{1}{64}$.

Roots

A number or variable that is raised to the second power is called a *square*. The opposite of a squared base is a *square root* (or *perfect square*), the number that, when multiplied by itself, equals that power.

For example, $10^2 = 10 \times 10 = 100$. If you want to find the square root of 100, you would indicate this with a radical sign, which would make your expression look like this:

$$\sqrt{100} = 10$$

When you're under time constraints on a standardized test, knowing the squares of the first 20 natural numbers will help you quickly get to your answer:

$1^2 = 1$	$\sqrt{1} = 1$
$2^2 = 4$	$\sqrt{4} = 2$
$3^2 = 9$	$\sqrt{9} = 3$
$4^2 = 16$	$\sqrt{16} = 4$
$5^2 = 25$	$\sqrt{25} = 5$
$6^2 = 36$	$\sqrt{36} = 6$
$7^2 = 49$	$\sqrt{49} = 7$
$8^2 = 64$	$\sqrt{64} = 8$
$9^2 = 81$	$\sqrt{81} = 9$
$10^2 = 100$	$\sqrt{100} = 10$
$11^2 = 121$	$\sqrt{121} = 11$
$12^2 = 144$	$\sqrt{144} = 12$
$13^2 = 169$	$\sqrt{169} = 13$
$14^2 = 196$	$\sqrt{196} = 14$
$15^2 = 225$	$\sqrt{225} = 15$
$16^2 = 256$	$\sqrt{256} = 16$
$17^2 = 289$	$\sqrt{289} = 17$
$18^2 = 324$	$\sqrt{324} = 18$
$19^2 = 361$	$\sqrt{361} = 19$
$20^2 = 400$	$\sqrt{400} = 20$

When you're asked to find a square root of a number you're unfamiliar with, knowing the squares of the first 20 natural numbers can help you quickly zero in on the correct square root answer.

Roots are not always so nice and neat, however. You may encounter different types of roots on your exams, so here are a few other things you can do with roots:

1. **Add or subtract them.** You can add or subtract roots that have the same number inside the radical sign and coefficients outside. Add or subtract the coefficients, not the numbers inside the radical: $3\sqrt{6} + 5\sqrt{6} = 8\sqrt{6}$

   You can't add or subtract roots with different numbers inside the radicals.

2. **Multiply or divide them.** Unlike with addition and subtraction, you can multiply and/or divide the coefficients and the numbers (or variables) inside the radicals, even if they're different: $2\sqrt{7} \times 3\sqrt{2} = 6\sqrt{14}$ or $\frac{6\sqrt{a}}{3\sqrt{b}} = 2\sqrt{\frac{a}{b}}$

3. **Simplify them.** Roots can be simplified if the number under the radical sign has a factor that is a perfect square. Factor out the square and place it outside as a coefficient. The remaining factor stays inside the radical sign:

   $$\sqrt{72} \rightarrow \sqrt{36 \times 2} \rightarrow \sqrt{6 \times 6 \times 2} \rightarrow 6\sqrt{2}$$

Polynomials

Any expression involving one or more terms that may be separated by an operation is called a polynomial. A term with more than three terms is referred to only as a polynomial and does not have a special name. You should be aware of three basic types of polynomials:

▶ **Monomial.** This is a polynomial that has just one term: 5, $10x$, and $4xy^2$ are all monomials.

▶ **Binomial.** This is an expression with two terms joined by an operation: $8xy + 4$ and $6 - 2$ are binomials.

▶ **Trinomial.** These are expressions with three terms joined by operations, such as $x^2 + 6y + 4$.

Most nursing school entrance exams ask you to add, subtract, multiply, and divide much more complicated polynomial expressions and equations than the ones you've seen so far.

Remember a few rules when you're dealing with polynomials:

▶ **Simplify before you solve.** Combine like terms. To do this, simply add the coefficients.

▶ **Multiply or divide.** Where you can, apply multiplication and/or division operations. To do this, multiply or divide coefficients like you normally would. Then do the same to the variables and exponents.

▶ For multiplication, you can multiply and combine unlike bases: $(8x)(2xy^3)$ $= 8 \times 2 \times x \times x \times y \times y \times y = 16x^2y^3$.

▶ With division, treat the operation like a fraction:

1. For example, with $\frac{36a^3}{10a^2}$, you would reduce the coefficients like you would any fraction: $\frac{18a^3}{5a^2}$

2. Next, reduce the exponents. An easy way to do that is to write out the base the number of times indicated in the exponent: $\frac{a \times a \times a}{a \times a}$. In this example, the bottom two a's cancel out two of the a's on the top: $\frac{a \times a \times a}{a \times a}$, leaving none behind in the denominator.

3. Your final reduction would be $\frac{18a}{5}$.

▶ **Use FOIL when multiplying or dividing binomials.** FOIL stands for "First, Outer, Inner, and Last," or the order in which you would multiply or divide terms (most often multiplication). Try it with this example: $(4x - 3)(3x - 6)$

1. Multiply *First* terms $4x \times 3x$, *Outer* terms $4x \times -6$, *Inner* terms $-3 \times 3x$, and *Last* terms -3×-6, and then add. The resulting equation looks like this:

   $(4x - 3)(3x - 6) = (4x \times 3x) + (4x \times -6) + (-3 \times 3x) + (-3 \times -6)$

2. Now solve what's in parentheses:

   $(4x - 3)(3x - 6) = (12x^2) + (-24x) + (-9x) + (18)$

3. Finally, simplify the expression by combining like terms:

   $(4x - 3)(3x - 6) = 12x^2 + (-33x) + 18$

> **TEST TIP**
>
> The final expression you have in this example is a quadratic expression. We explain more about this later in this chapter. For now, memorize this format so you can recognize it easily. It will save you a lot of time on the test.

Simple Polynomial Factoring

Factoring polynomials is a common algebraic task that challenges you to find out what smaller expressions make up a larger expression. This means you have to work backward to figure out what was multiplied to get the expression or equation you're given, but it's not as bad as it sounds. We break it down for you piece by piece.

Let's start with simple factoring. The first thing you need to do is figure out the greatest common factor or GCF (see Chapter 7) of the terms, or the largest factor that two or more terms share (variables included). If variables are also involved, you need to look for the variable term with the lowest common exponent. For example, if you're looking for the GCF for $27x^2$ and $15x$, your GCF would actually be $3x$, because 3 is the greatest factor 27 and 15 have in common and x^1 is shared by both terms.

After you've determined the GCF, divide each term by the GCF. Place the simplified terms separated by their operations in parentheses and place the GCF outside. Let's try it.

Factor the previous expression: $27x^2 + 15x$.

1. You know that GCF is $3x$, so start by breaking down each term into prime factors:

   $27x^2 = 3 \times 3 \times 3 \times x \times x$

   $15x = 5 \times 3 \times x$

   What do both of these have in common? One instance of $3 \times x$.

2. Simplify each of these by crossing out one $3 \times x$ in each expression:

   $27x^2 = 3 \times 3 \times \cancel{3 \times x} \times x$

   $15x = 5 \times \cancel{3 \times x}$

3. Now combine like terms and place the new expression in parentheses with $3x$ outside: $27x^2 + 15x = 3x(9x + 5)$.

To check to see if you're right, multiply each term in parentheses by $3x$: $3x \times 9x = 27x^2$ and $3x \times 5 = 15x$.

Quadratic Expressions

Now that you have a good idea of how to work simple factoring, let's move on to something a little more complicated: factoring quadratic expressions. If you're presented with an expression that has the following structure or if the expression

you're left with after factoring out the GCF has this structure, think quadratic expression: $ax^2 + bx + c$. Here, the x's can be any variable, a and b are coefficients, and c is a constant.

All of the following are quadratic expressions: $y^2 + 13y + 30$; $x^2 + 10x + 25$; $a^2 + 7a + 12$.

When you factor quadratic expressions, you're actually working FOIL backward to find the two binomials that, when multiplied, make up the quadratic. You do this in a few simple steps:

$$x^2 + 8x + 12$$

1. Create two sets of binomials, with the expression's variable as the first term: $(x\ )(x\ )$.

2. To figure out the second terms in each of the parentheses, list out the factors of the last term. Now find the pair that, when added together, equals the coefficient of the middle term.

   For this example, break 12 into factors: 1×12, 2×6, and 3×4. (It's a good idea to do this with negatives as well.) When you add 2 and 6, you have 8, which is the coefficient of the middle term.

3. Plug these numbers into the parentheses: $(x + 2)(x + 6)$.

4. Finally, figure out whether you need positive or negative signs and where. Because both 2 and 6 are positive, use an addition sign in both sets of parentheses (shown previously). If the 2, 6, or both had negatives, you would use a subtraction sign in the parentheses.

To check your work, FOIL the binomials you've made. The answer should be the original equation.

Term	Definition
Ray	Part of a line that has one finite endpoint but goes on infinitely in the other direction.

Geometry Review

Many people find geometry to be much easier to handle than algebra. This could be because there are more steadfast rules in geometry and fewer exceptions. Like algebra, geometry is meant to teach you logic. Unlike algebra, geometry has many more practical applications, such as figuring out how much flooring you need for a room based on its dimensions.

The type of geometry that's on nursing school entrance exams concentrates mostly on a handful of concepts that you need to brush up on to get you through. Familiarize yourself with the terminology in the following table.

Geometry Vocab

Term	Definition
Polygon	A closed two-dimensional shape made up of at least three sides. Examples are a triangle, a hexagon, and a quadrilateral.
Area	The space an object occupies. Usually measured in square units.
Perimeter	The distance around an object.
Vertex	The point where the two lines or line segments that make up an angle intersect.
Line	A 180° angle that stretches infinitely in two directions.

Lines

Lines form the basis of geometry, and you'll see them in many forms. The most important things to know about lines are that they're infinite (they stretch in either direction without end) and can be segmented, for the purposes of a test question. Some specific line types you should know include the following:

▸ **Line segment.** This is a part of a line with two endpoints. It's often broken up into several smaller segments that are labeled with letters. The midpoint is the marking directly in the center of the line.

Line segment

▸ You may be asked to identify certain parts of a line segment, such as its midpoint; calculate the length of a line segment based on information given; or apply properties of certain types of lines to figure out lengths or angle values.

▸ **Parallel lines.** These are special types of lines that run next to each other but never meet.

Parallel lines

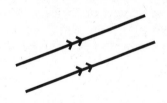

▸ **Perpendicular lines.** Two lines are perpendicular if they intersect at a point and the resulting angles are all 90°.

Perpendicular lines

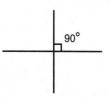

Angles

Angles are simply formed when two lines, rays, or line segments intersect at a common point; they are measured in degrees. Angles you should know include these:

▸ **Right.** An angle that looks like an *L*. It measures 90°; the lines are perpendicular.

▸ **Acute.** Any angle that is less than 90°.

▸ **Obtuse.** Any angle that is more than 90°.

▸ **Straight.** A straight line is actually a 180° angle. This is an important number to remember because it can help you calculate the degrees of other angles in a geometry question.

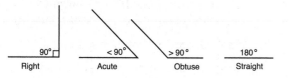

Now that you know the basics, memorize these special types of angles and their properties. Not only can you be asked to identify these types of angles on the test, but knowing the following rules associated with them will enable you to figure out missing values of angles in various questions:

▸ **Complementary.** Two angles that together make a right angle, so the sum of the angles equals 90°.

▸ **Supplementary.** Two angles that together make a straight line. The sum of the angles equals 180°.

▸ **Adjacent.** Two angles that share a common side. Adjacent angles look like one large angle that's split at the vertex. The sum of the two angles is equal to the larger angle.

▸ **Corresponding.** You'll often see these as a set of parallel lines with another line, called a *transversal*, running through both. This creates a set of angles with specific properties and relationships. Memorize the relationships outlined on the following diagram.

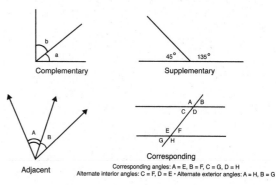

Triangles

Learning the types of triangles there are and the rules associated with them will help you through many types of questions. Often, questions involving triangles ask you to determine missing values before you get to the main part of the problem, which may be calculating area or some other task.

Memorize these basic rules about angle relationships in triangles. They'll help you quickly calculate missing values:

▶ Triangles have three internal angles. They also have external angles. Each internal angle is adjacent to an external angle (see the next diagram).

▶ The three internal angles of a triangle always add up to 180°.

▶ The sum of an internal angle and its adjacent external angle always is 180°.

▶ You can calculate the value of an internal angle if you know the value of the adjacent external angle. Simply subtract the value of the external angle from 180. In the following diagram, the external angle is 45°. 180 − 45 = 135, which means the adjacent internal angle is 135°.

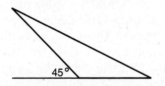

▶ You can figure out the value of an external angle by adding the two internal angles that do not touch the external angle. In the following diagram, you would add 88 + 42 to find the value of angle x (130°).

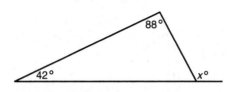

You should also be familiar with several special triangles:

▶ **Similar triangles.** These are two triangles that have internal angles that are equal to each other and therefore have proportional sides.

In the following diagram, the degrees of angles g, d, and f are the same in each triangle. This means that side a is proportional to side x, side c is proportional to side y, and side b is proportional to side z.

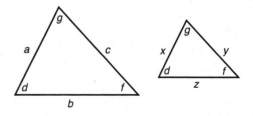

▶ **Congruent triangles.** Two triangles whose corresponding side lengths and angles are the same values.

Congruent

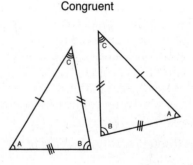

To test if two triangles are congruent, ask the following questions. If the answer to any of these is yes, you have congruent triangles:

▶ Are all three corresponding side values equal?

▶ Are two corresponding sides and the angle they make equal?

▶ Are two corresponding angles and the side they share equal?

▶ Are two corresponding angles and a side they don't share equal?

Common types of triangles you'll find on nursing school entrance exams include:

- ▶ **Isosceles.** A triangle with two sides of equal length, and therefore two angles that are equal.

- ▶ **Equilateral.** A triangle with all side lengths and angles equal. Angles are always 60°.

- ▶ **Right.** A triangle with one angle equal to 90°.

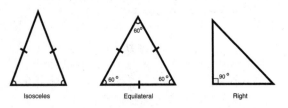

Now that you're familiar with common triangles and their properties, let's talk about what you'll be asked to do with this information on the test. Most often you'll need to find the perimeter (value of the length around), area (value of the space within), or a missing value. Here's what you do:

- ▶ **Perimeter.** Add the lengths of all three sides.

- ▶ **Area.** Determine the length of the base of a triangle, divide by half, and then multiply by the height using the equation $A = \frac{1}{2}bh$. Take a look at the following diagram.

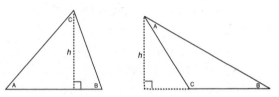

- ▶ The base of a triangle is the length of the bottom line, and the height is the distance between the triangle's highest point and the base. Often you'll see this indicated as a dotted line running from the base to the top angle. A triangle's area is represented in square units (cm², ft.²) when units of measure are given in the problem.

- ▶ **Missing value of an angle(s).** Determine what type of triangle you're looking at, and label the diagram with the values you're given in the problem. Then use the rules discussed earlier in this section to calculate the values you need. For instance, if you're given a right triangle and told that one angle is 30°, you know the other is 60°.

- ▶ **Missing side of a right triangle.** When you know the value of any two sides of a right triangle, you use the Pythagorean Theorem to calculate the other: $a^2 + b^2 = c^2$. In this equation, c is always assigned to the hypotenuse (the longest side) of the right triangle. Memorize this formula and the following diagram. Substitute the two sides for the corresponding letters in the equation. Then solve for the missing side.

Pythagorean Theorem

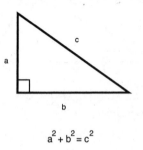

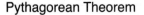

$$a^2 + b^2 = c^2$$

When you solve for the missing side of a right triangle, you have to figure out the square root to get the actual length of the side, because in the equation, each of the sides is squared. If the square root of that value does not result in a whole number, you can usually just list the answer within a radical.

Quadrilaterals

Quadrilaterals are polygons that have four sides and corners. You need to know these quadrilaterals:

▶ **Parallelograms.** These are quadrilaterals that have opposite sides that are parallel and equal in length. This makes the opposite angles also equal. Rectangles, rhombi, and squares are all parallelograms.

▶ **Rectangles.** These are parallelograms with four right angles. The sides that run parallel to each other are equal.

▶ **Squares.** All four sides are congruent, and angles are right angles. A square is a special type of rectangle.

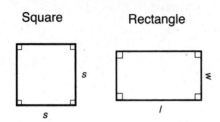

As with triangles, you should know how to calculate area and perimeter for each of these. With perimeter, you add the values of all the sides. With area, you multiply the value of the length times the value of the width. In the previous rectangle, if length = 4 in. and width = 2 in., you'd multiply 4 by 2 and find that the area is 8 in.².

For a parallelogram, you'd multiply the base times the height. The height is found in the same way as for a triangle.

You should know two special types of quadrilaterals:

▶ **Rhombus.** This is a parallelogram that has two sets of parallel lines that are all the same length but whose corners are not necessarily right angles. (A square is one type of rhombus.) Opposite angles, however, are equal. Take a look at the following diagram:

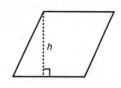

To calculate the area of a rhombus, you multiply the base by the height. For example, if the height line in the previous diagram is 10 in. and the base (which can be any side) is 8 in., the area would be 80 in.².

- ▶ **Trapezoid.** This is a quadrilateral with just one pair of parallel sides. To calculate the area of a trapezoid, you use the following formula:

$A = \frac{1}{2} \times h \times (b_1 + b_2)$. In this case,

b_1 and b_2 are the values of the bases (which are the top and bottom lines of the following figure).

Trapezoid

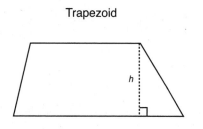

In the previous diagram, if b_1 = 12 in., b_2 = 18 in., and h = 6 in., this is how you would work the equation:

$$A = \frac{1}{2} \times 6 \times (12+18)$$

$$A = \frac{1}{2} \times 6 \times 30$$

$$A = \frac{1}{2} \times \frac{6}{1} \times 30$$

$$A = \frac{6}{2} \times 30$$

$$A = 3 \times 30$$

$$A = 90 \text{ in}^2$$

Circles

Circles are a lot easier to work with than you might think. Memorize a few essential bits of information, and you'll do fine:

- ▶ **Radius (*r*).** This is a segment that's drawn from the center of a circle to the edge. A circle can have an infinite number of radii. This term may also refer to the length of such a segment.

- ▶ **Diameter (*d*).** This is a segment whose endpoints are on the circle and that goes through the center of the circle. Double the value of any radius, and you get the diameter.

- ▶ **Circumference (*c*).** This is the distance around a circle.

- ▶ **Chord.** This is a line segment in a circle that touches any two points of the edge. A diameter is a special type of chord.

- ▶ **pi (≠).** This is a mathematical constant that appears in many formulas involving circles. All you need to know is that it equals about 3.14 or $\frac{22}{7}$, which is enough to get you through your test calculations.

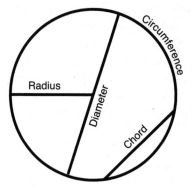

These gems of wisdom about circles and the following formulas should help you tackle just about any circle question on your exam:

- ▶ Circumference: $C = 2\pi r$
- ▶ Area: $A = \pi r^2$

Solid Figures and Volume

If you see a solid figure on your exam, it will likely be either rectangular or cylindrical. You're most often asked to figure out volume or surface with rectangular solids (think cubes).

Cube

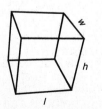

The two main tasks you'll be asked to complete with solids are volume and total surface area:

▸ **Rectangular solids.** Use the following formula to figure out volume: $V = l \times w \times h$. Plug in the values for length, width, and height, or solve for a missing value based on the information given in the question. These values will always be notated with l, w, and h. To calculate surface area, use the following formula: $2lw + 2wh + 2lh$.

▸ **Cylindrical solids.** For cylindrical solids, the formula for volume is $V = \pi r^2 h$. Plug in the values of the radius, pi, and height to get your answer, or solve for a missing value based on the information given in the question. To calculate total surface area, use the formula $TSA = 2\pi r(r + h)$.

Practice Questions

For each question, choose the best answer.

1. If $a = 5$ and $b = 4$, then $(a^2 - 9) + b^2 + a =$

   (A) 5
   (B) 16
   (C) 32
   (D) 37

2. $\frac{a^7}{a^9} =$

   (A) a^2
   (B) a^{-2}
   (C) $2a^{16}$
   (D) a^{16}

3. $(3x - 3)(4x - 2) =$

   (A) $12x^2 + (-18x) + 6$
   (B) $12x^2 + 18x + 6$
   (C) $12x^2 + (-6x) - 6$
   (D) $12x^2 + (-8x) + 6$

4. The radius of a barrel is 6 feet and its height is 15 feet. How much water can it hold?

   (A) 90.5 ft.^{3}
   (B) 540.25 ft.^{3}
   (C) 1,695.5 ft.^{3}
   (D) 1,822.5 ft.^{3}

5. If $7x - 12 > 3x + 8$, then $x >$

   (A) 5
   (B) –5
   (C) 20
   (D) –20

6. Two triangles with internal angles that are equal to each other and have proportional sides are

   (A) isosceles.
   (B) right.
   (C) similar.
   (D) congruent.

7. On line segment AC, point B is located 4 away from points A and C. Point B is the

   (A) midpoint.
   (B) vertex.
   (C) radius.
   (D) ray.

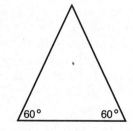

8. What is the value of the third angle in the previous triangle?

   (A) 36°
   (B) 45°
   (C) 60°
   (D) 90°

9. Factor $y^2 - 13y + 30$.

   (A) $(y - 3)(y - 10)$
   (B) $(y - 6)(y - 12)$
   (C) $(y + 3)(y + 10)$
   (D) $(y + 3)(y - 10)$

10. You're laying carpet in a room that is 12 feet long by 30 feet wide. You have only half the amount of carpet needed to complete the job. How many more square feet of carpet do you need to get?

   (A) 50 ft.²
   (B) 80 ft.²
   (C) 95 ft.²
   (D) 180 ft.²

11. Solve for y: $gy - n = x$

   (A) $y = x + n$
   (B) $y = \frac{x+n}{g}$
   (C) $y = \frac{x-n}{g}$
   (D) $y = x - n$

12. $\sqrt{324} =$

   (A) 16
   (B) 17
   (C) 18
   (D) 19

13. What is the value of the hypotenuse if a right triangle has the following values: $a = 5$; $b = 12$?

   (A) 13
   (B) 25
   (C) 144
   (D) 169

14. $\frac{6a^2}{5b} \div \frac{2b}{9a} =$

   (A) $\frac{12a^3}{45b^2}$
   (B) $\frac{27a^3}{5b^2}$
   (C) $\frac{27ab}{5ab}$
   (D) $\frac{12ab}{45ab}$

15. $3\sqrt{2} \times 4\sqrt{5} =$

   (A) $7\sqrt{7}$
   (B) $7\sqrt{10}$
   (C) $12\sqrt{7}$
   (D) $12\sqrt{10}$

Answers and Explanations

1. **D.** When you plug in the numbers given in the question, you have: $(5^2 - 9) + 4^2 + 5$. Follow order of operations to solve:

   ▸ Parentheses: $5^2 - 9 = 25 - 9 = 16$

   ▸ New expression: $16 + 4^2 + 5 =$

   ▸ Exponents: $4^2 = 4 \times 4 = 16$

   ▸ New expression: $16 + 16 + 5 =$

   ▸ Addition left to right: $32 + 5 = 37$

2. **B.** When you divide exponents, you actually subtract one from the other. So for this problem, you would subtract $7 - 9$ to get -2. Your answer should look like a^{-2}.

3. **A.** Use FOIL here:

   $(3x - 3)(4x - 2) = 12x^2 + (-6x) + (-12x) + (6)$

   Now combine like terms:

   $12x^2 + (-18x) + (6)$

4. **C.** Use the volume formula for cylindrical solids here:

   $V = \pi r^2 b \rightarrow 3.14 \times 6^2 \times 15 \rightarrow 3.14 \times 36 \times 15 = 1{,}695.6 \ \text{ft}^3.$

5. **A.** Solve this inequality like an equation. Start by isolating the x to one side:

   $7x - 12 > 3x + 8$

   $7x - 3x - 12 > \cancel{3x - 3x} + 8$

   Combine like terms and add 12 to each side:

   $4x - 12 > 8$

   $4x \ \cancel{-12 + 12} > 8 + 12$

   $4x > 20$

   Now divide both sides by 4:

   $\frac{4x}{4} > \frac{20}{4}$

   Because you did not multiply or divide the inequality by a negative number, the symbol stays the same. The final answer is $x > 5$.

6. **C.** An isosceles triangle has two sides of equal length and therefore two angles that are equal. Right triangles have one side that is equal to 90°. Congruent triangles have corresponding side lengths and angles with the same values. Similar triangles have internal angles that are equal to each other and therefore have proportional sides. The lengths of the sides are likely to be different from the first triangle, though.

7. **A.** Because point B is equidistant from the two endpoints, it marks the midpoint.

8. **C.** The two sides on the bottom are 60°, which means the other angle has to be 60° as well. This makes the triangle equilateral.

9. **A.** This is a quadratic expression. You can either FOIL the answer choices or factor the expression: $y^2 + 13y - 30$:

   $(y \ )(y \ )$

   List factors of 30:

   1×30

   2×15

   3×10

   If you add 3 and 10, you get 13, which is the middle term. Because the middle term in the original expression is negative, both signs in the final binomials will be negative. The final answer is $(y - 3)(y - 10)$.

10. **D.** Calculate the area of the room. Because you know it's a rectangle, multiply the length times the width to get 360 ft.². Then divide by half to find the missing amount: 180 ft.².

11. **B.** This one may look scary, but it's really just an equation that uses variables instead of numbers. The same rules apply and the name of this game is to move the variables around until you have y isolated on one side of the equal sign. Start by adding n to both sides:

$gy - n = x$

$gy - n + n = x + n$

Divide both sides by g and you're done!

$gy = x + n$

$\frac{gy}{g} = \frac{x+n}{g} \rightarrow \frac{\cancel{g}y}{\cancel{g}} = \frac{x+n}{g} \rightarrow y = \frac{x+n}{g}$

12. **C.** This is a square root. $18 \times 18 = 324$

13. **A.** Use the Pythagorean Theorem for this question: $a^2 + b^2 = c^2$. Plug in the values and solve:

$5^2 + 12^2 = c^2$

$25 + 144 = c^2$

$169 = c^2$

$\sqrt{169} = c$

$13 = c$

14. **B.** You're dividing fractions here, so start by changing the division sign to a multiplication sign and flipping the second fraction: $\frac{6a^2}{5b} \div \frac{2b}{9a} \rightarrow \frac{6a^2}{5b} \times \frac{9a}{2b}$.

Now multiply across and simplify:

$\frac{6a^2}{5b} \times \frac{9a}{2b} = \frac{54a^3}{10b^2} = \frac{27a^3}{5b^2}$

15. **D.** Multiply and/or divide the coefficients and the numbers inside the radicals: $3\sqrt{2} \times 4\sqrt{5} = 12\sqrt{10}$

Scientific Method

Of course, any nursing school entrance exam is going to have some kind of evaluation of your science knowledge. After all, you are applying for entrance into a program that's all about science. But not every exam tests the same subjects, nor does every program require that candidates complete the same science sections of the exam. Don't worry, though. We've got you covered.

In this part, you'll get some great review in high school biology, earth and life sciences, chemistry, and physics. Essential concepts are explained in each area, so in case you're not up on the difference between meiosis and mitosis, you can brush up in time for your exam. You'll also find practice questions, answers, and explanations for each of these disciplines.

Science of Life

Nursing school entrance exams test your abilities in three main subjects: math, language, and science. So far, we've walked you through the different verbal and math concentrations most often found on these exams. The rest of this book will concentrate on the sciences.

Some exams have specific sections dedicated to chemistry, anatomy and physiology (A&P), biology, and physics. We'll get more in depth with these topics in the next few chapters. However, many exams also mix in a variety of general life- and earth-science questions.

This chapter introduces you to some of the topics these questions have been known to cover and provides you with some essential review to make sure you're prepared for just about anything. Then you can practice what you've learned until it all makes perfect sense.

What to Expect

You'll find a wide variety of topics covered on the science sections of the various nursing school entrance exams. First, every exam covers different areas that can range from subject-specific subtests to an overall science section within the greater exam. For example:

▶ **NLN PAX.** This includes 60 questions covering general biology, anatomy and physiology, chemistry, health, and physics.

▶ **HESI A².** There are 30 questions each for chemistry, anatomy and physiology, and biology. Some programs may not require the science sections, so make sure to double check if yours does.

- ▸ **ATI TEAS.** Includes 53 questions covering anatomy and physiology, life and physical sciences, and scientific reasoning.

- ▸ **Psychological Services Bureau, Inc. Registered Nursing School Aptitude Exam.** Has 90 questions covering general high school science topics, such as biology, chemistry, physics, health, and earth science.

Second, most of these exams come in various versions to reduce the possibility of cheating. This means that within your state, region, or even the testing center where you're taking your exam, the questions you see on your exam are not necessarily what someone else is seeing.

For these reasons, it's impossible for us to tell you exactly what topics you are going to see on your test. What we can do is give you a general idea of what areas have come up in the past. And because these questions are pretty straightforward, your best bet is to use the general approach described in Chapter 3 when you get to this section of your exam.

Life Science Review

Life science is a branch of science that encompasses a diverse array of sciences relating to all *organisms* on Earth. These include biology (and all of its subdivisions), zoology, botany, physiology, ecology, genetics, medical sciences, and others.

> **DEFINITION**
>
> The word **organism** is the formal scientific way of saying something is a living thing.

Earth science is also included in the study of life science. Why? The environment in which organisms live is just as much a part of life science as the organisms themselves. And within the realm of earth science, you also have topics that you might not expect, like weather and astronomy.

Because there's no telling exactly what subjects you're going to be tested on—we've heard tales of test-takers having tons of geology and other earth- and life-science topics, and only a few A&P questions—we've provided a little of everything in this chapter.

Cells

Cellular biology is a science all on its own, and we go into more detail about cells in Chapter 10. Here are some general concepts to get you started.

A cell is the basic unit of life. It is an enclosed structure that contains a variety of components that work together to make the cell perform some specific purpose. For complex, eukaryotic cells (explained later in this section), these components include …

- ▸ **Plasma membrane.** This is the outer structure that holds everything else inside.

- ▸ **Cytoplasm.** This term refers to the whole of a cell's internal components that are suspended within cytosol, a fluid that makes up the majority of a cell. Cytosol is made up of electrolytes, proteins, carbohydrates, and organelles.

- ▸ **Organelles.** These are subcellular structures that perform a specific function in the lifecycle of a cell. Organelles are contained within membranes separate from the plasma membrane.

- **Nucleus.** This is a very specialized organelle located at the center of a cell. It is responsible for housing the cell's genetic information and controlling how the genetic code is expressed by the cell.

- **Proteins.** These are chemicals found within a cell that control its metabolism (chemical reactions that occur within the cell) and how the cell interacts with its surroundings.

An easy way to think about cells is to picture a capsule you'd take to relieve a headache. The gelatin casing holds in the right proportion of chemical particles that make up the medicine that will make your headache go away. Separately, these components will not achieve their intended purpose, but when they are packaged together and taken correctly, they will take that headache away.

An organism can be made up of a single cell or groups of cells that work together to form a structure (like an organ) or cause something to happen (like healing a wound).

Though there are many structures and variations of cells, there are two main types of cells that make up living organisms. These cell types are defined by the absence or presence of a true nucleus:

- **Prokaryotic cells.** These cells usually make up single-celled organisms, such as bacteria. The following diagram shows a type of bacterial prokaryotic cell:

Prokaryotic Cell

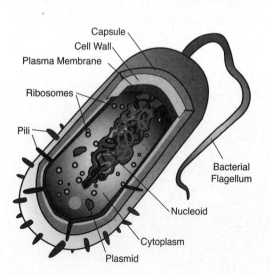

- Prokaryotic cells have no defined nucleus encased in a membrane. Instead, their genetic material (as both chromosomes and plasmids) is generally found in the nucleoid (the squiggly stuff in the middle of the diagram). Plasmids are similar to chromosomes in that they hold genetic information, but are a different type of DNA molecule that replicates independent of chromosomes. Some plasmids may lie outside of the nucleoid.

- The contents of most prokaryotic cells are contained within a capsule. A cell membrane acts as a buffer between the contents of the cell and the capsule, which may also have *flagella* attached. Our diagram shows a bacterial prokaryote with a single flagellum.

> **DEFINITION**
>
> **Flagella** (or *flagellum* in singular form) are tiny tail-like protrusions that wiggle in order to move a cell.

- You may also recognize some of the other parts of the cell, such as cytoplasm and plasma membrane. These are common to most types of cells.

- **Eukaryotic cells.** These cells are found primarily in more complex organisms, such as plants and animals (See Chapter 10 for an example of an animal cell, which is eukaryotic). Eukaryotes have a defined nucleus that is encased in a membrane. The contents of a eukaryotic cell are like those described earlier in the chapter: cytoplasm, membrane-bound organelles, and chemicals that perform metabolic functions for the cell.

Taxonomy

With all of the millions of forms of life on Earth, scientists would have a very hard time studying them without a system of classification. That is what taxonomy is all about.

Though there have been varying systems of taxonomic classification used throughout the years, the Linnaean system is what is most commonly studied in high school and college life-science courses. This system breaks down organisms into eight divisions (*taxa*) that can be used to identify an organism. From largest to smallest, the *Linnaean taxa* are:

- **Domain.** There are only three domains: Eukaryota (living things with cells that have a nucleus), Bacteria (single-cell prokaryotes with no nucleus and a cell membrane made of unbranched fatty acid chains), and Archaea (single-cell prokaryotes, similar to both eukaryotes and bacteria with different rRNA, cell wall, and membrane chemistry).

- **Kingdom.** What used to be two large categories of life (plants and animals) now encompasses five major groups of organisms: Animalia (animals, vertebrates, invertebrates), Plantae (plants, mosses), Fungi (mushrooms, molds), Protista (slime molds, some algae), and Monera (bacteria, some pathogens).

- **Phylum.** This classification is based on one of two things: either the physical characteristics of an organism (such as having a spine or a shell) or the degree of its evolutionary relationship to others of its population. Each kingdom has its own list of phyla.

- **Class.** After an organism is defined by kingdom and phylum, it is placed into a class. Classes are usually defined by history and a general consensus among the scientific community and are generally described as a major group of organisms. Think mammals, reptiles, insects, etc. Within a class, there can be a variety of subclassifications.

- **Order.** Orders describe groups of organisms based on more specific characteristics than class does. Primates (prosimians, simians), Lepidoptera (mothlike insects), and Carnivora (predators, like lions, tigers, and bears, oh my!) are all orders. As with class, taxonomists decide what qualifies to be placed in one order or another, with no hard-and-fast rules that are agreed upon universally.

- **Family.** Organisms within an order are further defined into families. Hominidae is a family within primates that includes apelike animals, such as chimpanzees and gorillas (humans, too). Canidae is a family within Carnivora that includes doglike animals, such as foxes and wolves.

- **Genus.** This is the first of the final two classifications of an organism. Genus and species work together to make a specific identification of an organism. For example, *Homo* is the genus that people fall into, while wolves fall into the *Canis* genus. Both are genera of *Hominidae* and *Carnivora*, respectively.

- **Species.** Organisms are differentiated from others within their genus by their species classification. Wolves and dogs are differentiated from their genus name by the addition of their species name. Wolves are *Canis lupus*, and dogs are *Canis familiaris*.

TEST TIP

Try to make up a mnemonic that is familiar to you to remember the order of the Linnaean system. Or better yet, run a Google search for some common mnemonics. We found Dear Kevin's Poor Cow Only Feels Good Sometimes; Dumb King Phillip Cried Out For Good Soup; and Daddy Kirby Picks Crude Objects From Gooey Snouts.

Plants

Organisms fall into two categories:

- **Autotrophs.** Organisms that make their own food by converting the radiation they receive from the sun and nutrients from the surrounding environment into organic compounds. They are known as producers.

- **Heterotrophs.** Organisms that need to consume carbon-based substances, such as autotrophs and other heterotrophs, in order to survive. They are known as consumers.

As autotrophs, plants serve an important function in the world's ecological balance. They provide nourishment for heterotrophs, and because of their ability to convert energy from the sun into chemical energy, they are an invaluable source of energy and nutrients that are used by the surrounding environment.

Plants are made up of eukaryotic cells, which look something like this:

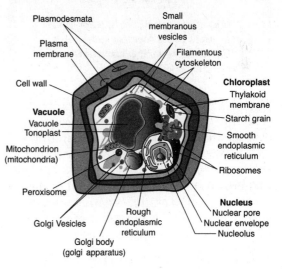

The organelles that make up a plant cell are the same as an animal cell's, with two exceptions. First, plant cells have a cell wall made of cellulose encasing the cell membrane. The other more significant difference is the presence of chloroplasts, the organelles that make photosynthesis possible. Chloroplasts have chlorophyll, which looks green because it reflects wavelengths of green light while absorbing red and blue light. As producers, plants make their own food, which is accomplished through photosynthesis.

So how does photosynthesis work and what makes it so special? All cells have to be able to produce energy in some way by making a chemical called adenosine triphosphate (ATP). We will go into how other types of eukaryotic cells produce ATP through *aerobic cellular respiration* in Chapter 10. For plants, however, ATP is made through the process of photosynthesis, which is a form of *anaerobic cellular respiration*.

> **DEFINITION**
>
> The process of making ATP is called *cellular respiration*. **Aerobic cellular respiration** needs oxygen for ATP production. **Anaerobic cellular respiration** does not need oxygen for ATP production.

During photosynthesis, a plant (or some types of algae and bacteria) takes carbon dioxide and water from the surrounding environment, and photons (energy from the radiation that comes from the sun), and uses them to create a chemical reaction in the chloroplasts that produces carbohydrates such as glucose. This process is represented by the following chemical equation:

$$6CO_2 + 6H_2O \text{ (+ light energy)} \rightarrow C_6H_{12}O_6 + 6O_2$$

The actual process of photosynthesis takes place in two parts:

▸ **Light-dependent reactions.** When light reaches a plant cell, molecules in the chlorophyll absorb wavelengths of red and blue light (among others, but these are the most effective for photosynthesis). This influx of energy starts a reaction with the electrons and protons of the molecules, which then kick-starts the production of adenosine triphosphate (ATP), nicotinamide adenine dinucleotide phosphate (NADPH), and oxygen.

▸ **Light-independent reactions.** Sometimes called *dark reactions*, this process does not actually take place in the dark; they just don't need photons to take place. During this stage of photosynthesis, the energy and products of the light-dependent reactions (ATP, NADPH, and oxygen) are used to convert carbon dioxide and water into carbohydrates and oxygen that nourish the plant and heterotrophs that eat the plant.

Now that you have a basic understanding of plants on a cellular level, let's talk about the anatomy of a plant:

▸ **Roots.** These are protrusions that span out underground. They anchor the plant within the soil and provide a large amount of surface area that can absorb water and nutrients the plant needs from the soil.

▸ **Shoot.** This is the part of the plant that is above ground.

▸ **Stem.** This is the main structural component of the plant. Water and nutrients are transported through a vascular system that runs up the stem and out to the branches and leaves that shoot off of it.

- **Leaves.** Photosynthesis takes place in leaves, which are built to allow for the exchange of carbon dioxide, oxygen, and water.

- **Flowers.** Flowers are the sexual organs of a plant. Plants are sexual reproducers, as strange an idea as that may seem. Important parts of a flower include:

- **Stamen.** These are the male reproductive organs. They are long, thin shoots topped with pollen—the plant equivalent of sperm.

- **Pistil.** This is the female reproductive organ, usually found in the center of the flower. The pistil contains the ovary of the flower and ovules that are fertilized by the pollen. Fertilized ovules become seeds that remain safe within the ovary until maturation. When a mature seed is scattered from the flower, it takes root in the ground and grows into another plant.

Ecology

Ecology is the study of the environment and how organisms live and interact within different habitats. All life on Earth depends on keeping a careful balance within and among these habitats, which is why global warming is such a concern. Even slight changes in abiotic (nonliving, like a rise in temperature) and biotic (living, like increased populations of predators) conditions can have devastating consequences for a habitat and all those who interact with it.

A few key concepts about ecology (besides the definition) you should be familiar with for your test include the following:

- **Biomes.** These are essentially large habitats that are defined by the type of weather, vegetation, and organisms that inhabit them. There are two main types of biomes: terrestrial and aquatic. Terrestrial biomes are those that are on land, and aquatic biomes are underwater.

- Within these two main biomes are various others that you may be more aware of, including:

- **Freshwater.** These are aquatic biomes that are characterized by the lack of salt in the water. They include lakes, streams, rivers, and wetlands.

- **Marine.** Another aquatic biome, but this one has a high concentration of salt in the water. They include the oceans, coral reefs, and estuaries, and cover about three quarters of the Earth's surface. Aside from providing a habitat for millions of species of life, marine biomes also provide most of the oxygen for the world and process a large amount of carbon dioxide from the air.

- **Desert.** A habitat is considered a desert if it experiences less than 50 cm of rain a year. There are four types of deserts on Earth: hot and dry (the Sahara, Death Valley), semiarid (Red Rock Canyon in Nevada), coastal (Namibia's coastal desert), and cold (Greenland, Antarctica). Animals and vegetation that live in these climates are specially adapted to the lack of water and sometimes extreme temperature.

- **Forest.** This habitat is characterized by heavy vegetation in the form of trees and plants. Forests are found all over the world and come in three main types: tropical (rainforests of South America and Africa), temperate (the Adirondack and Rocky Mountains), and boreal or taiga (Denali National Park, Alaska; Jasper National Park, Alberta, Canada).

▸ **Grassland.** Grasslands are wide, flat expanses of land that are mostly populated by grasses, shrubs, and a few trees. The two types of grasslands are savanna (the Serengeti Plains in Africa) and temperate (the Great Plains in the United States).

▸ **Tundra.** This describes the very cold, mostly barren lands—think of them as frozen deserts, because very little vegetation or animal life exists there. The Arctic tundra is found throughout the Arctic Circle and runs south until it meets taiga. Alpine tundra is the other type and is found on mountains that go above an altitude that can sustain the growth or trees. Think of the mountains that always have snow at the top.

▸ **Food web.** In grammar school, you probably learned about the food chain. We've already discussed the food chain a little when we talked about autotrophs and heterotrophs—producers and consumers. To that, we're going to add decomposers, which are organisms that break down dead organic matter and recycle it within an *ecosystem*.

DEFINITION

An **ecosystem** is the biological environment of a specific area that encompasses all of the biotic and abiotic factors that affect it.

▸ Producers, consumers, and decomposers are very important links in the food chain: producers provide nutrition for consumers, and decomposers break down the organic wastes producers and consumers leave behind. An example of this is an ear of corn (producer) being eaten by Farmer Jim (consumer). Farmer Jim throws the outer leaves of the corn into his compost pile and then eats the kernels off the cob and throws the cob in the pile as well. Decomposers in the compost break down all of that waste and turn it into rich soil. Farmer Jim later takes that soil and uses it to fertilize his corn field, so he can grow more corn.

▸ In reality, though, this cycle of survival is more complex than that. After all, Farmer Jim isn't the only one who eats his corn; so do birds, rodents, pigs, bacteria, and other organisms. That's where the concept of the food web comes in. A food web takes into consideration all of the different food chains within an ecosystem or environment and looks at how they all affect each other.

▸ **Ecosystem relationships.** Relationships among organisms within any given ecosystem are symbiotic: what affects one affects the others in some way and there is some benefit to the populations as a result of these interconnected relationships. Types of symbiotic relationships within an ecosystem can be ...

▸ **Mutual.** All organisms in the relationship benefit.

▸ **Parasitic.** One or a group of organisms benefits while another is harmed.

▸ **Commensal.** One or a group of organisms benefits while another is not affected at all.

Evolution

Evolution is the study of how life forms have changed over time through natural selection. Within any community of organisms, there is going to be a natural amount of variety in the physical and genetic makeup of the population (see the discussion of genetics in Chapter 10).

Look at the population of the United States, for example. There's a reason the United States is called the melting pot of the world; there is so much diversity in our population. The same is true of other populations of organisms on the planet.

Now if the environment in which we live changed significantly, our ability to survive in the new environment could depend on which traits we have. This is basically the idea behind natural selection.

> **NURSING NOTES**
>
> The process of natural selection is also sometimes called survival of the fittest and is the defining factor of evolution. Organisms do not "choose" to evolve. Changes in a population are the result of changes to the environment in which the population lives.

Antibiotic resistance is a great example of natural selection. Before the introduction of antibiotics into the general population during the early twentieth century, bacterial infections, such as staph (*Staphylococcus aureus*), were often fatal because the body's immune system has a hard time defeating these types of bacteria. But as scientists developed stronger and more varied types of antibiotics, strep and staph bacteria were easily killed when they infected a human body.

Over time, like with any population, genetic mutations within the populations of strep bacteria enabled some strains to resist the effects of antibiotics. While other strains were killed off, these resistant strains lived and reproduced new populations, which also changed over time.

This cycle of killing off the bacteria that could not fight off the antibiotics and the reproduction of bacteria with the genetic changes that enable it to resist the effects of the antibiotics has caused a shift in our ability to fight some strains of staph. The increase in prevalence of the methicillin-resistant *Staphylococcus aureus* (MRSA) bacteria is a real cause for concern in the medical community because very few treatments work in killing off populations of this deadly bacteria when it infects the body.

This example also illustrates just how natural selection works and how organisms evolve over time. In addition to random genetic mutations that take place in cells, sexual reproduction (described in Chapter 10) plays a big role in natural selection as well.

The blending of genetic material through the fertilization of an egg results in random pairing of physical traits, some of which are expressed (dominant) and some of which are not expressed, but still present in the organism's genetic code (recessive). Recessive traits can be passed down through future generations and can play a role in those generations' ability to adapt to new environments.

Earth Science Review

So far, we've covered all kinds of topics relating to life on Earth. Now let's talk about the Earth itself. Earth science is a branch of study that encompasses what makes up the Earth, the sky, and the universe in which all of this is contained.

The Earth

The study of the Earth itself is called *geology*. If that word makes you think of rocks, you're right! The Earth is really not much more than one great big ball of rock, right on down to its core. Geologists know this, and they spend their time studying all of the different layers of rock and soil that make up the planet we call home.

Specifically, the Earth is made up of four main layers, which can then be subdivided into more layers:

▸ **Lithosphere.** You probably know this as the *crust*. It encompasses the solid, rocky top layer of the planet (the one on which we live) and part of the upper mantle. On the surface, you have the Continental crust (the land that makes up the continents) and the Oceanic crust (the land under the oceans). The entire lithosphere is only about 125 miles deep, and the crust only about 45 miles of that!

▸ The entire lithosphere is divided into tectonic plates, which pretty much float on top of the asthenosphere, which is made up of semiliquid rock. Because of this, tectonic plates shift, which results in earthquakes, volcanic eruptions, and the occasional sinking or creation of an island. The grooves where tectonic plates meet are called *fault lines*.

> **CODE RED!**
>
> Questions about plate tectonics (the study of how tectonic plates behave) have shown up on some exams. Keep that in mind when studying this section.

▸ **Mantle.** This is the next layer down. It's about 1,800 miles thick and makes up about 85 percent of Earth's total volume. The mantle is divided into several layers: the upper mantle (which is made up of the lithosphere and asthenosphere); transition region; lower mantle; and D" layer.

▸ The rock in the mantle is made up mostly of ferromagnesium silicates and the layer changes in texture from very rigid for a few miles, to soft and hot for several more miles, and then back to rigid again.

▸ Pressure and temperature in this layer are both very high. In fact, the majority of the Earth's heat comes from this layer and the movement of convection currents (heat) through the mantle is believed to be responsible for the movement of tectonic plates.

▸ **Outer core.** The outer core is about 1,400 miles thick and is made entirely of molten rock. Though you may associate molten rock with lava, when it's underground, it's called magma. The two main elements found in the outer core are iron and nickel.

▸ **Inner core.** This is the final layer of the Earth. It's about 800 miles thick and made of solid iron and nickel. Temperatures and pressure in the inner core are higher than anywhere else on the planet, yet the metals that make it up remain solid.

Rocks

More than 3,700 known mineral rocks are present in the Earth's crust. These rocks are divided into three main categories:

▸ **Igneous rock.** This type of rock is formed as a result of molten lava that has cooled and hardened. All rocks on Earth are originally created as igneous rock.

▸ **Sedimentary rock.** Over time (say millennia), igneous rocks get worn down (eroded) into particles not much larger than dirt. Weather patterns and movements of organisms scatter these particles far and wide. Though not really visible to the eye, this process results in layers of sediment that form on the bottom of lakes, streams, and oceans. As these layers interact with other minerals, the particles that make them up get heavier and more closely bonded. Eventually, they form solid layers of sedimentary rock. *Fossils* are usually found in these layers.

DEFINITION

Fossils are skeletons of living organisms that have been preserved over time by rock. Soft sedimentary rock, such as shale, often houses fossils.

▸ **Metamorphic rock.** This type of rock results when igneous or sedimentary rock is "cooked" by the Earth's interior, causing the finished product to look very different than its original version. Shale, marble, and quartzite are all metamorphic rock.

Rocks are often classified based on their hardness. This is determined by testing a rock's resistance to scratching and comparing the results to the Mohs scale of mineral hardness, which gives a 1 to 10 rating (1 being the softest and 10 the hardest). Soft rock, like talc or graphite, scores a 1. Minerals such as feldspar, quartz, and topaz are toward the middle (scoring 6, 7, and 8, respectively). Diamonds top the scale, at 10, as they're the hardest known mineral on Earth.

Atmosphere

When we talk about the atmosphere, we are mostly discussing meteorology, the science of weather and the air around us. Let's take a look at some of the factors that come into play when dealing with the atmosphere.

Atmospheric Layers

The atmosphere itself is a series of layers of varying gases in varying proportions. It has a lot of jobs that all equal one result: it enables carbon-based life to exist on Earth. Among its functions are:

▸ Filtering out radiation from the sun

▸ Regulating the planet's temperature

▸ Transporting energy from region to region around the planet

▸ Protecting the Earth from space debris that might otherwise pelt the planet

▸ Providing gases essential for breathing and metabolic respiration

▸ Filtering and disposing of waste gases

To accomplish all of these tasks, the atmosphere needs to be layered. These layers are:

▸ **Troposphere.** This is the layer closest to Earth and extends up into the sky where clouds form; the upper part/transition layer of the troposphere is called the *tropopause*. The entire layer extends up to 12 miles high, is the only layer of our atmosphere that can support life, and is also known as the *lower atmosphere*.

▸ **Stratosphere.** This is the layer above the troposphere and is about 12 miles high as well. Ozone and about 19 percent of the atmosphere's total gases are present in this layer. The higher up in the stratosphere you get, the higher the temperature rises. This results in the formation of ozone, which helps deflect solar radiation from reaching the lower atmosphere.

▸ **Mesosphere.** This layer extends about 53 miles above the planet. The mesosphere has the opposite effect of the stratosphere in that the higher you go, the colder it gets. It's in this layer that smaller meteorites and other space debris that make it through the top layer of the atmosphere burn up.

TEST TIP

The root *meso* means middle. The mesosphere and stratosphere together are known as the *middle atmosphere*.

▸ **Thermosphere.** This layer extends about 430 miles above the planet and is also known as the *upper atmosphere*. It is also the hottest layer, reaching up to 3,600°F. This is caused by the heavy absorption of solar radiation by the molecules in the very thin air.

▸ **Exosphere.** This is the final layer of the atmosphere, and extends to about 6,200 miles above the surface of the planet. It marks the barrier between the Earth's atmosphere and space and is where satellites orbit.

Barometric Pressure

Barometric pressure is a measure of the weight of the air as it pushes down on an area of Earth. This has a significant effect on the weather we experience and weather patterns around the world. The two main things about barometric pressure you should know are:

High pressure = good or improving weather

Low/falling pressure = poor or worsening weather

Clouds

Clouds are formations of gaseous water. In English, this means that when water evaporates from the Earth, it changes states from liquid to gas (see our physical science discussion). As the water reverts to a liquid state and settles in the atmosphere, clouds begin to form. Once the clouds begin to take shape, meteorologists can identify the type of cloud based on how high it is in the sky and how it looks. That's why most clouds have two parts to their name: the first part deals with their height, the second with their appearance.

Here are some cloud names and descriptions you should know:

▸ **Cumulus.** Puffy like cotton balls; often appear in groups.

▸ **Cirrus.** Wispy, like shreds of cotton; made of ice crystals.

▸ **Cumulonimbus.** Tall and thick; sometimes called thunderheads because they often bring thunderstorms.

▸ **Stratus.** Look like a thick, flat blanket; all one color, but can look pink or orange during sunrise or sunset.

The Moon and Stars

Astronomy is the study of matter in outer space, including celestial bodies and the universe as a whole. Because Earth is a part of this, it's considered an area of focus in earth science. A few general concepts you should familiarize yourself with follow.

Planets

Our solar system consists of eight planets. In 2006, Pluto was designated as a dwarf planet and no longer qualified for full planetary status. Therefore, the eight planets in our solar system in order from proximity to the sun are Mercury, Venus, Earth, Mars (all considered inner planets), Jupiter, Saturn, Uranus, and Neptune:

▸ **Mercury.** The hottest planet because it's closest to the sun.

▸ **Venus.** The brightest planet.

▸ **Earth.** That's us, third rock from the sun.

▸ **Mars.** Known as the Red Planet, but is more of a reddish marble color. Its climate is volatile, known for violent dust storms.

▸ **Jupiter.** The largest planet; looks like a reddish-white marble. Its signature feature is the Great Red Spot, which is a storm that is three times the size of Earth and has been raging for at least 300 years!

▸ **Saturn.** This one is most well-known for its large rings made of ice, dust, and rock (other planets have rings that are much less visible). Saturn's structure is very similar to Jupiter's.

▸ **Uranus.** If you ran an imaginary stick vertically through our planet, from the North Pole to the South Pole, you would have the axis around which the Earth rotates. Uranus, though, spins on a horizontal axis. It is also known as a gas planet, like Jupiter, Saturn, and its sister planet, Neptune, because its atmosphere is made

primarily of hydrogen, helium, methane, and ammonia.

▸ **Neptune.** Scientists question the composition of Neptune, and speculate that the planet is mostly made up of hydrogen with no real surface to speak of.

Planetary Motion

In the 1600s, astronomer Johannes Kepler discovered patterns in the way that the planets move in space. More than 100 years later, these patterns Kepler reported were called Kepler's Laws in Voltaire's *Elements of Newton's Philosophy*. Today, they explain the basic principles of motion among the planets in our solar system:

1. The sun is the center of the galaxy and all of the planets move around the sun in elliptical orbits.

2. Like the axis upon which the Earth rotates, the planets revolve around the sun attached to imaginary lines that extend out from the center of the sun. This means that the planets never move any closer or farther from the sun than the path of the ellipse they follow when rotating the sun brings it.

3. The amount of time it takes a planet to make one full trip around the sun depends on how far away the planet is from the sun. Based on this law, the time it takes Mercury to travel around

the sun a single time is less than the time it takes Earth to make a single trip around the sun.

In addition to Kepler's Laws, you should know that planets can have satellites (moons), which revolve around the planet, not the sun. Some planets, like Jupiter and Saturn, have multiple moons. Earth only has one.

As the Earth revolves around the sun, the moon revolves around the Earth, which results in only parts of the moon being visible to us. These are known as the phases of the moon, and they change on a predictable schedule throughout the month. Phases of the moon should not be confused with an eclipse of the moon, explained next.

Eclipses

An eclipse happens when our view of either the sun or the moon is blocked by either another object or Earth's shadow.

A solar eclipse happens when the moon moves between the Earth and the sun. The moon's blockage of the sun's light places the area of the Earth affected by the eclipse in shadow until the Earth revolves enough to move out of the shadow.

When the moon passes behind the Earth, the planet blocks the path of the sun from reaching the moon. This casts the moon in shadow and creates a lunar eclipse.

Lunar Eclipse

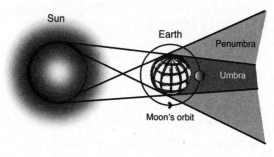

Not to scale

Solar Eclipse

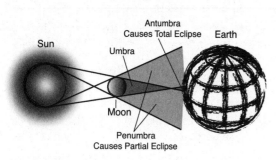

Not to scale

Practice Questions

For each of the following questions, choose the best answer.

1. The DNA of a eukaryotic cell is located in the

   (A) plasma membrane.
   (B) organelles.
   (C) nucleus.
   (D) cytoskeleton.

2. The phase of photosynthesis that processes photons into ATP, NADPH, and oxygen is called

   (A) cellular respiration.
   (B) aerobic cellular respiration.
   (C) light-independent reactions.
   (D) light-dependent reactions.

3. Nevada's Red Rock Canyon is an example of a

   (A) cold desert.
   (B) semiarid desert.
   (C) taiga.
   (D) hot dry desert.

4. A parasitic relationship in an ecosystem is one where

   (A) one or a group of organisms benefits while another is harmed.
   (B) one or a group of organisms benefits while another is not affected at all.
   (C) all organisms in the relationship benefit.
   (D) none of the above

5. Evolution is the study of

   (A) plants.
   (B) how life-forms have transformed themselves throughout history.
   (C) how life-forms have changed over time through natural selection.
   (D) life.

6. The outer core of the Earth

   (A) is nearly 3,000 miles deep.
   (B) contains mostly nickel and iron.
   (C) is composed of magma.
   (D) all of the above

7. The atmospheric layer closest to Earth is the

   (A) troposphere.
   (B) stratosphere.
   (C) mesosphere.
   (D) thermosphere.

8. Giant masses of Earth's crust that sit on top of the asthenosphere and move as a result of shifts in stability and temperature in this layer of softer rock are called

   (A) continents.
   (B) mountains.
   (C) tectonic plates.
   (D) plateaus.

9. When the moon appears between Earth and the sun, temporarily casting Earth in shadow, we experience a

   (A) supernova.

   (B) solar eclipse.

   (C) lunar eclipse.

   (D) meteor shower.

10. Proteins in a cell

   (A) remove wastes.

   (B) suspend the contents of the cell.

   (C) control the cell's metabolism.

   (D) none of the above

11. Cumulonimbus clouds

   (A) are puffy and often appear in groups.

   (B) are wispy and made of ice crystals.

   (C) are tall and thick.

   (D) look like a blanket.

12. The highest order of *Linnaean taxa* is

   (A) order.

   (B) phylum.

   (C) kingdom.

   (D) domain.

13. The purpose of a flagellum is to

   (A) provide nutrition for a cell.

   (B) move a prokaryotic cell.

   (C) communicate with other cells.

   (D) differentiate a eukaryotic cell from a prokaryotic one.

14. Another word for a producer is

   (A) autotroph.

   (B) heterotroph.

   (C) decomposer.

   (D) none of the above

15. Freshwater is what kind of biome?

   (A) terrestrial

   (B) aquatic

   (C) tundra

   (D) forest

Answers and Explanations

1. **C.** The nucleus holds all of the genetic material in a eukaryotic cell.

2. **D.** Photons are energy that is derived from light. Light is needed for light-dependent reactions to take place in photosynthesis.

3. **B.** The climate in Red Rock Canyon is rocky, dry, and arid, with little vegetation and a less extreme temperature than a hot or cold desert.

4. **A.** Answer B describes a commensal relationship; Answer C describes a mutual relationship.

5. **C.** Evolution is all about natural selection. Life-forms do not choose to change themselves; change happens through changes in the environment and the organism's physical ability to adapt to those changes.

6. **D.** Each of these is true.

7. **A.** These are listed in order from closest to farthest from the Earth.

8. **C.** The Earth's crust is segmented into tectonic plates that slide over the asthenosphere.

9. **B.** When the moon blocks the sun from view, it is a solar eclipse. When the moon passes into the Earth's shadow, it is a lunar eclipse.

10. **C.** Proteins are chemicals found within a cell that control its metabolism (chemical reactions that occur within the cell) and how the cell interacts with its surroundings.

11. **D.** Choice A describes cumulus clouds, B describes cirrus, and C describes stratus.

12. **D.** The order from highest to lowest: domain, kingdom, phylum, class, order, family, genus, species.

13. **B.** A flagellum or flagella are like little tails that move prokaryotes.

14. **A.** Producers are autotrophs. Consumers are heterotrophs. Decomposers are decomposers.

15. **B.** Freshwater is an aquatic biome characterized by the lack of salt in the water.

Bio Basics

The human body is an incredible chemical machine. Every part of our bodies—from the smallest droplet of blood to the skin that covers us from head to toe—is made up of cells. Billions of these microscopic structures are working around the clock to ensure that all of our systems run the way they should and get all of the nutrients and energy they need.

As a nurse, you will need to have a firm grasp of how cells work and the chemistry that makes the human body perform the way it does in order to help your patients. Though you will take courses in cellular biology and biochemistry during your nursing education, some programs want to gauge your readiness to handle those courses. Enter the biology section of a nursing school entrance exam.

In Chapter 9, we had a short introduction to what cells are and some of what makes them up. We take you further into that discussion in this chapter. Here, you look at the anatomy of a cell, its main functions, and how genetics work. And of course, you'll be able to test your knowledge against questions at the end of the chapter.

What to Expect

The biology sections of most nursing school entrance exams focus primarily on basic biochemistry concepts, cellular biology, and genetics. As with most of the material on your exam, this section covers high school–level concepts. If you've ever taken a high school Biology I or Biology II course, the material in this chapter will be somewhat familiar to you.

Before we dive into the biology of cells, take a look at the following vocabulary list. We will be using these terms throughout the chapter, and they're also important concepts to know going into the exam in general.

Biochemistry Vocabulary

Term	Definition
ADP	Stands for *adenosine diphosphate*. When energy is released from an ATP molecule, it becomes an ADP molecule.
ATP	Stands for *adenosine triphosphate*. This type of molecule stores energy that can be released through chemical means. ADP is turned into ATP during the electron-transfer chain process of cellular respiration.
Carbohydrate	An organic compound that contains carbon, hydrogen, and oxygen often in a 1:2:1 ratio. Carbohydrates are a main source of energy and structure for cells. Common carbohydrates are simple sugars (monosaccharides) and starches (polysaccharides).

Term	Definition
Enzyme	A chemical, often a protein, that acts as a catalyst to speed up a reaction by lowering a reaction's activation energy (see Chapter 12).
$FADH_2$	Stands for *flavin adenine dinucleotide*. It's an oxidation-reduction molecule used in cellular respiration.
Inorganic compound	A chemical compound that does not have carbon in its makeup.
NADH	Stands for *nicotinamide adenine dinucleotide*. It is a coenzyme used in cellular respiration.
Nucleic acids	These are the basic units that make up DNA and RNA. They are made of chains of nucleotides, which are the structural units of DNA. These include adenine, guanine, thymine, and cytosine.
Organic compound	A chemical compound that has carbon as part of its chemical makeup.
Protein	Long chains of amino acids joined by peptide bonds. Contains oxygen, hydrogen, nitrogen, and sulfur. They are enablers for cells, allowing them to perform a variety of functions. Enzymes, hormones, and even antibodies that help you fight off infections are proteins.

Term	Definition
Lipid	This is basically a fat. Lipids have a lower concentration of oxygen in their chemical makeup and hold more energy than carbohydrate molecules. Fats store energy, serve as a structural component of cells, and aid in communication between cells.

What's in a Cell?

We mentioned in Chapter 9 that a cell is the basic unit of life. It is an enclosed structure that contains a variety of components that work together to make the cell perform some specific purpose. Here's a review of the two types of cells:

▶ **Prokaryotic.** Usually single-celled organisms. Main differentiators are that prokaryotes have no defined nucleus, have contents that are contained within a capsule, and have a cell membrane that acts as a buffer between the contents of the cell and the capsule.

▶ **Eukaryotic.** Found primarily in more complex organisms. Eukaryotes have a defined nucleus encased in a membrane. Contents include cytoplasm, membrane-bound organelles, and chemicals that perform metabolic functions for the cell.

In this chapter, we discuss eukaryotic cells, such as this animal cell:

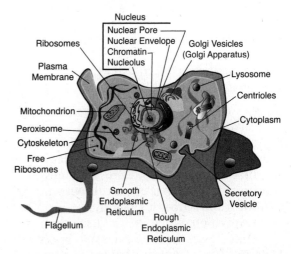

The organelles in this cell are …

▶ **Cytoskeleton.** Like our own skeleton, a cell's cytoskeleton helps give it structure. Cytoskeletons are made of strands of protein that also anchor the structures inside the cell.

▶ **Centrioles.** These are little tubelike structures whose only purpose is to assist in cell division, whether through asexual or sexual reproduction.

▶ **Endoplasmic reticulum (ER).** These are winding canals of thin tubes, sacs, and membranes; they look like a maze. There are two types of ER. Rough ER has ribosomes attached to its outer structure, giving it a rough texture. This type of ER assists ribosomes in creating proteins. Smooth ER does not have ribosomes attached and acts as a storage center for ions and steroids.

▶ **Golgi apparatus.** This is a series of thin discs that pack molecules together and either store them for later use or send them out into the cytoplasm for some function. Golgi also produce lysosomes and are thought of as the transportation system of the cell.

▶ **Lysosomes and peroxisomes.** We talk about these two together because they are so similar. Lysosomes are created by golgi and hold enzymes that the cell creates. These enzymes break down other chemicals within the cell, such as during cellular respiration. When the cell itself dies, enzymes in the lysosomes will break down the chemicals that make it up. Hydrolytic enzymes, which protect cells against bacteria, are also present in lysosomes. All of these types of enzymes work best in environments where there is little oxygen. Peroxisomes, however, hold enzymes that need oxygen to function. The enzymes they carry absorb nutrients, break down alcohols and cholesterols, and enable the synthesis of amino acids.

▶ **Mitochondria.** Mitochondria break down carbohydrates and fats to provide energy for the cell in the form of ATP. The Krebs Cycle and electron transport chain phases of cellular respiration (explained later in this chapter) take place in mitochondria.

▶ **Nucleus.** The nucleus is the controlling body of the cell. Not only does it contain all the genetic information needed for reproduction, it also regulates all of the cell's functions. The nucleus is contained within the nuclear envelope, which has pores that allow proteins and other chemicals to pass through to and from the nucleolus, the dense center of the nucleus that contains protein and RNA. The DNA, RNA, and nuclear proteins needed for reproduction are in the chromatin surrounding the nucleolus.

▶ **Ribosomes.** Ribosomes either make or synthesize proteins for use in the cell. They are found either floating in the cytoplasm or as part of rough ER.

▶ **Vacuoles.** These are just storage containers within a cell. They might store nutrients or wastes.

All of these structures are common to most animal cells you'll find on Earth. Plants are a little different; you can see a diagram of a plant cell in Chapter 9. If you compare it to the animal cell we just looked at, you'll find that most of the organelles are the same, with the exception of the following:

▶ **Chloroplasts.** These are only found in plant cells. Chloroplasts are specialized organelles within which photosynthesis takes place. See Chapter 9 for more information.

▶ **Cell wall.** Cell walls are made of cellulose, a complex carbohydrate that is used for structural purposes in a cell. In this case, it takes the place of the plasma membrane as a containing structure for a plant cell.

Moving In and Out of a Cell

Before we can talk about cellular functions, we first need to understand how chemical substances get into and out of cells. The reason for this is that most cellular processes involve the passage of proteins, carbohydrates, or enzymes from one type of cell or organelle to another.

This kind of movement means these chemicals have to cross membranes without altering the chemical composition of the membrane itself. Because maintaining the right chemical balance in a cell is a delicate business, cells have to control what's allowed to cross its membranes and how they're able to make that trip. There are a couple ways this can happen.

Diffusion

Diffusion is simply the passing of molecules across a plasma membrane. This can happen in the form of active or passive diffusion.

Passive diffusion. When the difference in concentrations of substances on both sides of the membrane causes movement, you have passive diffusion. For example, if the concentration of oxygen is high on the outside of the plasma membrane but low on the inside of the membrane, that difference in concentration enables oxygen molecules to enter the cell. This is what happens in the alveoli when blood from the heart goes to the lungs for oxygen. (See Chapter 11 for discussion of the circulatory system.) Facilitated diffusion is a type of passive diffusion where special transport proteins guide molecules through channels in the membrane and into the cell; no energy is used in the process.

Active diffusion. This process involves movement from a low concentration to a

high one. Think of trying to walk against the current in a stream: you have to expend much more energy to move. The same is true with active diffusion. To move from a low concentration to a high one, a cell needs to use energy to enable the transport proteins to move the molecules across the barrier. The other two types of diffusion do not need to use energy to transport the molecules.

Osmosis

In a solution, whichever substance there is more of proportionally is called the *solvent*. The solute is whatever substance there is less of proportionally. For example, if you dissolve salt into water, water is the solvent and salt is the solute.

When you have water-based solutions that have different concentrations of solute on both sides of a semipermeable membrane (like a plasma membrane), water can flow freely across the membrane, but solute may not be able to pass through the openings of the membrane. This creates a *hypertonic* to *hypotonic* balance between the two sides of the membrane.

> **DEFINITION**
>
> A **hypertonic** solution has a high concentration of a substance in a solution, while a **hypotonic** solution has a low concentration of a substance.

So where does osmosis come in? *Osmosis* is what we call the flow of water across a membrane from a hypertonic to a hypotonic (or vice versa) environment. Let's say you have a cell that has a saltwater solution inside it. Then you surround the cell with unsalted water. The cell membrane does not allow salt molecules to pass, thus creating a hypertonic/hypotonic situation.

The water on the outside of the cell has a high concentration of water molecules and no concentration of salt molecules, making it hypertonic for the water molecules. Inside the cell, there is a lower concentration of water molecules because they are sharing space with the salt molecules. This makes the inside of the cell hypotonic for the water molecules. As a result, the water molecules are going to try to equalize themselves out and will then flood the cell.

However, you still have the salt to deal with. Inside the cell, you have a hypertonic environment in regard to salt because of the higher concentration of salt molecules. Outside the cell is a hypotonic environment because there are no salt molecules. This means that the salt molecules will try to cross the membrane to get out—only they can't because they won't fit (that doesn't mean they're not going to try, though). So the salt molecules end up blocking the passages out of the membrane, and no or very little water can get out.

But remember, there's nothing stopping the water from flowing in. When the concentration of water inside the cell becomes too much for it to handle, the cell wall will bulge and then burst. If the conditions were reversed and water was flowing out of the cell while none could get in, the cell would dehydrate. If the solute concentrations on both sides of the membrane were equal, the water would be in balance and the water would not flow in either direction; this is also known as an *isotonic state*.

Cellular Respiration

Probably the most important cellular process to us as humans is cellular respiration. Why? This is what enables us as heterotrophs—consumers of carbon-based substances—to turn the autotrophs and other heterotrophs that we eat into energy.

Cellular respiration is the process of breaking down chemical nutrients into energy that can be used by a cell or the organism in which the cell lives. When we talk about cellular respiration, we usually discuss the process in terms of breaking down glucose (simple sugar) and turning it into ATP or stored energy.

Optimally, for every molecule of glucose that is processed, 38 molecules of ATP are produced. The following list outlines the process that takes place within a cell to accomplish this:

1. **Glycolysis.** This is the beginning phase of cellular respiration. During this anaerobic process, glucose ($C_6H_{12}O_6$) in the cytoplasm of a cell is broken down from a 6-carbon molecule chain into two 3-carbon chains called *pyruvates*. Two molecules of ATP are used to generate the energy needed to complete this process. (When a molecule of ATP is used in glycolysis, it changes into ADP. ADP is later used to create ATP.)

   Each of the 3-carbon chains then produces 2 ATP molecules, 1 NADH molecule, and 1 pyruvate. The net by-products of glycolysis are ...

   ▸ 2 ATP (because 2 are used in the first part of the process)

   ▸ 2 NADH

   ▸ 2 pyruvates

2. **Krebs cycle.** Sometimes also called the *citric acid cycle*, this is the aerobic phase of cellular respiration which takes place in the mitochondria of a cell. The cycle begins with the *oxidation* of one of the pyruvates. This results in the creation of carbon dioxide, acetyl-coenzyme A (acetyl-coA), and NADH.

The acetyl-coA blends with a 4-carbon molecule chain which reacts to create citric acid, a 6-carbon molecule chain. The citric acid then oxidizes and creates carbon dioxide, ATP, NADH, and $FADH_2$. When both pyruvates complete the Krebs cycle, the following are created:

- ▸ 2 ATP
- ▸ 8 NADH
- ▸ 2 $FADH_2$

3. **Electron transport chain.** This is where the majority of ATP is created during cellular respiration. The NADH and $FADH_2$ molecules oxidize within the inner membrane of a mitochondrion (called the *matrix*), and proteins pump resulting hydrogen protons through the matrix wall into the outer portion of the mitochondrion. When the protons re-enter the matrix, they travel through ATP synthase proteins and this motion turns ADP from the matrix into ATP. This process nets 34 ATP molecules.

If you add together the 2 ATP from glycolysis, the 2 ATP from the Krebs cycle, and the 34 from the electron transport chain, you have a total of 38 ATP produced from one molecule of glucose.

Another important step in the cellular respiration process is fermentation. When glycolysis takes place in an environment that doesn't have oxygen, pyruvates are oxidized to create other kinds of substances, such as lactic acid.

Cellular Reproduction

There are two ways that cells reproduce or make new cells. The first is asexual reproduction or *mitosis*, meaning that new cells are formed without the fusion of two different nuclei. The second is sexual reproduction or *meiosis*, which involves the nuclei of two different cells combining to create new cells.

Mitosis: Asexual Reproduction

The process of mitosis occurs in every type of cell except those used for sexual reproduction (gametes). So when you get a cut on your hand, your skin cells go through mitosis to replace the ones that were severed or killed off by the cut. When these new cells are put into place, your cut has healed.

Mitosis occurs during the course of several steps, only the last of which is actually called *mitosis*. The first three steps in mitosis take place during one long phase called *interphase*. During interphase, the following happens:

- ▸ **G_1 stage.** This is called the *first gap phase*, during which the cell creates all the carbs, lipids, proteins, and enzymes needed to reproduce at some stage. New organelles that will be passed on to the daughter cells created at the end of mitosis are also formed and stored. G_1 is a growth stage and can last years in slow-growing cells.

▸ **S stage.** *S* stands for *synthesis* in this phase. Proteins are synthesized and spindle structures will pull the cell apart during stage M. Human cells normally have 46 *chromosomes*. During S stage, they replicate to form 92 chromosomes—46 for each new cell. You can't actually see the chromosomes at this point. That will come during prophase of active mitosis. S stage can last anywhere from 8 to 10 hours.

▸ **G₂ stage.** This is a preparation stage for M stage. More proteins are synthesized and any other structures that are needed to divide the cell into two genetically identical cells are made.

The end of G₂ stage marks the beginning of M stage, which is broken up into the phases of mitosis most people are familiar with: prophase, metaphase, anaphase, and telophase:

▸ **Prophase.** The chromosomes become visible as the DNA becomes denser. The nuclear membrane disintegrates and the chromosomes are released into the cell's cytoplasm, along with the rest of the nucleus's contents. The cell's two centrioles begin to move to opposite sides of the cell, and the spindle structures begin to elongate while the chromosomes line up to the spindles in the center of the cell.

▸ **Metaphase.** The spindles finish elongating and the chromosomes attach themselves along the length of the spindle apparatus (just a name for all of the spindles together). The centromeres anchor the chromosomes to the spindle apparatus and a line of chromosomes forms through the middle of the cell.

▸ **Anaphase.** When anaphase begins, the fibers that make up the spindle apparatus start pulling the chromosomes apart at the centromere. This results in half of the paired chromosomes going to one side of the cell and the other half going to the other side.

▸ **Telophase.** This is the finishing touch. You now have two cells, still connected by a strand of plasma membrane. Inside each cell, the nuclear membranes re-form, the spindles break down, and the chromosomes uncoil and go back to the state they stay in when the cell is not replicating. Cell division ends when the cells go into cytokinesis, which is just a fancy way of saying that the plasma membrane connecting the two cells breaks off, leaving two completely independent, genetically identical cells.

Mitosis

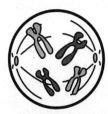

Prophase
DNA condenses into chromosomes,
nucleus breaks down

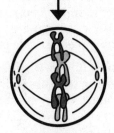

Metaphase
Chromosomes line up,
attach to mitotic apparatus

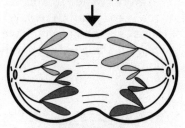

Anaphase
Mitotic apparatus
pulls chromosomes away

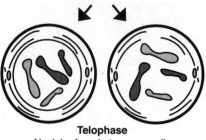

Telophase
Nuclei reform in two new cells

Meiosis: Sexual Reproduction

Meiosis is a little more involved because you are joining the genetic material of two independent cells to create a new one (of four, as you'll see) that is genetically unique.

Meiosis is a process that occurs exclusively with gametes, special cells whose sole purpose is to mix with another gamete during fertilization to create a completely new cell that has a blending of genetic information from both parent cells. Sound familiar? It should. This is exactly how a human male's sperm and a human woman's eggs are produced.

A gamete only has 23 single chromosomes (not paired ones like in mitosis), as opposed to the 46 present in other cells. This is so that when a gamete mixes with another gamete, the resulting cell has the 46 chromosomes it should instead of 92.

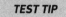

> **TEST TIP**
>
> When a gamete is by itself with its 23 chromosomes, it's called a *haploid*. When the number of its chromosomes doubles after fertilization, the resulting cell (zygote) is called a *diploid*.

Meiosis is broken down into two cycles of pretty much the same process as mitosis, with a few tweaks:

▸ **Prophase I.** During interphase in meiosis, DNA replicates and the number of chromosomes doubles. In the case of the fertilization of an egg by a sperm, the chromosomes from each haploid cell combine to create a diploid cell. Either way, you have 46 single chromosomes floating around the nucleus of the cell.

- During prophase, the chromosomes start to join and form homologues; you have 23 homologues at the end of this process. The interesting thing that happens during this pairing up is that chromosomes that are genetically different from each other can exchange genetic information, or "cross over." The result of this is that the new homologues that are formed are now coded differently than both sets of the parent chromosomes.

- **Metaphase I.** The centrioles go to opposite sides of the cell while the homologues line up their centromeres to the spindle apparatus. The homologues line up in random order and attach to the spindle apparatus at their centromeres.

- **Anaphase I.** The spindle fibers start pulling the cell apart and the homologous pairs divide evenly between the two sides, sending 23 pairs to one and 23 pairs to the other.

- **Telophase I.** The cells continue separation into two haploid daughter cells, each with 23 paired chromatids.

- **Prophase II.** When Telophase I is complete, the two newly formed daughter cells will each begin to separate in what's called Meiosis II. The new nuclei break down, but the DNA doesn't replicate. Spindles form in preparation for cell division.

- **Metaphase II.** The chromosome pairs line up at the spindle apparatus and attach at their centromeres. The centrioles move to either side of the cell.

- **Anaphase II.** Like with anaphase in mitosis, the spindles pull the chromosome pairs apart at the centromere to create two sets of 23 single chromosomes.

- **Telophase II.** Each of the daughter cells that were created in Meiosis I is now ready to split into two. When cytokinesis is complete, you have 4 gametes, each haploid with only 23 chromosomes.

CODE RED!

Note that in Anaphase I, the paired chromosomes are pulled to each side. In mitosis, the paired chromosomes were split apart during anaphase. Don't confuse this. The chromosomes need to stay in pairs during Meiosis I so that they can later be separated in Meiosis II.

NURSING NOTES

When meiosis takes place for sperm cells, it's called *spermatogenesis*. When it takes place for egg cells, it's called *oogenesis*. Both begin with a special diploid cell created by the body.

Meiosis

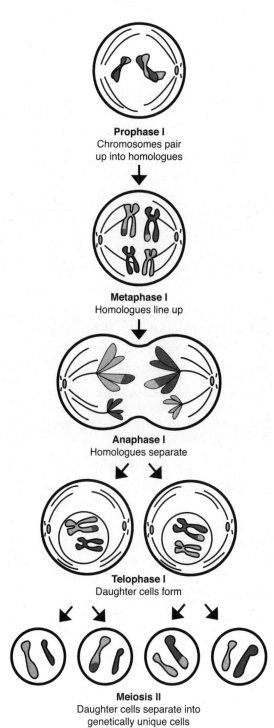

Prophase I
Chromosomes pair
up into homologues

Metaphase I
Homologues line up

Anaphase I
Homologues separate

Telophase I
Daughter cells form

Meiosis II
Daughter cells separate into
genetically unique cells

Genetics

Now that you know how cells replicate, let's talk about what exactly it is that replicates: genetic information. Genes are chemical codes for physical traits. What hair color you have or how tall you will grow to be—in some cases if you will create cancer cells— all depend on your genes.

We already know that when sexual reproduction takes place, genetic information is blended and reproduced. This is a lot of what gene theory is about. Genetic information is located in chromosomes in the form of DNA.

The offspring of two gametes reproducing through meiosis will have genetic information from both gametes. It's the way that the chromosomes mix during meiosis that determines which genes are expressed and which are not. More on that in a minute. First, let's look at what DNA is all about.

DNA

Deoxyribonucleic acid (DNA) is a nucleic acid made up of sequenced pairs of two types of nucleotides: purines (adenine and guanine) and pyrimidines (cytosine and thymine). When they are sequenced together, they form base pairs.

> **TEST TIP**
>
> Adenine can only pair with thymine. Guanine can only pair with cytosine. You will never see these nucleotides in a strand of DNA without these pairings. It is the sequence in which these base pairs are placed that makes each of our DNA unique identifiers.

These base pairs are held together by two 5-sugar and phosphate spines, one on the outside edge of each nucleic acid, to form a kind of ladder structure (if you were to lay a strand of DNA flat). But DNA isn't flat. It is twisted into a double-helix structure.

The most important concept to understand with DNA is how it replicates:

1. Within the chromatin of a cell, the tightly coiled double helix unwinds to form a ladder structure or maybe more accurately, a zipper structure.

2. An enzyme in the chromatin causes the double strand to "unzip," breaking the bonds between the base pairs and generating two single strands of DNA.

3. Ribonucleic acid (RNA) in the form of messenger RNA, which is also present in the chromatin, copies the DNA's sequence in a process called *transcription*.

4. Enzymes then work to pair up free nucleotides in the chromatin with their partner nucleotide on the two single DNA chains that are formed through unzipping the double helix.

5. When all of the pairing is complete, the two new strands of DNA coil into separate double helixes and will eventually replicate as well.

> **CODE RED!**
>
> The exact transcription of the nucleic acid sequence is vital to DNA replication. Any variation in that sequence results in mutation of the gene.

This is a very high-level look at the process of DNA replication. There is much more involved with this process, but this amount of knowledge should be enough to get you through your exam.

Mendel

If you took biology in high school, you probably learned all about Gregor Mendel (1822–1884). He was an Austrian monk and scientist who, through his studies of genetic traits in pea plants, figured out that the genes that we carry are not always expressed.

By "expressed," we mean seen or manifested. For example, some people are said to be "carriers" of genes that can cause certain illnesses, such as sickle cell disease. This means that the information that causes this condition is written in their genetic code but does not affect the person who carries that code. Because the gene is not expressed, it is carried. This is an example of genotype: information about your physical structure coded into your DNA that may or may not be expressed.

Of course, you have lots of genes that are expressed. We call this your *phenotype*, or the physical expression of your genetic code. For example, your genes might say that your hair will be blond or your eyes will be green. These are examples of phenotype.

> **TEST TIP**
>
> An easy way to remember the difference between genotype and phenotype is to associate the meaning with the beginning sounds of the words: genotype = genetic; phenotype = physical.

Mendelian Theory

Mendel came up with this idea of genotype and phenotype as a way to explain why tall plants that were mated with short plants resulted in a whole generation of tall plants. The results of his experiments include the following findings:

▶ **Genes vary.** Mendel figured out that an organism's genes are generally the same, but the coding for how they are expressed varies. For example, every human has genetic coding to form a nose—which is a trait. However, the shape and size of that nose varies from person to person.

- Mendel named the genetic coding of a trait an *allele*, and theorized that one inherited allele from each parent is needed for a trait to be expressed. How those alleles converge into gene pairs determines how the trait will be expressed. This is known as the *Law of Segregation*, which also explains that when gametes reproduce, only one copy of each allele goes to each cell that's produced.

- **Gene pairs form randomly in meiosis.** In addition to the Law of Segregation, Mendel theorized the Law of Independent Assortment. This states that when one gamete is fertilized by another, the gene pairs that result from the union form independent of each other. For example, the formation of the gene pair for hair color has nothing to do with the gene pair for height.

- **Some genes are dominant.** Mendel figured out that some alleles mask others. The offspring of his paired tall and short plants were all tall. But the alleles that coded for shortness in the height of the plant had to still be in the genetic coding somewhere. To explain this, Mendel categorized the "tall" allele as being dominant over the "short" allele, meaning that when both are present, only the tall allele is expressed.

- **Some genes are recessive.** Mendel called the short gene *recessive* because it was dominated by the tall gene, but still present in the allele for height.

Predicting Genetic Inheritance

Mendel noticed that when he crossbred his tall and short plants, the ratio of tall plants to short plants was 3:1. For every breeding of purely tall plants with purely short plants (no hybrids), three tall plants and one short plant would be produced.

In the early twentieth century, Reginald C. Punnett built on Mendel's genetic theories and devised a way of predicting the probability that a trait would be inherited based on gene pairs from a mother and a father. What resulted is now known as the Punnett square.

The idea behind the Punnett square is very simple. Take a look at the following example.

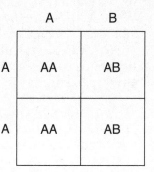

This Punnett square shows the alleles for the blood types of a mother and a father. The father's gene pair is shown on top: AB (an A allele from his mother and a B allele from his father produced this blood type). The mother's allele is shown on the side: AA (both her parents passed A alleles to her, resulting in an AA blood type).

In this example, the father's blood type is considered heterozygous, meaning that it is made up of two different alleles. The mother's blood type is homozygous, or made up of two of the same alleles.

You can use this square to predict what blood type a child of these two people might be. To do this:

1. Place the letters on the left side of the square in the first position in each box in the row next to them. As shown in the figure, A goes in all four boxes.

2. Place the letters on the top of the square in the second position of each box in the column under them. As shown in the figure, the first two vertical boxes have As and the second two vertical boxes have Bs.

3. Evaluate the results. This Punnett square says that if these two people had a baby, its blood type would be either AA or AB. These are the only two possibilities presented in the box. From here, you can calculate the probability of this couple having an AB baby as 50 percent.

Practice Questions

For each of the following questions, choose the best answer.

1. A prokaryotic cell contains

    (A) a plasma membrane.
    (B) a nucleoid.
    (C) cytoplasm.
    (D) all of the above

2. The phenotype of an organism is

    (A) the physical expression of its genotype.
    (B) the genetic constitution governing a heritable trait.
    (C) the changes in a population gene pool.
    (D) the mutation of a gene.

3. Which of the following is true about meiosis?

    (A) It's a mechanism in which the diploid number of chromosomes is reduced to the haploid number for sexual reproduction.
    (B) It's a mechanism by which a single nucleus gives rise to two nuclei that are genetically identical to each other and to the parent nucleus.
    (C) DNA is replicated before meiosis.
    (D) Each chromosome acts independently.

4. Which type of metabolism releases the maximum amount of energy from food molecules and stores it as ATP?

    (A) photosynthesis
    (B) fermentation
    (C) cellular respiration
    (D) glycolysis

5. Major products of glycolysis are

    (A) ATP, pyruvates, and NADH.
    (B) glucose, AMP, and NADH.
    (C) glucose, pyruvates, and NADH.
    (D) none of the above

6. Which of the following is not true regarding Mendel's work?

    (A) He observed patterns of inheritance and proposed mechanisms to explore them.
    (B) He identified dominant and recessive traits.
    (C) He proposed that hereditary carriers are present as discrete units that retain their integrity in the presence of other units.
    (D) He developed the Punnett square.

7. The passing of molecules through a plasma membrane from a high concentration area to a low concentration area is called

    (A) diffusion.
    (B) osmosis.
    (C) hypertonics.
    (D) hypotonics.

8. A person is homozygous recessive for a particular trait if he or she has

   (A) two dominant alleles for the trait.
   (B) two recessive alleles for the trait.
   (C) one dominant and one recessive allele for the trait.
   (D) more than two alleles for the trait.

9. The electron transport chain requires oxygen to

   (A) produce ATP.
   (B) form lactic acid.
   (C) produce calcium.
   (D) form acetyl-coA.

10. The function of meiosis is

    (A) to promote genetic diversity.
    (B) to ensure that each of the four products has a complete set of chromosomes.
    (C) to reduce the chromosomes from diploid to haploid.
    (D) all of the above

11. The process of mitochondria in a eukaryotic cell using energy from food substances to produce ATP is known as

    (A) cellular respiration.
    (B) cellular metabolism.
    (C) cellular reproduction.
    (D) mitochondria matrix.

12. Which of the following is not true about sexual reproduction?

    (A) It produces a clone that has genotypes identical to its own.
    (B) It provides for genetic diversity.
    (C) It eliminates genetic recombination.
    (D) It has the ability to exploit a stable environment.

13. Glycolysis

    (A) is the pathway in which food molecules are converted to a compound that can be used in cellular respiration.
    (B) is the first part of fermentation.
    (C) takes place in the cytoplasm.
    (D) all of the above

14. The Krebs cycle is significant in the production of

    (A) adrenaline.
    (B) energy.
    (C) insulin.
    (D) ketone bodies.

15. Using the Punnett square, what is the blood type of an offspring if both parents are AO blood type?

    (A) type A only
    (B) type O only
    (C) type A or O
    (D) all ABO types are possible

Answers and Explanations

1. **D.** A prokaryotic cell contains a plasma membrane, a nucleoid, and cytoplasm.

2. **A.** Genotype is the genetic constitution governing a heritable trait. Microevolution is the changes in a population gene pool.

3. **A.** All other answers relate to mitosis.

4. **C.** Photosynthesis uses light energy to synthesize food compounds. Fermentation releases energy from food compounds in the absence of oxygen. Glycolysis is the pathway in which food molecules are converted to a compound that can be used in cellular respiration and is also the first part of fermentation.

5. **A.** Glycolysis produces four ATP molecules (although two are used in the first part of the process), two NADH molecules, and two pyruvates.

6. **D.** Mendel did not develop the Punnett square. British geneticist Reginald Crundall Punnett devised this square.

7. **A.** Diffusion can happen in the form of facilitated diffusion, where proteins guide molecules through channels in the membrane and into the cell; or passive diffusion, where a difference in concentrations of substances on both sides of the membrane causes movement.

8. **B.** Homozygous for a trait means that the person has two of the same alleles.

9. **A.** ATP is the final product of the electron transport chain, which passes high-energy electrons to oxygen.

10. **D.** All of the answers relate to meiosis.

11. **A.** *Cellular metabolism* refers to the total of all the biochemical reactions that take place within a cell. *Cellular reproduction* refers to the replication of cells. The mitochondria matrix is the inner membrane of a mitochondrion.

12. **A.** All of the other answers are true.

13. **D.** All of the answers relate to glycolysis.

14. **B.** The Krebs cycle is the second step in cellular respiration, which turns carbohydrates into energy in the form of ATP. Adrenaline and insulin are hormones created by the endocrine system. Ketone bodies are by-products of the breakdown of fatty acids in the body.

15. **C.** The possibilities are type AA, AO, or OO.

Anatomy and Physiology Check-Up

There's really no mystery as to why a nursing school entrance exam may include a section on anatomy and physiology (A&P). After all, being a nurse is all about dealing with the human body, and that is what A&P is: a study of the parts of the human body and how those parts work.

You may already have a background in this particular subject. If so, that's great! This chapter will be a good refresher for you and may even teach you a thing or two you didn't know. If you're planning on taking A&P once in nursing school, this chapter will give you a lot of information that will help you prepare for the course.

But even if you've never taken an A&P course in your life, this chapter will help get you through this section of your nursing school entrance exam. We cover each of the main systems of the human body, explain what makes them up and how they work, and give you an introduction to some of the terminology that you'll become very familiar with throughout your nursing studies.

What to Expect

Basics, basics, basics. This is the name of the game for most A&P sections of nursing school entrance exams. You'll find questions asking you to identify different parts of the body, systems that make the body work, how they work together, and how the body works as a whole.

Some nursing programs will not allow you to take the entrance exam until you have already taken certain college-level science courses, A&P included. Still, others allow high school graduates to take the entrance exams. This means that most questions on an A&P test will be geared toward the student who has taken high school anatomy or other science that covers anatomy in some way.

As we've said in every other science chapter in this book, make sure that it is absolutely necessary for you to take the A&P section of your entrance exam. Many nursing schools only require the math and verbal sections; the subject-specific sections may not be required. If you just finished an A&P course before taking your entrance exam and feel strong in this subject, you can complete the section to try to raise your score. Beware, though: if you do poorly on the section, it will lower your score.

Basic Terminology

The field of medicine has its own language. Luckily, that language is based on Greek and Latin roots, just like much of English. Also, the prevalence of medical-based shows on television has brought many of the words used by health-care professionals into the mainstream lexicon.

So what does this mean for you? Knowing some medical terminology will help you a great deal when preparing for an A&P exam, because you're dealing with the structure and workings of the human body. To help you out, we've provided a few tables of word roots and general terminology that will broaden your familiarity with words you may encounter on the test. They will also help you get clues about the meanings of words you're not sure of, so that you can either eliminate them as possible answers or include them as a correct answer choice.

Anatomy and Physiology Roots

Root	Related Body Part
arteri/arterio	Arteries
cardio/cardiac	Heart
cerebr	Brain
cervic	Neck
crani/cranio	Skull
derm	Skin
gastro	Stomach
gluco/glyco	Glucose
hemat	Blood
hist/histo	Tissue
hyper	Extreme beyond
hypo	Extreme below
nephr/nephro/ren/reno	Kidney
ocul/oculo/ophthalm/opthalmo	Eyes
or(o)	Mouth
ost/osteo/ossi	Bones
ot	Ear
pneum/pneumo/pulmon/pulmo	Lungs
rhin/rhino	Nose
somat/somato	Body
trache(o)	Trachea
tympan(o)	Eardrum
vascular	Blood vessels
ven	Veins

Common Spatial Vocab

Term/Root	Meaning
Anterior	Front; opposite of posterior
Ascending	Travelling upward
Bilateral	On two sides
Descending	Travelling downward
Distal	Farther away from the beginning; opposite of proximal
Dorsal	Pertaining to the human back; opposite of ventral (think dorsal fin on a shark)
Endo	From inside
Epi	On the surface
Exo	From the outside
Inferior	Below; opposite of superior
Lateral	One side of the body; opposite of medial
Medial	Middle or inside; opposite of lateral
Peri	Surrounding
Posterior	Back; opposite of anterior
Proximal	Close to the beginning; opposite of distal
Superior	Above; opposite of inferior
Unilateral	On one side
Ventral	Pertaining to the abdomen; opposite of dorsal

Circulatory System

The circulatory system deals with the transport of blood throughout the human body. It is a *closed system* made up of many components that work together in order to provide the body with oxygen and nutrients to all the cells in the body.

DEFINITION

The circulatory system is considered a **closed system** because it is completely contained within blood vessels. Unless a vessel is severed, blood cannot flow outside of the system. However, substances within the blood, such as oxygen and nutrients, can pass through the vessel wall into the tissues in a process called *diffusion*. It is through this process that the blood picks up wastes, such as carbon dioxide.

The circulatory system also carries waste products to the kidneys and lungs, organs that filter the blood and get rid of those wastes. Let's take a look at the different components that make up this vital system.

Blood

Blood has long been held as a symbol of life in cultures throughout the world. And for good reason. It is our blood that carries the energy our cells need to live and reproduce. It takes away the waste our tissues produce and contains cells that help us fight off infection. Without blood, there is no life.

Blood contains a careful balance of cells, fluid, chemicals, and nutrients. Blood, for the most part, is produced in bone marrow (long bones in children, flat bones in adults), though some is produced in the spleen.

The main components you should be aware of include:

▸ **Plasma.** This fluid (mostly water, proteins, and dissolved salts) makes up between 55 and 60 percent of blood's volume. The other components of blood are suspended in plasma.

▸ **Red blood cells (RBCs).** Also called erythrocytes, these are flat, disc-shaped cells that are made up mostly of hemoglobin, a protein that enables RBCs to carry oxygen to tissues. RBCs make up around 40 percent of blood's volume.

- **White blood cells (WBCs).** Also called leukocytes, these protect the body against infection by attacking invading parasites, viruses, bacteria, and sometimes allergens, in addition to helping dispose of dead or damaged cells. They do this through phagocytosis, a process of surrounding another cell and breaking it down. RBCs outnumber WBCs by a ratio of about 600 to 700:1.

- **Platelets.** Also called *thrombocytes*, these particles clump together (clot) to stop bleeding and release chemicals that also promote clotting.

Heart

The heart is the driving force of the circulatory system. It's kind of like the home base for blood within the system, so when we start talking about the path of blood later, we start there.

The heart is unique in that it is both an organ and a muscle made of a special type of muscle tissue called *cardiac muscle*, which is only found in the heart. Its only function in the body is to pump blood through the circulatory system, so the fact that it is a muscle makes sense. This pumping action is initiated by the sinoatrial node, or pacemaker, which emits an electrical impulse that makes the heart contract.

When the heart pumps, it creates pressure in the blood vessels, which causes the blood to move throughout the system. A contraction of the heart increases the pressure, while the relaxation of the heart decreases the pressure. Blood pressure is measured by a ratio of contraction pressure (systolic reading) to relaxation pressure (diastolic reading).

The heart is largely hollow inside and is divided into four chambers that hold blood:

- **Atria.** These are the two upper chambers of the heart. They allow blood to enter the heart from the body (through the vena cavae) or the lungs (through the pulmonary vein).

- **Ventricles.** These are the two lower chambers of the heart. They allow blood to exit the heart to the lungs (through the pulmonary artery) or the body (through the aorta).

Within the heart, blood moves from one chamber to the next through a series of valves. These are important to ensure that blood cannot flow backward and continues in a forward motion throughout the system. Each chamber of the heart has one intake valve and one outlet valve.

The entire heart is encased in a "bag" of connective tissue called *pericardium*. The pericardium is made up of two layers. The fibrous pericardium is the outer layer. Its job is to anchor and protect the heart within the chest, as well as prevent the heart from filling up with too much blood. The second layer is the serous pericardium, which lies between the heart and the fibrous layer. Its purpose is to lubricate the heart and prevent friction.

Blood Vessels

Blood vessels are tubes through which blood flows throughout the body. They are segmented with a series of one-way valves that prevent the backflow of blood in the system.

The following diagram shows the three types of blood vessels in the human body:

- **Arteries.** These blood vessels take oxygen-rich blood away from the heart and into the major parts of the body, which is why they are the darker ones in the diagram. Arterial blood is a deep crimson color. The largest artery is the aorta, which stems from the left ventricle of the heart and branches into three arteries that carry blood to the brain and arms before extending down into the abdominal cavity. There, the aorta splits into two arteries that bring blood to the legs. From there, smaller arteries bring blood to the capillaries within the tissues.

Circulatory System

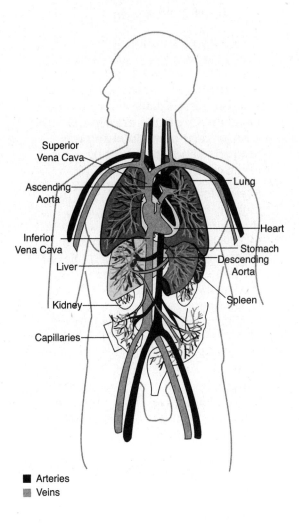

Superior
Vena Cava

Ascending
Aorta

Inferior
Vena Cava

Liver

Kidney

Capillaries

Lung

Heart

Stomach
Descending
Aorta

Spleen

■ Arteries
▦ Veins

▶ **Veins.** Veins bring blood that has been depleted of oxygen and has picked up waste products back to the heart. They are the lighter-colored vessels in the diagram, and the blood that flows through them is often a bluish color due to the lack of oxygen. The vena cava is the vein equivalent of the aorta. It brings blood to the heart through two openings in the right atrium.

▶ The superior vena cava connects to the heart at the top of the right atrium and then branches off into two major veins (subclavian) that go into the arms. The subclavian veins then branch off into veins that go into the head.

▶ The inferior vena cava brings blood through another connection to the right atrium from the lower part of the body. It runs down from the heart into the abdomen, just like the aorta and then splits into two veins that go into the legs. From there, smaller veins take blood to the capillaries within the tissues.

▶ **Capillaries.** These are tiny blood vessels that serve as an intermediary between arteries and veins. It's in the capillaries that water, oxygen, wastes, and nutrients are exchanged in the tissues. In a healthy body, blood flows through these vessels with little problem. However, blood vessels can be damaged, which impedes the flow of blood through the body. This can occur as a result of ...

▶ **High blood pressure.** Higher-than-normal blood pressure can damage the cells in your arteries, making them vulnerable to stiffening and hardening, bulging, or rupture. It also can damage the heart, brain, and other organs, as well as lead to more serious conditions, such as coronary artery disease and stroke.

▶ **High cholesterol.** Blood contains fats in the form of cholesterol, which comes in three types: LDL (bad), HDL (good), and VLDL (triglycerides). Too much "bad" cholesterol in your blood can lead to build-up of fat deposits (plaque) in the arteries, which can lead to blockages.

> **TEST TIP**
>
> Remember, veins bring blood into the heart. Arteries take blood away from the heart. Also, the pressure of blood is stronger in arteries than it is in veins.

Path of Blood

The path blood takes to reach every part of the human body really consists of a series of smaller routes. We begin our discussion with the heart, which directs the flow of oxygen-rich and oxygen-poor blood simultaneously:

▶ **Pulmonary circulation.** This is the process of reoxygenating blood that has travelled through the body and spent its oxygen while picking up waste products. The path of pulmonary circulation is as follows:

1. Blood enters the right atrium through two large veins called the vena cavae.

2. The right atrium pushes the blood through a one-way valve into the right ventricle.

3. The blood is then pushed through another valve into the pulmonary artery, which brings the blood to the lungs and is the only artery in the body that carries deoxygenated blood.

4. Within the capillaries of the lungs, the carbon dioxide in the blood is exchanged for oxygen.

5. The reoxygenated blood is then carried through the pulmonary vein (the only vein in the body that carries oxygen-rich blood) back to the heart and fills the left atrium.

6. The left atrium pushes the blood through a one-way valve to the left ventricle, which then pushes the blood out of the heart through the aorta.

▶ **Coronary circulation.** The heart itself also has a series of arteries and veins that takes nourishment from the blood that travels through it. These vessels deliver oxygen-rich blood directly to the muscle and take away oxygen-poor blood and waste products to be filtered out by the rest of the circulatory system.

▶ **Systemic circulation.** Oxygen-rich blood is carried from the heart through the aorta and into a system of arteries that bring the blood to the other organs, systems, and tissues in the body. One very important stop is the kidneys, which filter out all of the wastes in the blood, except for carbon dioxide, and turn them into urine.

As arterial blood flows through the tissues, nutrients and wastes are exchanged in the capillaries. Then the now oxygen-poor, waste-rich blood travels back to the heart. After the blood gets back to the heart, the whole process starts again.

Respiratory System

The respiratory system deals with the intake of air into the lungs and the exchange of that air with carbon dioxide. The following diagram shows both the upper and lower parts of the respiratory system.

Respiratory System

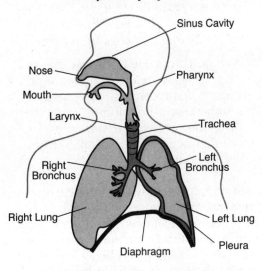

Upper Respiratory System

Air enters the body through the upper respiratory system. It consists of the …

▶ **Nose.** This airway includes the nasal cavity, which connects to the sinus cavity and runs down to the top of the back of the mouth. It is lined with tiny hairs and cilia, and also contains some amount of mucus. Its purpose is to warm the air going into the body and filter out particles.

▶ **Mouth.** This is the other opening through which air enters the respiratory system. It is beneath the nasal cavity and connects to the pharynx.

▶ **Pharynx.** The pharynx is what most people think of as the back of the throat. It is the tubular airway that runs from the nasal cavity, down the throat, and to the larynx. At the bottom of the pharynx, the tube splits into the trachea (air tube to the lungs) and esophagus (food tube to the stomach).

▶ **Larynx.** This is the voice box, but also serves as protection for the trachea. It's located just below the pharynx. A small flap of tissue called the *epiglottis* covers the entrance of the larynx when you swallow. The flap closes the trachea so that what you're swallowing can go into the esophagus and not the lungs.

Lower Respiratory System

The lower respiratory system is what most people think of when you mention this bodily system. It consists of the following:

▶ **Trachea.** This is the tube that brings air from the upper part of the respiratory system to the lower part. It runs from the base of the throat and into the chest before branching off into two bronchi. The trachea is lined with cilia to help filter the air more and to also help in the removal of mucus from the lungs.

▶ **Bronchi.** These tubes connect the trachea to the lungs, and they branch off into smaller tubes called bronchioles. Bronchioles further branch off (like tree branches) into an intricate web of alveoli, which are little capillary-dense sacs that hold air.

- **Lungs.** These are spongy organs that inflate and deflate with air through the process of respiration. Each lung is separated into lobes. The left lung has two lobes; the right lung has three lobes.

NURSING NOTES

The left lung is smaller than the right lung because the heart is also situated toward the left side of the chest. The two have to share a small space with the heart inside the rib cage, which accounts for the difference in size.

- **Diaphragm.** This is a thin band of fibromuscular tissue that is situated below the lungs and separates the chest cavity from the abdomen. When it expands and contracts, it enables the lungs to inhale and exhale. The diaphragm's movement is controlled primarily by the involuntary nervous system (discussed later in this chapter).

Path of Air

When you inhale, air enters your body through the upper respiratory system. The cilia and mucus in your nasal cavity filter out bacteria and debris and warm the air before it travels down the pharynx, through the larynx, and into the trachea. From there, it goes through the bronchi and bronchioles to fill the alveoli.

When there, the oxygen passes (diffuses) into the rich concentration of capillaries in the alveoli, where it's picked up by the blood. In return, the alveoli fill with carbon dioxide waste from the blood. The carbon dioxide is released from the air sacs and the lungs when you exhale.

Nervous System

Everything you feel, see, and do is controlled by one system: the nervous system. This is essentially a combination of several systems that route electrical signals from the brain to the rest of the body.

Before we start our discussion of the parts of the nervous system, it's important to understand a few things about the basic unit of the system: the neuron or nerve cell. This is a special type of cell that sends and receives electrical impulses.

A neuron has two types of fibers that extend from one large cell body:

- **Dendrites.** These receive impulses from the brain or other neurons. They extend off of all sides of the rounded cell body like branches from a tree.

- **Axons.** This is one long fiber that extends from the cell body to the muscle that receives the impulse. Axons transmit the impulse that the dendrites receive to tissues, muscles, or other neurons. They look like tails on the neuron.

When an impulse travels from neuron to neuron, axons secrete chemicals called neurotransmitters, which travel the space between the axon and surrounding dendrites. This space is called a synapse. The neurotransmitters cross the synapse and trigger the dendrites in surrounding neurons to pick up the impulses it's sending and then react.

Now that you have a basic understanding of how neurons work, let's look at the subsystems that make up the body's greater nervous system.

Nervous System

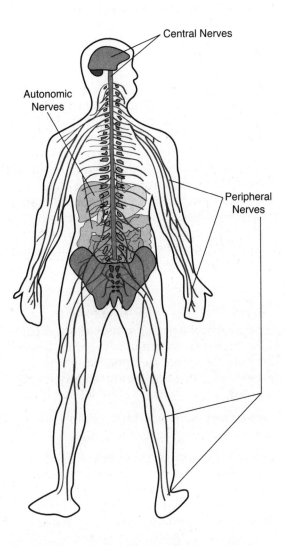

Central Nerves

Autonomic Nerves

Peripheral Nerves

Central Nervous System

We start our discussion with the brain and spinal cord, which make up the central nervous system (CNS). The brain is the source of all of the electrical activity that goes on in the nervous system. It is the central processor of every action we perform (voluntarily or not) and every experience we have. It enables our bodies to function by controlling all of our functions and senses,

and it enables us to experience and make sense of the stimuli we receive.

The brain is a very special organ, dense in neurons. It requires continuous nourishment from oxygenated blood and is protected by what's known as the blood-brain barrier. This is a layer of capillaries that cannot accept certain chemicals from the blood, such as certain types of medicines, toxins, and proteins. The brain is also encased in three layers of tissue called *meninges*. The meninges provide both the brain and spinal cord with a cushion of cerebrospinal fluid and protect them from trauma due to movement of the body.

Generally, the brain is broken down into three main parts, each of which has smaller portions responsible for specific bodily functions. They are the ...

▶ **Cerebrum.** When you think of the brain, this is the part that stands out. That's because it's the largest part, divided into two main hemispheres that are joined in the middle by a set of nerve fibers called the *corpus callosum*. Each hemisphere is made up of lobes that are responsible for specific functions:

▶ **Frontal lobes.** Control some voluntary actions, learned motor skills, and higher brain functions—language, thought, planning, etc.

▶ **Parietal lobes.** Process incoming stimuli, movement, perception, and language; performs calculations, spatial memories, and orientation.

▶ **Occipital lobes.** Process vision and visual memories, visual and spatial orientation.

▶ **Temporal lobes.** Control memory and emotions, short-term/long-term memories; process sound and vision.

- The outer layer of the cerebrum is called the *cerebral cortex* (commonly known as *gray matter*) and is the home of the most neurons in the nervous system. The layer underneath the cerebral cortex is made up of nerve fibers that act as a connection between the neurons in the cerebral cortex and the basal ganglia, thalamus, and hypothalamus. These are nerve centers in the brain that perform specific tasks:

- **Basal ganglia.** Helps control motor function.

- **Thalamus.** Routes sensation information to and from the cortex, so that you feel when something is hot or cold, etc.

- **Hypothalamus.** Regulates some involuntary functions, such as body temperature and appetite.

- Finally, we have the limbic system, which is a cluster of nerves located at the base of the cerebrum and connects the hypothalamus with the frontal lobes. The limbic system helps control emotion and involuntary functions.

NURSING NOTES

Ever hear someone say they're "left brained" or "right brained"? They're talking about which hemisphere of the cerebrum they favor. The right brain has the centers that are more artistic and intuitive. The left brain has the centers that are more analytical and logical.

- **Cerebellum.** This part of the brain is much smaller than the cerebrum and is the center of balance and coordination for the body. It's located just below the cerebrum, but above the brain stem.

- **Brain stem (medulla oblongata).** This is the part of the brain that connects to the spinal cord. It's responsible for consciousness and the body's vital functions: breathing, heartbeat, blood pressure, and swallowing.

All of these varied portions of the brain act as the center for the messages that are transmitted to the rest of the body. A message originates from the brain and is transmitted through the nerves to the spinal cord. This is a long, thick rope of nerves that route messages from the brain to the peripheral nervous system. Conversely, it takes messages that are transmitted from the body through the peripheral nervous system up to the brain.

Peripheral Nervous System

The peripheral nervous system (PNS) is basically the entire system of nerves that extend out from the spinal cord and into the rest of the body. The PNS contains two types of neurons:

- **Sensory neurons.** Brings information about a stimulus to the CNS.

- **Motor neurons.** Takes information from the CNS to muscles and glands that perform some kind of action.

The PNS is divided into two subsystems:

- **Somatic nervous system.** Neurons in this subsystem control the cranial and spinal nerves. This is also known as the *sensory-somatic nervous system* because it connects the CNS to the body's sensory organs, such as the ears, eyes, and mouth. They also carry sensory information from outside and within the body to the CNS for processing. It's through the somatic nervous system that the brain can regulate blood pressure, sense pain, or signal that you need to use the bathroom. Many of the messages carried to and from the brain through the somatic nervous system are voluntary commands, such as moving your hand or walking.

▸ **Autonomic nervous system.** This controls largely involuntary bodily functions, such as breathing and digestion. These neurons run from the CNS to various internal organs and systems. The autonomic nervous system is divided into two subsystems:

▸ **Sympathetic.** This system provides a response to stress, often referred to as *fight or flight*. When a stressor, such as a scare or sexual arousal, affects the body, the nerves in this system react by generating more energy, hormones, and efficient blood flow to vital organs to prepare your body to handle the stress. In a sympathetic response, adrenaline flows, your heart rate increases, your temperature goes up, and your respiration increases.

▸ **Parasympathetic.** This system contains nerves that send signals to the CNS to counter the sympathetic responses. It's responsible for calming bodily functions, slowing respiration and heart rate, resuming digestion, and normalizing other functions that are sped up during a sympathetic response.

Endocrine System

Your body's chemistry has to be carefully balanced at all times to maintain *homeostasis*. This is where the endocrine system comes in.

The endocrine system helps regulate the body's internal environment by controlling the amount of hormones that are secreted from the various glands in the body. Hormones are chemical messengers that tell different systems what they should be doing.

Endocrine System

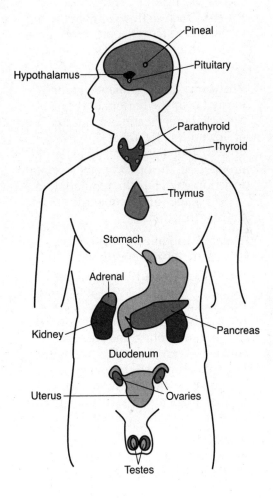

Here is a look at the different glands that make up the endocrine system:

▶ **Hypothalamus.** This is the largest endocrine gland in the brain and secretes human growth hormone (HGH), parathormone, oxytocin, and vasopressin. HGH regulates the growth of the body, and parathormone regulates the release of another hormone (thyroxine) from the thyroid. Oxytocin is important in facilitating and recovering from childbirth, as it affects contractions of the uterus. Vasopressin regulates how the kidneys absorb water from the blood.

▶ **Pineal.** This is a tiny gland at the top of the brain stem that produces melatonin, which regulates your sleeping patterns.

▶ **Pituitary.** This pea-shaped gland located near the bottom of the hypothalamus secretes a variety of hormones that affect skin tone, growth, blood pressure, breast milk production, the onset of labor, sexual function, metabolism, regulation of water balance and temperature, and thyroid function.

▶ **Thyroid and parathyroid.** These glands are located together around the outside of the throat. The thyroid secretes thyroxine and triiodothyronine, which help regulate the body's metabolism, growth, and sensitivity to other hormones. The parathyroid glands are a set of four glands located behind the thyroid glands. They secrete parathormone, which regulates calcium and phosphate concentrations in the blood and bones.

▶ **Adrenal.** These are located just above the kidneys and secrete fight-or-flight stress hormones:

epinephrine, norepinephrine, and cortisol. Epinephrine (also called *adrenaline*) facilitates a sympathetic response to a stressor (see the earlier discussion of the sympathetic nervous system). Norepinephrine counters this response by triggering the parasympathetic nervous system. Cortisol exerts some control over fats and carbohydrate metabolism, response to stress, and suppression of the immune system.

▶ **Pancreas.** The pancreas is located in front of and just below the stomach. It produces insulin and glucagon, hormones that control the regulation of glucose in the blood. Insulin causes levels of glucose in the blood to go down, while glucagon causes them to rise.

▶ **Ovaries.** These are important parts of the female reproductive system and also the endocrine system. Ovaries produce estrogen and progesterone, which contribute to the development of sexual organs and menstruation. Estrogen affects the development of secondary female characteristics, promotes growth of the reproductive organs, and helps preserve bone mass and elasticity within the body. Progesterone maintains the lining of the uterus (the endometrium) for pregnancy and regulates menstruation.

▶ **Testes.** These are part of the male reproductive system and the source of testosterone, the primary male sexual hormone. Testosterone is responsible for the development of secondary male sexual characteristics, libido, and sperm production.

Digestive System

The digestive system has a few jobs. First, it breaks down the food that you eat. Then, it processes the food into chemicals that the body can use. Finally, it filters out what's needed and what's not and then gets rid of the waste.

There are many different parts of the digestive system, also known as *the gastrointestinal (GI) system*. Take a look at the following diagram as we start our discussion of this complex system and follow the path of food through the upper and lower GI tracts.

Upper GI Tract

The digestive system begins in the mouth (oral cavity). As the teeth chew (masticate) a piece of food, saliva produced by the salivary glands mixes with the food and begins the chemical breakdown:

▸ **Salivary glands.** The submandibular glands are located under the lower jaw, while the sublingual are located on top of the submandibular glands and just under the tongue. The largest salivary gland is the parotid gland, which is located behind the throat.

> **NURSING NOTES**
>
> About 70 percent of saliva is produced by the submandibular glands.

▸ **Esophagus.** When food is soft enough to swallow, the tongue pushes it into the throat, where the epiglottis closes off the larynx and trachea so that the food is routed into the esophagus, the tube leading to the stomach. The esophagus is lined with muscles that expand and contract to keep the food moving, a process called *peristalsis*. At the bottom of the esophagus is a valve called the esophageal sphincter. Its job is to keep stomach content from backing up into the esophagus.

Digestive System

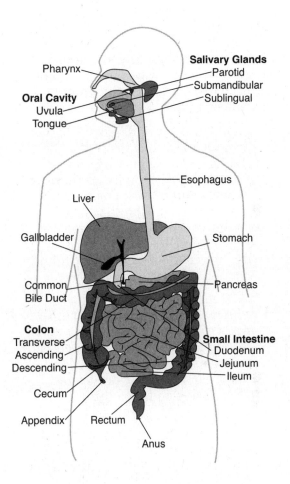

▸ **Stomach.** After the food enters the stomach, it is further digested by a rhythmic motion that grinds the contents of the stomach and mixes it with gastric juices. Hormones trigger the release of these juices by the lining of the stomach. Gastric juices consist primarily of mucus, hydrochloric acid, and pepsin, an enzyme that breaks down proteins. When these juices are mixed with food, a mixture called *chyme* is formed. This process not only prepares food to go into the lower GI tract, but also kills bacteria due to the high acid content of the stomach.

Lower GI Tract

The lower GI tract begins with the small intestine, which is broken up into several distinct parts: the duodenum, jejunum, ileum, liver, gallbladder, and colon.

▸ **Duodenum.** When the chyme in the stomach is of a consistency that the small intestine can manage, it passes through the pyloric sphincter (a valve at the bottom of the stomach that protects the small intestine from coming in contact with stomach contents) into the duodenum. It also prevents too much chyme from entering the lower GI tract at one time.

▸ When in the duodenum, the chyme mixes with juices from the liver, gallbladder, and pancreas, as well as enzymes secreted from the duodenum itself. Within the duodenum, fats, proteins, and carbohydrates (ones not already processed by saliva or the stomach) are broken down further by this mixture of juices so that the next part of the intestine can absorb the nutrients.

▸ **Jejunum and ileum.** After being further processed by the duodenum, the mixture of semidigested food is moved through the remainder of the duodenum, into the jejunum through the ileum by villi—thin fingerlike projections that line part of the duodenum and all of the jejunum and ileum. The villi not only move the

mixture through the small intestines, they also absorb nutrients through epithelial cells and convert them into forms that are moved into the blood and sent to the liver through the hepatic portal vein.

▸ **Liver and gallbladder.** The liver is a huge filter for the blood. Nutrient-rich blood from the small intestine travels to the liver, which basically sorts through the nutrients, breaking them down further into forms that can be used by the body and sending them where they need to go. The liver removes wastes, toxins, and bacteria that transferred into the bloodstream from the intestine. It also removes excess glucose from the blood and turns it into glycogen; then, it stores the glycogen and releases it as glucose into the blood as needed.

> **TEST TIP**
>
> Guess where about half of the body's cholesterol comes from? You got it: the liver. Keep that in mind on the test.

▸ The liver secretes bile as a waste product and stores it in the gallbladder. Bile contains salts and enzymes that help the body process fats and removes dead red blood cells and excess cholesterol from the body.

▸ **Colon.** When all of the processes of the small intestine are complete, what's left is a liquid chyme mixture that moves into the large intestine, or *colon*, to be processed as waste. The ileum connects to the large intestine at the cecum and has yet another valve that controls the flow from one side to the other. (The appendix hangs off of the bottom of the cecum. It's a fleshy protrusion shaped like an elongated teardrop that serves no known function in the body.)

- The chyme travels through the cecum and up the ascending colon, across the transverse colon, and finally down through the descending colon. While in these passages, water and salts are absorbed through the lining and what's left is processed by the more than 700 species of bacteria that live in the colon, such as E. coli, and compacted for excretion through the rectum and anus as feces.

- Intestinal bacteria are prokaryotic microorganisms that serve an important function in turning substances in the colon into vitamins needed by the body. For instance, vitamin K, B_{12}, thiamine, and riboflavin are all by-products of bacterial processing of chyme in the colon. These vitamins are absorbed by the blood and used to nourish the body.

Urinary System

The urinary system consists of the kidneys, bladder, and the tubes that connect them and lead out of the body. The system's function is to filter wastes, salts, and water out of the blood.

Here's a closer look at how the urinary system works:

- **Kidneys.** When we discussed the circulatory system earlier in this chapter, we talked about systemic circulation and how arterial blood went to the kidneys to be filtered. The aorta provides oxygen-rich blood to the renal arteries running into the kidneys.

- From there, the arteries branch off into between five and seven smaller arteries, and then again so that they lead through the interior of the kidney to the millions of nephrons. We call the nephrons the functional units of the kidney because it is here that filtration takes place. Each nephron has a glomerulus that removes excess fluid and wastes from the blood and turns them into urine.

Urinary System

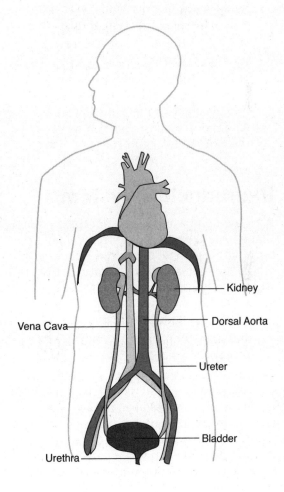

Kidney

Dorsal Aorta

Vena Cava

Ureter

Bladder

Urethra

- When this process is complete, the urine collects in the center of the kidney (the renal pelvis) and the filtered blood travels through a series of veins before going to the renal vein and up the inferior vena cava.

- **Ureters.** The urine in the renal pelvis empties into the ureters—long, thin tubes that connect the kidneys to the bladder.

- **Bladder.** This is where urine is stored. Kidneys produce urine; the ureters move it from the kidneys to the bladder; the bladder holds on to it. This is the only function of this organ.

- **Urethra.** This is the tube through which urine is released from the body. It is a short tube inside the body in a female. In a male, it runs the length of the penis and also serves as the exit point for semen.

Reproductive System

Both men and women have specific systems that enable them to reproduce. Women are born with a store of ova (often called *eggs*), which are special cells that contain all of the woman's genetic information. Men create sperm, millions of little cells that contain all of the man's genetic information.

Sperm are propelled by long, thin tails and released into a woman during sex. After they are released, the sperm swim through the woman's reproductive organs until they reach an egg that has been released. Then, the sperm try to break into the egg during a process called fertilization. Only one can make it through, and when it does, it sets off a whole chain reaction of cellular reproduction, which we discuss in Chapter 10.

Now that you have the condensed version of how humans reproduce, let's take a look at the components of both systems.

Male

Men have both internal and external organs that work together to produce, sustain, and release sperm in order to reproduce.

Male Reproductive System

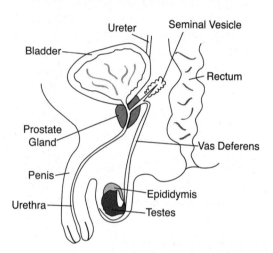

Here's a closer look at how the male reproductive organs work:

- **Testes.** These are two rounded structures that hang in the scrotum, between the legs and behind the penis. Each testis produces sperm, which are released into the epididymis until they are mature enough to fertilize an egg. The testes also produce testosterone, the primary sex hormone discussed in our section about the endocrine system.

- **Vas deferens.** When sperm is ready to be released, it travels up the vas deferens, two tubes that connect to the epididymis. The vas deferens brings the sperm to the connecting tubes of the seminal vesicle and prostate gland, which secrete fluid that makes up semen through the ejaculatory duct. The sperm are bathed and nourished in the semen as they make their way out of the male's body and into the female's.

▸ **Penis.** Blood flows to the penis during sexual arousal and stimulation, making the long cylindrical structure firm enough to enter the female body. The urethra runs through the center of the penis and attaches not only to the bladder, but also the ejaculatory duct. When a male reaches orgasm, semen is forcefully ejected from the ejaculatory duct, through the urethra, and out of the penis.

Female

The female reproductive system is a little more complex. Take a look at the following diagram to see the two main parts of the female reproductive system.

Here's a closer look at how these organs work and what happens as the body prepares for reproduction:

▸ **Ovaries.** These are where ova are created and stored. During fetal development, a female generates all of the eggs she will ever have. They are stored in the ovaries, two round sacs that protrude off of either side of the uterus. These eggs remain dormant until a woman enters puberty. Then one ova will begin a process of maturing every month.

Female Reproductive System

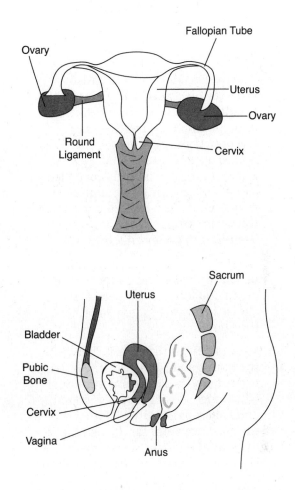

▸ The ovaries produce the female sexual hormones estrogen and progesterone, as well as a small amount of testosterone. Progesterone facilitates the development of the egg, which, when mature and ready to be fertilized, is then released through a follicle into the fallopian tube.

- **Fallopian tubes.** Because an egg can be released from either ovary, there are two tubes that connect the ovaries with the uterus. When an egg is released from the ovary, it travels into the fallopian tube, where it waits to be fertilized.

- **Uterus.** Each month, a release of progesterone causes the endometrial lining of the uterus to thicken in preparation for a fertilized egg (zygote). If an egg is not fertilized within a certain amount of time, it travels to the uterus and is expelled along with the lining through menstruation. If it is fertilized, the zygote travels to the uterus and implants itself in the endometrial lining.

- **Cervix.** This is the opening of the uterus located at the bottom of the organ and leads to the vagina. It closes during pregnancy to protect the uterus.

- **Vagina.** This is the passage between the uterus and cervix and the outside of the body. It is the canal through which menstrual tissue is excreted and babies pass during birth. It is also the entrance point for the penis during sexual intercourse. When a man ejaculates into the vagina, the sperm travel in semen through the vagina and cervix, into the uterus and up to the fallopian tubes. It is only in the fallopian tubes that an ovum can be fertilized.

Muscular System

So far, we've talked about what makes the body work, but not much about how it moves. We know that the nervous system controls movement through neurons. Now let's look at the actual muscles that perform that movement.

The muscular system is made up of three types of muscles:

- **Cardiac.** This is the type of muscle that makes up the heart. It is only found in this organ.

- **Smooth.** As the name suggests, this type of muscle is smooth in comparison to the striated muscle. Its cells are narrow and only have one nucleus. Smooth muscles perform involuntary movements, such as organ movements during digestion and the flexing of blood vessels in circulation.

- **Striated.** These are often called skeletal muscles because they are attached to the bones of the skeleton through tendons. They are made up of long, multinucleated fibers that give them the appearance of being striped. Striated muscles are used in voluntary movement, such as walking and talking. The following diagram shows the major striated muscle groups in the body.

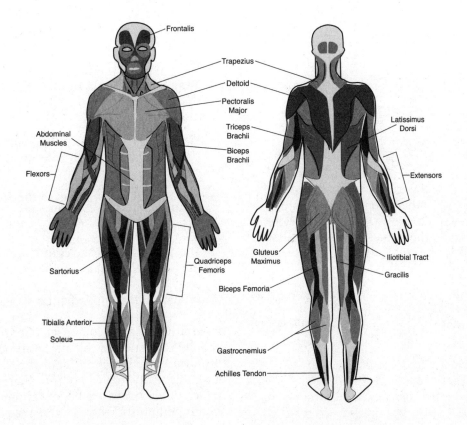

Muscles create movement by contracting and relaxing. They often work in pairs to create specific movements. For example, the quadriceps in the thigh contract to lift the leg up, causing the biceps femori (commonly known as the *hamstring*) on the back of the thigh to relax. When you put your leg down, the hamstring contracts and the quadriceps relax. This is a flexor/extensor relationship.

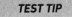

TEST TIP

Muscle cells need a lot of energy to function properly. They consume massive amounts of adenosine triphosphate (ATP), which we describe in Chapter 10, to react to neural signals to contract.

Skeletal System

Our discussion of human anatomy and physiology ends with the skeleton. You may think that the skeleton's only purpose is to provide structure for the body. However, it also feeds the blood supply, provides protection to vital organs (like the heart and lungs), stores minerals needed for proper function, and gives muscles something to hold on to.

On your exam, you are likely to come across names of different types of bones. The following diagram shows the major bones and their names. It's a good idea to memorize them.

Skeletal System

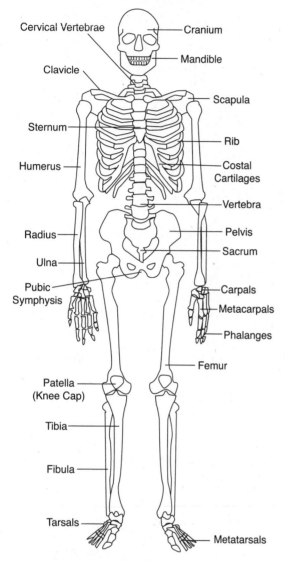

Cervical Vertebrae
Cranium
Mandible
Clavicle
Scapula
Sternum
Rib
Humerus
Costal Cartilages
Vertebra
Radius
Pelvis
Sacrum
Ulna
Pubic Symphysis
Carpals
Metacarpals
Phalanges
Femur
Patella (Knee Cap)
Tibia
Fibula
Tarsals
Metatarsals

Here are some interesting facts about the skeletal system:

▸ The adult body has 206 bones.

▸ Spinal bones are called vertebrae (singular is vertebra).

▸ The spine is divided into three sets of vertebrae: the top 7 are the cervical vertebrae; the middle 12 are the thoracic vertebrae; the lower 5 are the lumbar vertebrae.

▸ There are 18 ribs total, which join at the sternum in the front of the body and at the spine at the back of the body.

▸ Long bones (femur, humerus) in children have marrow that produces red blood cells.

▸ Flat bones (pelvis, scapula) in adults have marrow that produces red blood cells.

▸ The axial skeleton refers to the 28 bones that make up the skull and the 33 vertebrae.

▸ The appendicular skeleton refers to the bones that make up the rest of the body. If it's not a head or spinal bone, it's part of the appendicular skeleton.

Bones are primarily composed of hard mineral deposits, such as calcium. But though the surface of a bone may appear to be hard, it is really made of porous material. In fact, many bones are hollow and in their spongy center (marrow) produce red blood cells. Blood vessels can be found throughout bones, delivering nutrients that bones provide the body and taking away wastes.

NURSING NOTES

If a pregnant woman is not getting enough calcium from her diet, the body will take calcium from the bones to preserve the pregnancy.

Bones connect at joints through ligaments and are cushioned in the joint by cartilage. There are a few types of joints you should be familiar with:

▶ **Ball and socket.** These are joints like the hips and shoulders. The rounded top of a bone fits into the hollow of a socket to produce circular movement.

▶ **Hinge.** Like a door hinge, two bones connect in such a way that only an up-and-down or in-and-out movement is possible. Elbow and knee joints are hinge joints.

▶ **Sutures.** These are only found in the skull and connect the 28 bones that make up this part of the body. Sutures do not move in any way, they just connect one bone to another.

Practice Questions

For each of the following questions, choose the best answer.

1. What substance in blood carries oxygen to the cells?

   (A) neutrophills
   (B) lymphocytes
   (C) hemoglobin
   (D) monocytes

2. What organ produces insulin?

   (A) liver
   (B) gallbladder
   (C) pancreas
   (D) spleen

3. What structure of the male urinary system is common to the reproductive system?

   (A) ureter
   (B) bladder
   (C) urethra
   (D) epididymis

4. The functional unit of the kidney is/are the

   (A) renal artery.
   (B) nephron.
   (C) Bowman's capsule.
   (D) kidney receptors.

5. Urine is stored in the

   (A) kidney.
   (B) bladder.
   (C) ureter.
   (D) urethra.

6. In which structure is the ovum (egg) fertilized?

   (A) ovary
   (B) fallopian tube
   (C) uterus
   (D) endometrium

7. Upper respiratory structures

   (A) warm the air entering the nose.
   (B) filter the air entering the nose.
   (C) exchange carbon dioxide and oxygen gases.
   (D) A and B

8. The path of blood through the heart is

   (A) superior and inferior vena cava to the left atrium, left ventricle, pulmonary artery, lungs, pulmonary vein, right atrium, left atrium, aorta.
   (B) superior and inferior vena cava to the right atrium, right ventricle, pulmonary artery, lungs, pulmonary vein, left atrium, left ventricle, aorta.
   (C) superior and inferior vena cava to the right atrium, right ventricle, pulmonary vein, lungs, pulmonary artery, left atrium, left ventricle, aorta.
   (D) superior and inferior vena cava to the left atrium, left ventricle, pulmonary vein, lungs, pulmonary artery, right atrium, right ventricle, aorta.

9. During internal respiration, oxygen moves into the cells by

    (A) diffusion.

    (B) osmosis.

    (C) condensation.

    (D) equalization.

10. What structure prevents food from entering the larynx during swallowing?

    (A) uvula

    (B) tongue

    (C) epiglottis

    (D) soft palate

11. An accessory organ of digestion is the

    (A) esophagus.

    (B) liver.

    (C) large intestines.

    (D) rectum.

12. Which gland secretes saliva?

    (A) parotid

    (B) pituitary

    (C) adrenal

    (D) thyroid

13. The respiratory control center is located in which part of the brain?

    (A) cerebellum

    (B) parietal lobe

    (C) medulla oblongata

    (D) temporal lobe

14. The walls of veins

    (A) have the same elasticity as the walls of the arteries.

    (B) have more elasticity than the walls of the arteries.

    (C) pump under lower pressure than arteries.

    (D) have thicker walls than arteries.

15. All of the following statements about blood are true except:

    (A) Blood transports oxygen and nutrients to the body cells.

    (B) Blood carries carbon dioxide and waste materials from the body cells.

    (C) Blood is produced in the stem cells of the red bone marrow.

    (D) Leukocytes are not an element of blood.

Answers and Explanations

1. **C.** All of the others are types of white blood cells.

2. **C.** Insulin is one of several hormones the pancreas produces.

3. **C.** Answers A and B are part of the urinary system. Answer D is part of the reproductive system.

4. **B.** Nephrons are called the functional units of the kidney because it is here that filtration takes place. Each nephron has a glomerulus that removes excess fluid and wastes from the blood and turns them into urine.

5. **B.** Urine is made in the kidney. It travels through the ureter to reach the bladder, where it is stored and then gets released through the urethra.

6. **B.** While all of the other answers name parts of the female reproductive system, fertilization only takes place in the fallopian tubes.

7. **D.** The upper respiratory structure both warms and filters air entering the nose.

8. **B.** The path of blood is through the superior and inferior vena cava to the right atrium, right ventricle, pulmonary artery, lungs, pulmonary vein, left atrium, left ventricle, and aorta. Remember, arteries go away from the heart and veins go toward the heart.

9. **A.** Answers C and D do not describe movement of oxygen into cells. Answer B describes movement of water across a membrane from a hypertonic to a hypotonic (or vice versa) environment.

10. **C.** The epiglottis covers the opening of the trachea when you swallow to prevent food from being inhaled.

11. **B.** Food passes through each of the other organs mentioned, making them primary organs for digestion.

12. **A.** All of the other glands secrete hormones as part of the endocrine system.

13. **C.** This part of the brain is responsible for consciousness and the body's vital functions: breathing, heartbeat, blood pressure, and swallowing.

14. **C.** The walls of arteries are thicker than those of veins, and also contain more elastic fibers. Arteries are also under more pressure, since they receive blood pumped directly from the heart, which they then pass on through veins.

15. **D.** Leukocytes are white blood cells. All of the other statements are true.

The Right Chemistry

A good portion of the study of medicine is centered on chemistry. As you learned in Chapter 9, even the most basic unit of life—a cell—is made up of chemicals and subject to reactions that enable the cell to function properly. Now think of the entirety of the various organs and systems within the human body and how many chemical reactions take place within the cells that make them up. The number is astronomical.

It's no wonder that nursing schools want to evaluate your ability to know and understand basic concepts in chemistry before deciding whether to grant you entrance. Knowing the basic properties of certain chemicals, how they work together and against each other, what makes them up, and what laws govern them are all topics you can expect to cover during the pursuit of your nursing degree.

This chapter provides you with lots of basic high school–level chemistry concepts often found on nursing school entrance exams. This includes discussions about atoms, matter, chemical elements, reactions, solutions, equations, and more. At the end of this chapter, you'll find practice questions, answers, and explanations to help you better understand these concepts.

What to Expect

The subject of chemistry encompasses a variety of different topics: biochemistry, organic and inorganic chemistry, physical chemistry, theoretical chemistry, material chemistry, neurochemistry, nuclear chemistry, astrochemistry, and so on. No one book could possibly cover every single one of these.

The good news is that nursing school admissions committees only really want to see that you have a general knowledge and understanding of basic chemical principles and applications at the high school level. Chances are if you are applying to a nursing program, you've already graduated high school. And having graduated high school, you most likely have taken a chemistry class. So the topics and information that follow should be relatively familiar.

If for some reason you skipped chemistry in high school, the information we've provided should be simple and clear enough for you to understand and help prepare you for the types of questions you may see on your nursing school entrance exam.

[
CODE RED!

Make sure that it is absolutely necessary for you to take the chemistry section of your entrance exam. Many nursing schools only require the math and verbal sections; the subject-specific sections may not be required.
]

Keep in mind that every exam is different and that what you study here may or may not actually be on the test you take. Your best bet is to brush up on the concepts you are familiar with and get a strong understanding of those areas. After you've done that, move on to the topics that are less familiar and get as much of a grasp on them as you can before you take your exam.

To start you off, here's a list of chemistry vocabulary that anyone taking an entrance exam for a nursing program should know.

Basic Chemistry Vocabulary

Term	Definition
Atom	The basic unit of matter. It is also the smallest component of an element that retains all of the element's chemical properties. An atom is electrically neutral, though its nucleus contains at least one proton and neutron, and at least one electron outside of the nucleus. The lone exception to this rule is elemental hydrogen, H, which in its natural form contains no neutrons.
Chemical Property	How a substance reacts when mixed with other substances.
Compound	Atoms of two or more different elements that are combined in a specific proportion defined by mass. Compounds are joined by chemical bonds and the atoms within a compound can't be physically separated. Water is a compound of hydrogen and oxygen.
Electron	A particle that circles an atom's nucleus and has a negative charge. An electron's mass is about $\frac{1}{1,837}$ of a neutron or a proton.
Element	A pure substance that consists of only one type of atom and can't be broken down into smaller particles by chemical means. Hydrogen and oxygen are elements.
Ion	An atom that has an electrical charge due to the addition or subtraction of electrons.
Isotope	Two atoms of the same element that contain different numbers of neutrons.

Term	Definition
Mass	The amount of matter an object has. Measured in grams or kilograms.
Matter	Anything that occupies space and has mass.
Molecule	A combination of two or more atoms. These atoms can be from either the same or different elements.
Neutron	A particle in the nucleus of an atom that has a neutral electrical charge and a mass of about 1 *atomic mass unit* (*amu*).
Physical property	A property that can be measured or quantified through physical means.
Proton	A particle within the nucleus of an atom that has a positive electrical charge and a mass of about 1 amu.

> **DEFINITION**
>
> **Atomic mass unit (amu)** is the standard unit of measure for an atom. It equals about the mass of one proton.

Matter

Any discussion about chemistry has to begin with matter, which is defined as anything that takes up space and has mass. That pretty much encompasses everything in the universe—pretty simple, right?

Well, not so much. Any type of matter—whether they are simple atoms or entire human beings—is composed of various things. Chemistry is a science that looks at what makes up matter, how those components of matter behave, and how they can be changed. Now, for some specifics.

Breakdown of Matter

Atoms are the basic units of matter and chemical elements are pure substances made up of a single type of atom with specific properties. When elements are changed through either *chemical change* or *physical change,* they take on different properties and behaviors.

> **DEFINITION**
>
> **Chemical change** happens when a substance is converted into something else completely. (Your body turns a banana into glucose during digestion.)
> **Physical change** happens when a substance converts from one form of matter to another, but its chemical composition stays the same. (Your ice cream melts.)

Matter is generally classified into three states. Though you may find that some sources point to five states of matter, the ones most relevant to your exam are ...

▸ **Solid.** Atoms in this state are very close together (dense), so much so that the substance has a definite shape and volume. A major force is needed to change the shape of a solid.

▸ **Liquid.** Atoms in this state are not as closely bonded and tend to move so that a liquid takes the shape of whatever is containing it. However, it does have a measurable volume. Heat has the greatest effect of change on a liquid.

▸ **Gas.** Atoms in this state are very loosely bonded and will fill the entirety of any container that holds it (think of helium inside a balloon).

Gases do not take on any form of their own, nor do they have any measurable volume.

One state of matter can often be converted into another. Think of the example before about the frozen ice cream (a solid) melting into a liquid. This happens when heat is added to the atoms and molecules that make up that solid bit of ice cream matter—we all know that. So how does that work exactly?

Conversion of Matter

The atoms in any state of matter are constantly moving and therefore have kinetic energy, and as a result, heat. In our example of ice cream, we have a solid that is relatively soft, indicating that the atoms are packed closely together, but not as tightly as something more dense and rigid, such as stone. The atoms have room to move and create enough heat to maintain that soft-frozen state.

When you add heat (which is essentially energy) to the atoms and molecules that make up the ice cream, they begin to move more quickly, which weakens the bonds holding them together. Those bonds won't break, but become like elastic bands connecting the atoms instead of the plastic straws they were in solid form. This change in how the atoms are connected results in greater movement between atoms and molecules and creates the liquid form you are familiar with.

When matter goes from a liquid to a gas state, there needs to be enough heat to completely break the bonds holding the atoms together, resulting in a state where atoms are just floating around and bumping into each other. Think about water. To turn water from a liquid to a gas, you must heat it until it boils, which happens at 100°C or 212°F. This is the temperature at which water changes from liquid to gas.

It's important to note that no matter what state of matter is changing, there is a period where the temperature remains the same, even though more heat is applied. This is called *dynamic equilibrium*. During this time, two states of matter exist at the same time while the excess energy is being used to change the phase of matter from one state to another.

Changes in states of matter can be endothermic (achieved by adding energy) or exothermic (achieved by taking energy away). Some changes you should know:

▸ **Liquid to gas:** Endothermic change called *vaporization*.

▸ **Liquid to solid:** Exothermic change called *freezing*.

▸ **Gas to liquid:** Exothermic change called *condensation*.

▸ **Gas to solid:** Exothermic change called *deposition*.

▸ **Solid to liquid:** Endothermic change called *melting*.

▸ **Solid to gas:** Endothermic change called *sublimation*.

Composition of Matter

The following diagram shows the two main divisions of matter: substances and mixtures.

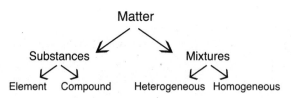

Substances, or pure substances, are always *homogeneous* and have specific chemical compositions that can't be changed. Pure substances are found in the form of elements and compounds, which we discuss later in this chapter.

> **DEFINITION**
>
> **Homogeneous** refers to something that has a uniform composition. Think of the milk in your refrigerator. If milk that comes straight from a cow is allowed to sit, a layer of high-fat cream will rise to the top. If that milk is homogenized, it is processed so that the cream remains an indistinguishable part of the milk. This results in the uniformly smooth liquid you put on your cereal in the morning.

Mixtures refer to matter that can be separated into two or more substances without a chemical reaction. They can be either homogeneous or heterogeneous:

▸ **Homogeneous mixture (also called a *solution*).** As the definition says, this is a blending of substances that results in a uniform type of matter. The substances retain their specific chemical properties (not necessarily the physical), but can be physically separated. The air we breathe is a homogeneous mixture because it is made up of different gases that make one uniform substance.

▸ **Heterogeneous mixture.** This is a mixture of two or more substances that retain all of their distinct physical and chemical properties. Think of a bottle of Italian salad dressing, which has layers of oil, vinegar, water, and seasoning. This is why we shake it right before adding it to our salad bowl.

Density

Matter is defined in terms of space and measured in terms of mass, but not in terms of how much space that substance occupies. For example, there is a big difference between a gram of aluminum and a gram of lead. To reach that gram of mass, you would need a lot more space for a gram of aluminum (the light metal your soda cans are made of) than you would a gram of lead. This is because the density of aluminum (about 2.706 g/cm³) is much less than that of lead (about 11.3437 g/cm³).

Likewise, you've probably heard the trick question, "Which weighs more, a pound of lead or a pound of feathers?" Of course, you know they both weigh exactly the same, since a pound is a pound (is a pound …). However, what this little riddle illustrates is that it's going to take a lot more feathers, space-wise, to weigh the same as that pound of lead. Again, this is because feathers as a material are far less dense than the metal.

To calculate the density of a substance, use the following formula: $d = \frac{m}{V}$. Here, density (d) is equal to mass (m) divided by the volume (V) of the containing structure. The standard unit of measure for density is kilogram per cubic meter (kg/m³).

Atoms

Now that we know a little bit about matter, we can start to look into what makes matter possible: the atom. In 1808, British scientist Jonathan Dalton defined the four main concepts upon which modern atomic theory is based:

1. All matter is composed of atoms. During Dalton's time it was thought that atoms were indivisible; we know now that they can be divided through nuclear fission.

2. All atoms of a given element are identical, but atoms of different elements are not. For example, all oxygen atoms are identical to each other, but hydrogen atoms are not identical to oxygen atoms; they are identical to other hydrogen atoms.

3. In chemical reactions, atoms are combined, not destroyed.

4. Compounds are formed as a result of elements reacting with each other, in prescribed whole-number ratios.

> **CODE RED!**
>
> These are important basic concepts to understand when talking about atoms. Memorize them.

Subatomic Particles

We know that pure substances are classified as elements and compounds. An element is a pure substance made up of only one type of atom that has specific properties. These properties depend on the particles that make up the atom, more specifically called subatomic particles. Take a look at the following diagram to get a better idea:

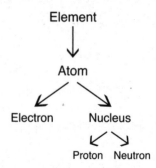

As you can see, an atom of a given element is first made up of electrons and a nucleus. Inside the nucleus are protons and neutrons. Let's explore each of these:

▶ **Nucleus.** As with the cells discussed in Chapters 9 and 10, the nucleus is of great importance. It is the dense portion of the atom and holds all of the protons and neutrons, which make up the majority of the atom's mass.

▶ **Electron.** Electrons carry a negative charge and revolve around the outside of the nucleus, forming "clouds" called *orbitals*. Orbitals are made up of empty space and contain only electrons, which account for the remainder of the atom's mass. An electron's contribution to an atom's mass is negligible, about $\frac{1}{1,837}$ of a neutron's or proton's mass.

▶ **Proton.** Protons are located inside the nucleus of an atom. They carry a positive electric charge and have a mass of about 1 amu. Atoms are electrically neutral, so the number of protons matches the number of electrons in order to balance out the charge created by both.

▸ **Neutron.** Neutrons do not carry any electrical charge and reside with protons in an atom's nucleus. The mass of a neutron is approximately equal to that of a proton.

Even though atoms in their natural form are electrically neutral, they often gain or lose electrons in an effort to become more stable, like those of inert gases. When this happens, the atom becomes an ion. More specifically, if the resulting charge is positive, the atom is a cation; if the resulting charge is negative, it is an anion.

You can easily spot the chemical symbol for an ion: a + or – sign is added to the element symbol as a superscript. For example, O^+ indicates one oxygen ion with a positive charge, meaning one electron was taken away from the atom. H^{-2} indicates a negative hydrogen ion that has had two electrons added.

Working with Subatomic Particles

There are a few things you can do with this information. First, you can find the atomic number and mass number of an element:

▸ **Atomic number (Z).** This is the number of protons (and thus also electrons) an electrically-neutral atom has. Atomic number for each element can be found on the Periodic Table of Elements, which is shown later in this chapter. It is denoted by the letter Z. Going back to Dalton's theory, all atoms of a given element will have the same number of protons and thus the same atomic number. This makes atomic number a good way to identify an element.

▸ **Mass number (A).** This is the total number of protons and neutrons (which together are called nucleons) in an atom. You can use the mass number of an element (which you can figure out based on the atomic mass numbers listed on the Periodic Table of Elements as well) to calculate the number of neutrons.

▸ Take a look at how this is done for an atom of argon (Ar), which has an atomic number of 18 and a mass number of 40 (we get this number by rounding the atomic mass for the element listed on the table, which is 39.948, to the nearest whole number). Subtract the atomic number from the mass number and you have the number of neutrons:

▸ 40 (total number of nucleons) – 18 (atomic number/number of protons) = 22 neutrons

▸ **Atomic weight (also called atomic mass).** This is not the same as a mass number. All elements have *isotopes*, and thus slightly different masses. What atomic weight measures is a weighted average of the masses of all of the known isotopes an element has based on each isotope's relative abundance in the natural world.

An **isotope** refers to when there are two or more atoms of the same element that contain different numbers of neutrons, which affects its mass. Because they retain the same number of protons (and thus the same atomic number), isotopes are still technically atoms of that element. Hydrogen has three known isotopes: protium (1 proton, 0 neutrons), deuterium (1 proton, 1 neutron), and tritium (1 proton, 2 neutrons).

This results in a whole number with a decimal, and it's this value that's listed on the Periodic Table. For example, krypton (Kr) has an atomic weight of 83.80, which takes into consideration the masses of all its 31 known isotopes. Its mass number is 84, the nearest whole number.

Elements

Earlier in the chapter, we talked about how matter is split into two main divisions: pure substances and mixtures. Pure substances are then further divided into elements and compounds.

Elements are substances that are made up of a single atom with specific properties that can't be chemically broken down into simpler parts. There are currently 118 known elements that are listed, detailed, and categorized on the Periodic Table.

In science, elements are described in specific terms, which you should be aware of:

▸ **Chemical symbol.** This is the scientific abbreviation for the name of the element. You'll find this in the middle of the box. Some letter combinations will make sense based on the element name (H = hydrogen; O = oxygen). Others, not so much (Au = gold; Sn = tin).

▸ **Superscripts.** These are notations that appear next to and above a chemical symbol. What those notations are and what they represent will tell you more about the element you're dealing with.

▸ **Before the symbol.** This indicates the total number of nucleons in an atom (i.e., protons and neutrons in the nucleus). You'll see this with isotopes because the number of nucleons will be different than in a regular atom of that element. Take the hydrogen example from the previous section. A single atom of hydrogen would be written as H. An atom of tritium would be ^3H, indicating that this isotope has two neutrons and one proton. Sometimes you will also see this after the symbol as well.

▸ **After the symbol.** This indicates a positive or negative charge for an ion, and the number of electrons that ion has. For example, N^{+2} indicates cation of nitrogen that has had two electrons taken away, giving it a positive charge (+2).

▸ **Subscripts.** These are notations that appear next to and below a chemical symbol. The most common type of subscript will tell you how many atoms of an element are present. The chemical formula for a molecule of water is H_2O. The $_2$ tells us that this molecule is made up of two atoms of hydrogen and one atom of oxygen. When there is no subscript present, you assume only one atom.

The Periodic Table

There have been various versions of the Periodic Table of Elements through the years. The Periodic Table on the following page includes both traditional and modern notations, because most exams you will take probably won't be up to speed on the most recent developments.

After looking at the Periodic Table we provide, you may ask yourself, "How am I supposed to read this?" It's easier than you think. First, each column is known as a group (or family) and generally lists elements that have similar chemical and physical properties. These groups include, starting from the far left column of the table:

▶ Hydrogen (stands as its own group)

▶ Alkali metals (Column 1 not including hydrogen)

▶ Alkaline Earth metals (Column 2)

▶ Transition metals (Columns 3–12)

▶ Borons (Column 13)

▶ Carbons (Column 14)

▶ Nitrogens (Column 15)

▶ Oxygens (Column 16)

▶ Halogens (Column 17)

▶ Noble gases (Column 18)

You may have also noticed that there are both Roman numerals and regular numbers at the top of each group. The Roman numeral notations are the more traditional group assignments, while the numbers represent the modern group assignments. Whichever one you choose to look at, these notations will help you determine the charge an atom of an element in that group will have as an ion in a solution or in a compound. The easiest way to do that is to remember a few things:

▶ Columns 1–8 have positive charges that correspond to the column number. Example: Elements in Column 1 will acquire a +1 charge. Elements in Column 2 will take on a +2 charge.

▶ To figure out the charges of elements in Columns 9–17, subtract 18 from the column number. Example: Elements in Column 9 will acquire a charge of –9 because 9 – 18 = –9. Elements in Column 10 take on a charge of –8 because 10 – 18 = –8.

▶ Elements in Column 18 are noble gases, which are inert and have a neutral charge.

Second, each row is known as a period. The elements in a row don't really have much in common other than their electron configurations, which is the number of electron orbitals (distinct clouds around a nucleus where the atom's electrons are most likely to be found most often) they have, and how many electrons are located in each orbital. The number of the period corresponds to the number of orbitals each element in the period has.

For example, hydrogen and helium are in the first period. They each have one orbital that holds their electrons. Lithium, beryllium, boron, carbon, nitrogen, oxygen, fluorine, and neon are in the second period and each has two orbitals that contain the atom's electrons. The electrons on the outermost orbit are called *valence electrons*.

Periodic Table of the Elements

Group	1 IA 1A	2 IIA 2A	3 IIIB 3B	4 IVB 4B	5 VB 5B	6 VIB 6B	7 VIIB 7B	8	9 VIII 8	10	11 IB 1B	12 IIB 2B	13 IIIA 3A	14 IVA 4A	15 VA 5A	16 VIA 6A	17 VIIA 7A	18 VIIIA 8A
Period 1	hydrogen 1 H 1.008																	helium 2 He 4.003
2	lithium 3 Li 6.941	beryllium 4 Be 9.012											boron 5 B 10.81	carbon 6 C 12.01	nitrogen 7 N 14.01	oxygen 8 O 16.00	fluorine 9 F 19.00	neon 10 Ne 20.18
3	sodium 11 Na 22.99	magnesium 12 Mg 24.31											aluminium 13 Al 26.98	silicon 14 Si 28.09	phosphorus 15 P 30.97	sulfur 16 S 32.07	chlorine 17 Cl 35.45	argon 18 Ar 39.95
4	potassium 19 K 39.10	calcium 20 Ca 40.08	scandium 21 Sc 44.956	titanium 22 Ti 47.88	vanadium 23 V 50.94	chromium 24 Cr 52.00	manganese 25 Mn 54.94	iron 26 Fe 55.85	cobalt 27 Co 58.93	nickel 28 Ni 58.69	copper 29 Cu 63.55	zinc 30 Zn 65.39	gallium 31 Ga 69.72	germanium 32 Ge 72.59	arsenic 33 As 74.92	selenium 34 Se 78.96	bromine 35 Br 79.90	krypton 36 Kr 83.80
5	rubidium 37 Rb 85.47	strontium 38 Sr 87.62	yttrium 39 Y 88.906	zirconium 40 Zr 91.22	niobium 41 Nb 92.91	molybdenum 42 Mo 95.94	technetium 43 Tc [98]	ruthenium 44 Ru 101.1	rhodium 45 Rh 102.9	palladium 46 Pd 106.4	silver 47 Ag 107.9	cadmium 48 Cd 112.4	indium 49 In 114.8	tin 50 Sn 118.7	antimony 51 Sb 121.8	tellurium 52 Te 127.6	iodine 53 I 126.9	xenon 54 Xe 131.3
6	caesium 55 Cs 132.9	barium 56 Ba 137.3	lanthanum 57 La *138.9	hafnium 72 Hf 178.5	tantalum 73 Ta 180.9	tungsten 74 W 183.9	rhenium 75 Re 186.2	osmium 76 Os 190.2	iridium 77 Ir 192.2	platinum 78 Pt 195.1	gold 79 Au 197.0	mercury 80 Hg 200.5	thallium 81 Tl 204.4	lead 82 Pb 207.2	bismuth 83 Bi 209.0	polonium 84 Po [210]	astatine 85 At [210]	radon 86 Rn [222]
7	francium 87 Fr [223]	radium 88 Ra [226.0254]	actinium 89 Ac ~[227]	rutherfordium 104 Rf [257]	dubnium 105 Db [260]	seaborgium 106 Sg [263]	bohrium 107 Bh [262]	hassium 108 Hs [265]	meitnerium 109 Mt [266]	darmstadtium 110 Ds [269]	Roentgenium 111 Rg [272]	Copernigium 112 Cn [277]	ununtrium 113 Uut [?]	ununquadium 114 Uuq [285]	ununpentium 115 Uup [?]	ununhexium 116 Uuh [289]	ununseptium 117 Uus [?]	ununoctium 118 Uuo [?]

*Lanthanide series

cerium 58 Ce 140.1	praseodymium 59 Pr 140.9	neodymium 60 Nd 144.2	promethium 61 Pm [147]	samarium 62 Sm 150.4	europium 63 Eu 152	gadolinium 64 Gd 157.3	terbium 65 Tb 158.9	dysprosium 66 Dy 162.5	holmium 67 Ho 164.9	erbium 68 Er 167.3	thulium 69 Tm 168.9	ytterbium 70 Yb 173.0	lutetium 71 Lu 175.0

~Actinide series

thorium 90 Th 232.0	protactinium 91 Pa 231	uranium 92 U 238	neptunium 93 Np 237	plutonium 94 Pu 242	americium 95 Am [243]	curium 96 Cm [247]	berkelium 97 Bk [247]	californium 98 Cf [249]	einsteinium 99 Es [254]	fermium 100 Fm [253]	mendelevium 101 Md [256]	nobelium 102 No [254]	lawrencium 103 Lr [257]

Within these groups and periods, you have boxes, each of which contains a single element and the following information:

▶ **Atomic number.** This is the number at the top of the box. It serves as a main identifier for each element. Elements are listed in order of atomic number. The atomic number of each element equals the number of protons in one atom of that element. It also equals the number of electrons, because they have to balance each other out in order for the electrical charge of the atom to be neutral.

▶ **Atomic weight.** This is the number at the bottom of the box and accounts for the average mass of all of the element's known isotopes.

TEST TIP

If you want to get more in depth with your study of elements and the Periodic Table, Jefferson Lab has a great interactive page at education.jlab.org/itselemental/.

All of the elements on the Periodic Table are further broken down into three main categories based on their physical and chemical properties:

▶ **Metals.** There are more metal elements than any other element on the Periodic Table. They are defined by the following properties:

▶ Takes either solid or liquid form

▶ Conducts heat and electricity easily

▶ Can be shaped and thinned out through physical means

▶ Shiny, some kind of luster is usually present

▶ Corrodes when comes in contact with water

▶ There are fewer nonmetals and metalloids, so we'll list those and just say that if the element you're dealing with isn't on those lists, it's a metal.

▶ **Metalloids.** These elements are neither metals nor nonmetals. They're a substance in between that have some properties of both:

▶ Solid

▶ May be shiny or dull

▶ Does not conduct heat or electricity as well as metals, but better than nonmetals do

▶ Can be shaped and thinned out through physical means

▶ Metalloids are boron (B), silicon (Si), germanium (Ge), arsenic (As), antimony (Sb), tellurium (Te), polonium (Po), and astatine (At).

▶ **Nonmetals.** These are almost the complete opposite of metals. In fact many nonmetals are gases! Properties include:

▶ Bad conductor of heat and electricity

▶ Can't be shaped and thinned out through physical means (if you try this on a solid nonmetal, it will most likely break apart)

▶ Dull, no luster like metals

▶ Are often gases in their natural state

▶ Nonmetals include hydrogen (H), carbon (C), nitrogen (N), oxygen (O), phosphorus (P), sulfur (S), selenium (Se), and the noble gases helium (He), neon (Ne), argon (Ar), krypton (Kr), xenon (Xe), and radon (Rn).

Compounds

When one or more elements chemically bond together in a fixed ratio, a compound is formed. Unlike with elements, compounds can be broken down into simpler atoms through chemical means.

Compounds are described by molecular formulas, which show the atoms that are present in the compound, in what percent compositions, and sometimes in what form. For example, the molecular formula for glucose is $C_6H_{12}O_6$(aq), which means that one molecule of glucose has 6 carbon atoms, 12 hydrogen atoms, and 6 oxygen atoms that are bonded in some way. The (aq) notation after the formula tells us that this molecule is in an aqueous solution. Other such notations you may see are (g) for gas, (s) for solid, and (l) for liquid.

Now comes the fun part: playing with these molecular formulas to figure out specific relationships.

Molecular Mass

When you are asked to find the molecular mass or weight of a compound, you're calculating the sum of the atomic weights of the atoms in the molecules that form these compounds. You do this by calculating the mass of the individual elements that make up the molecule, and adding the amounts together. Let's try it with our molecule of glucose: $C_6H_{12}O_6$.

1. Find the atomic weight of each element and multiply by the number of atoms present:

   C = 12 amu, $12 \times 6 = 72$ amu

   H = 1 amu, $1 \times 12 = 12$ amu

   O = 16 amu, $16 \times 6 = 96$ amu

2. Now add the total masses of each element together: $72 + 12 + 96 = 180$ amu. One molecule of glucose has a molecular mass of 180 amu.

Moles

You've just learned how to calculate the mass of a molecule or chemical formula in amu. But what do you do if you're asked what the weight of a molecule is in grams? Some conversion has to happen here, and that's where the mole comes in.

A mole is actually a pretty simple concept to understand, but is often explained in very complex terms. Basically, a mole is another way of representing what's called Avogadro's number: 6.022×10^{23}. For the purposes of your nursing school entrance exam, you will not need to calculate that number.

All you really need to understand is how moles work in relation to elements and grams: A mole of one atom of an element is equal to that element's atomic weight and the element's mass in grams.

Let's see how this can be applied:

> If you have 4 moles of ^{35}Cl, how many grams of chlorine do you have?

1. ^{35}Cl tells us that we are dealing with an isotope of chlorine that has an atomic weight of 35. The Periodic Table lists the atomic weight for chlorine as 35.453, so if the example had just said Cl, we could find the atomic weight by rounding to the nearest whole number.

2. Now that we've determined the atomic weight, we know that 1 mole of Cl = 35 amu. In turn, 1 mole of Cl = 35 g.

3. Multiply 35 by 4 (the number of atoms you're dealing with) to find out how many amu are in 4 moles of chlorine: $35 \times 4 = 140$ amu.

4. Because 1 mole of ^{35}Cl = 35 g, 4 moles of ^{35}Cl = 140 g.

Bonds

We've talked about bonds among atoms throughout this chapter. What we're talking about is the way that atoms stick together to form compounds and molecules. Here are a few things to understand before we jump into our discussion:

- Positive and negative charges are attracted to each other. That's where the whole "opposites attract" saying comes from. So atoms that are negatively charged are attracted to those that are positively charged.

- Atoms can turn into ions only by gaining or losing electrons. The number of protons in an atom remains constant.

- In our discussion of the Periodic Table, we talked about valence electrons. These are electrons on the outermost orbital of an atom. The more orbitals an atom has, the farther removed the valence electrons are from the atom's protons. The farther away an electron is from its protons, the less attraction those protons have on it, and the easier it is for those valence electrons to leave its atom.

- You can tell how many valence electrons an element has based on its position on the Periodic Table. Those in the first column have 1; the second column has 2. The last six columns have them in ascending order: 3, 4, 5, 6, 7, and 8 in the last column. The columns in between have variable valences.

- Atoms are constantly trying to become more stable by trying to get eight electrons in their outer orbital. This is called the *octet rule*. On the Periodic Table, the elements on the left (the alkali metals) are much less stable than the elements on the right (the halogens). The final family of elements is the noble gases, which are the most stable elements, inert, and have eight electrons in their outer orbital.

NURSING NOTES

Think about electron valences this way. Noble gases have the most stable electronic configurations. The elements with the lowest number of valence electrons only need to lose that small number in order to reach their most stable state (the octet), so they lose electrons easily. Elements closest to the noble gases only need to gain a small number of electrons to reach that more stable octet, so they take on electrons more readily.

Now that you have some understanding of the electron behavior of atoms, let's talk bonds:

▸ **Ionic bonds.** These are formed when an atom loses electrons that are then picked up by another atom. The result is that one atom takes on a negative charge, while the other takes on a positive charge. The atoms are then attracted to each other because they are now ions of opposing charges.

▸ Sodium chloride (table salt) is a good example of this. The molecular formula for table salt is NaCl. Na gives up electrons easily. When it comes in contact with Cl, which takes electrons easily, the Na atom loses an electron and takes on a positive charge. The Cl atom picks up that electron and takes on a negative charge. As a result, the two become attracted to each other and bond.

▸ **Covalent bonds.** When two atoms of similar electron configuration come in contact with each other, they can form a bond by sharing electrons equally. For example, if you put two atoms of oxygen together, each of which has six valence electrons, a bond will form where the atoms share two electrons to become a more stable compound: O_2. Both atoms in the compound now take on the properties of an oxygen atom that has eight electrons.

The kind of bond we just described is known as a nonpolar covalent bond. This just means that the bond did not create any change to the charge of the atoms. This is not always the case with covalent bonds, however.

Say you join an atom of oxygen with two atoms of hydrogen. We know that O has six valence electrons, and H has one (because there's only one electron for hydrogen). When O and two H atoms come in contact with each other, they start to share electrons and bond; one hydrogen atom on either side of the oxygen atom. The O uses the two H electrons to make eight valence electrons.

The two H atoms, by each sharing an electron from the O atom, attain their most stable state as well. It's important to remember that the most stable state for a hydrogen atom has two valence electrons. The element hydrogen is the lone exception to the octet rule.

The difference is that these electrons are not being shared equally. The H electrons are closer to the O atom than the O electrons are to the H atom. This results in a polar bond, in which the H_2O molecule has a slight positive charge closer to the hydrogen ends of the molecule and a slight negative charge at the oxygen end.

Reactions

When you bring together different types of chemicals, they can react and form different compounds. These are reactions, and in chemistry are represented by equations with an arrow, such as: $H_2 + O \rightarrow H_2O$.

In this equation, the symbols to the left of the arrow are called reactants. Two atoms of hydrogen are added to one atom of oxygen. The arrow acts as kind of an equal sign pointing to the resulting product of the reaction, which in this case is water (H_2O).

There are a few types of reactions you should be aware of for your nursing school entrance exam:

▸ **Synthesis.** These are also known as combination reactions because that's exactly what they do, combine two reactants that break the existing chemical bonds and form new ones. The previous example of a reaction is a synthesis reaction.

▶ **Decomposition.** This is the opposite of a synthesis reaction. Instead of combining reactants to create a new product, you are taking a single reactant and breaking it down into simpler parts through some infusion of energy, usually heat:

▶ $6NaHCO_3 \rightarrow 3Na_2CO_3 + 3H_2O + 3CO_2$

▶ What this equation tells us is that sodium bicarbonate can be broken down into three compounds: sodium carbonate, water, and carbon dioxide. This happens when you heat sodium bicarbonate.

▶ **Single displacement.** In this type of reaction, an element reacts with a compound and replaces an element in the compound. In the following equation, you see that when two atoms of aluminum in solid form are added to the compound Fe_2O_3 in a solution, the aluminum replaces the iron in the compound, leaving the iron on its own:

▶ $2Al(s) + Fe_2O_3(aq) \rightarrow Al_2O_3(aq) + 2Fe(s)$

▶ **Double displacement.** When ionic compounds are added to an aqueous solution, each pair of elements in the compounds separate to become cations and anions. Within the solution, new ionic bonds are formed between ions of opposite charge, resulting in a swap of ions, when comparing the compounds that appear in the products and reactants:

▶ $NaCl(aq) + KNO_3(aq) \rightarrow KCl(aq) + NaNO_3(aq)$

▶ In the previous reaction, each compound would break down into the following ions: Na^+ Cl^- K^+ NO_3^-. Then the ions with an opposite charge form a bond: $K^+Cl^- + Na^+NO_3^-$. The charges balance each other out and the new compounds are neutral. This is called a neutralization reaction.

▶ A special type of double displacement reaction takes place when the compounds you're working with are acids and bases. We go into this in depth in the Acids and Bases section later in this chapter.

▶ **Combustion.** This is the reaction a compound has when combined with elemental oxygen, usually to form water and carbon dioxide. Combustion reactions are exothermic (produce heat):

▶ $CH_3OH + O_2 \rightarrow CO_2 + 2H_2O + heat$

▶ This equation shows how methanol (rubbing alcohol) reacts when it encounters elemental oxygen; water, carbon dioxide, and heat are formed.

Reaction Rates

Reactions have to meet two conditions in order to happen. First, the reactants have to come in contact with each other in some way. Second, there has to be enough energy present when they come in contact with each other for that contact to result in the breaking down of old bonds and the creation of new ones. Every reaction has a different amount of energy needed for this to happen. We call this *activation energy*.

You can manipulate both these conditions in order to increase or decrease the speed at which a reaction occurs:

▶ **Heat.** When you add heat to a reactant, you add energy. Add more energy and you increase the movement of the atoms in your reactants and increase the probability that they will meet, causing your reaction.

▸ **Surface area.** This increases the reaction rate by giving the atoms more space to interact. Now, we're not talking about making a reactant bigger, but cutting it down into smaller pieces so that more of the other reactant has greater contact with its atoms. For example, a crushed sugar cube will dissolve faster in water than a whole sugar cube because the water has access to more of the sugar cube molecules in the crushed form than in the cube form.

▸ **Concentrations.** Increasing the concentration of molecules reduces the space between them and increases the likelihood that they will come in contact and react.

▸ **Catalysts.** These substances reduce or increase the amount of activation energy needed for a reaction to occur. A positive catalyst increases the reaction rate by reducing the activation energy. A negative catalyst slows down the reaction rate by increasing the activation energy.

Balancing Equations

The final part of our discussion of reactions has to do with balancing chemical equations. Dalton's laws tell us that in chemical reactions, atoms are combined, not destroyed. They also state that compounds are formed as a result of elements reacting with each other in defined whole-number ratios. This means that the product of a chemical reaction has to have equal proportions of the same compounds involved in the reactants. A favorite chemistry question found on standardized exams is balancing chemical equations so that these proportions are equal on both sides of the arrow.

Balancing equations is a pretty simple concept, but it takes some practice to master.

Basically, it's a numbers game. You can't subtract atoms from an equation, but you can add them. And that's exactly what you do until both sides have the same number of atoms of each element that make up the reactants.

Let's try one. The following equation shows propane burning to produce carbon dioxide and steam:

$$C_3H_8(g) + O_2(g) \rightarrow CO_2(g) + H_2O(g)$$

1. Break down each of the reactants into the number of atoms present:

   C atoms: 3

   H atoms: 8

   O atoms: 2

2. Now break down each of the products the same way:

   C atoms: 1

   H atoms: 2

   O atoms: 3

3. The carbon in the product needs to increase from 1 atom to 3. We do that by writing 3 as a *coefficient* in front of CO_2, and keep in mind that 3 will apply to the oxygen atom as well:

   $$C_3H_8(g) + O_2(g) \rightarrow 3CO_2(g) + H_2O(g)$$

DEFINITION

As in algebra, a **coefficient** in chemistry is a number placed before a compound in an equation that multiplies the number of complete molecules, but leaves the relative number of atoms within that molecule (i.e., its chemical identity) alone. For example, a single molecule of water is H_2O. If we add a coefficient of 2 before that molecule, we have $2H_2O$, with 2 x 2 = 4 atoms of hydrogen and 2 x 1 = 2 atoms of oxygen.

4. Now look at the hydrogen atoms. The reactant has 8 and the product only has 2. If we multiply the H_2O by writing 4 as its coefficient, we raise the number of hydrogen atoms to 8:

$$C_3H_8(g) + O_2(g) \rightarrow 3CO_2(g) + 4H_2O(g)$$

5. Finally, you have oxygen to deal with. Originally, the reactants had two atoms of oxygen and the products three atoms. But more atoms of oxygen were added to the product when the coefficients were introduced and now have 10 atoms of oxygen to the right of the arrow (i.e., on the products side) and two to the left (i.e., on the reactants side). You can balance this out by adding 5 as a coefficient to the oxygen reactant:

$$C_3H_8(g) + 5O_2(g) \rightarrow 3CO_2(g) + 4H_2O(g)$$

You now have a balanced chemical equation.

CODE RED!

Sometimes when you balance equations, you will have a fraction as a coefficient. To get rid of the fraction or a decimal, multiply the whole equation by a number whose product with the fraction is a whole number. This will get rid of your fraction/decimal and keep the equation in balance.

Try it on your own with this equation:

$$Al + CuO \rightarrow Al_2O_3 + Cu$$

If you got $2Al + 3CuO \rightarrow Al_2O_3 + 3Cu$, you're right!

Stoichiometry

Yes, it is a big word, but it stands for a simple concept: the calculation of a relationship between reactants and products in a balanced chemical equation. So in other words, it's about proportion.

A common problem you'll see that uses stoichiometry looks something like this:

> How many grams of CuO would you need to use up 65 g of Al using our newly balanced chemical reaction: $2Al + 3CuO \rightarrow Al_2O_3 + 3Cu$?

1. Define a molar relationship between reactants. You can easily see that for every 2 atoms of Al, you need 3 molecules of CuO.

2. Find out how many moles of Al are in 65 g of Al:

   ▸ Figure out the atomic weight of Al by looking up the atomic weight on the Periodic Table. (It's 27.)

   ▸ This tells you that one mole of Al = 27 g.

3. Divide the number of grams in the problem statement by the number of grams that equals 1 mole of aluminum: $\frac{65}{27} = 2.4$. This means that 65 g of Al is equal to 2.4 moles of Al.

4. Because the chemical equation tells you there is a 2:3 ratio between Al and CuO, you would now multiply 2.4 moles of aluminum by the conversion factor (3 moles CuO / 2 moles Al). The result is 3.6 moles CuO.

5. Now look up the atomic weight of Cu (64) and O (16) and then add them together to determine the molecular weight of one mole of CuO: 64 + 16 = 80. So you now know that one mole of CuO is equal to 80 grams of CuO.

6. Finally, convert 3.6 moles of CuO back to grams of CuO by multiplying by this new conversion factor: 3.6 moles CuO × (80 g CuO /1 mole CuO) = 288 g CuO. This is your final answer to the original question, how many grams of CuO would be needed to react with 65 grams of Al.

Solutions

We touched on solutions in Chapter 10 when we talked about osmosis. In a solution, whatever substance dissolves (i.e., disappears, quite often) into the other substance is called the *solute*. The other substance, which "does the dissolving," is called the *solvent*. For example, if you dissolve salt into water, water is the solvent and salt is the solute.

To help keep the two terms straight, perhaps think of going camping. Your tent (like a sol-VENT) is what surrounds you at night and keeps you warm and dry.

Determining Concentration

An important concept when dealing with solutions has to do with calculating concentrations, or molarity, of the solute and/or the solvent. You do this by dividing the number of moles of solute that's added to the solvent by the volume of the solvent. Say you have 4 liters of water and to that you add 5 moles of salt (NaCl), you would calculate: 5 ÷ 4 = 1.25. The molarity of this solution is 1.25 M NaCl.

Dilutions, Emulsifications, and Tinctures

The concepts of dilutions, tinctures, and emulsifications are pretty basic, so we're addressing them all together:

▶ **Dilutions.** When you add volume to the solvent in a solution, you reduce the molarity of a solution. If you think about it, this makes sense because you calculate molarity based on the volume of solvent. Increase the solvent and you decrease the molarity because you have changed the proportions of the solution (i.e., increased the denominator, thereby causing the overall quantity to be smaller).

▶ **Emulsifications.** An emulsification joins two solutes that would not normally mix; for example, oil and water. But add some egg yolk to that solution, and you've added an emulsifier that will enable the oil and water molecules to mix completely. Then add in a little pepper and lemon juice and you have hollandaise sauce!

▶ **Tinctures.** Tinctures are solutions made with alcohol and not water. You can make herbal tinctures in your kitchen and use them as health supplements.

Acids and Bases

Acids are substances that produce hydrogen ions (H^+) when mixed with water. Bases produce hydroxide ions (OH^-) when mixed with water. There are a couple ways you can tell whether a solution is basic or acidic:

▶ **Chemically.** Litmus paper will change color when it comes in contact with an acidic or basic solution: red for acid, blue for basic (easy alliteration there). You can also use phenolphthalein, a chemical compound that when mixed with an acid does not change the solution any color, but when mixed with a base turns pink.

▶ **Physically.** You can use your senses to tell an acid from a base, though we wouldn't recommend it because strong acids and bases can be harmful to the body. Acids taste sour or burn the tongue or skin, depending on the concentration of acid. Bases taste bitter, can also burn the skin in high concentrations, and feel slippery to the touch when mixed with water. Soap is the product of a careful balance of oil (acid) and lye (base); the slippery feeling you get when you wash your hands with soap is actually the basic properties coming out.

The pH scale measures the strength of the acidity and basicity of substances:

▶ 0–6 = acidic

▶ 7 = neutral

▶ 8–14 = basic

In actuality, this is more of a spectrum than a scale. Acids at the low end of the scale are stronger than those closer to the neutral numbers. A 6 is still slightly acidic (milk); an 8 is slightly basic (egg whites). The far end of the spectrum has the strongest bases, such as lye.

Scientific Notation

It is common to deal with very, very large numbers when working with chemistry. To make these numbers easier to deal with, scientists often use scientific notation. This is just a way to use exponents to shorten a long number and still have it represent the correct value.

You see this with Avogadro's number, 6.022×10^{23}. The actual number this stands for is 602,200,000,000,000,000,000,000. Instead of having to write all of this out, it is referred to in terms of scientific notation.

To write a number in scientific notation, follow these steps:

1. Move the decimal point to the left until it is behind the first nonzero digit of the number. Try it with 248,500,000. You would move the decimal eight places to the left, to get 2.48500000.

2. Drop all the 0s at the end of the number: 2.485.

3. Multiply by the power of 10 the number of places you moved the decimal: 2.485×10^8.

Practice Questions

For each of the following questions, choose the best answer.

1. Which of the following is a true statement about the Periodic Table?

    (A) The position of elements in the Periodic Table is related to the arrangement of their electrons, and that determines the chemical and physical properties of the element.

    (B) Elements are arranged in order of increasing atomic number.

    (C) Vertical columns are referred to as groups or families and horizontal rows are called periods.

    (D) all of the above

2. A property exhibited by aqueous solutions of bases is that they

    (A) have a sour taste.

    (B) conduct an electric current.

    (C) have a bitter taste.

    (D) turn blue litmus paper red.

3. The accepted value of a mole, which is the SI unit for amount of substance, is

    (A) 6.022×10^{23}

    (B) 6.022×10^{-23}

    (C) 6.1×10^{23}

    (D) 6.1×10^{-23}

4. An atom or group of atoms that carry an electrical charge is known as a/an

    (A) molecule.

    (B) ion.

    (C) metal.

    (D) chemical composition.

5. What is mass?

    (A) A measure of the quantity of matter a body contains, which does not vary as position changes.

    (B) A measure of gravitational attraction of the Earth for the body.

    (C) A measure that varies with distance from the center of the Earth.

    (D) A standard unit of length.

6. What is the reaction in a chemical change?

    (A) One or more substances that are used up.

    (B) One or more new substances that are formed.

    (C) Energy that is absorbed or released.

    (D) all of the above

7. What is a compound?

    (A) A substance that cannot be decomposed into simpler substances by chemical changes.

    (B) A substance that can be decomposed by chemical means into simpler substances, always in the same ratio by mass.

    (C) A combination of two or more pure substances in which each substance retains its own composition and properties.

    (D) Something that cannot be further broken down by physical means.

8. The molecular mass of a substance is

   (A) the sum of the atomic weights of the elements in the formula, each taken the number of times the element occurs.
   (B) the atomic weight.
   (C) the percentage of composition.
   (D) none of the above

9. What is an acid?

   (A) A combination of hydrogen ions (H+) with hydroxide ions (OH−) in aqueous solution.
   (B) A substance that contains hydrogen and that produces H+ in aqueous solution.
   (C) A substance that contains the OH group and produces hydroxide ions (OH−) in aqueous solution.
   (D) A substance that is a proton acceptor.

10. What is an electrolyte?

    (A) A water-soluble substance whose aqueous solutions conduct electrical current.
    (B) A water-soluble substance whose aqueous solutions do not conduct electricity.
    (C) A process in which a solid ionic compound separates into its ions in solution.
    (D) A process in which a molecular compound separates to form ions in solution.

11. What is the charge on calcium in the compound $CaCO_3$?

    (A) +2
    (B) −2
    (C) +1
    (D) −1

12. Sulfur, argon, and krypton are all

    (A) acids.
    (B) metals.
    (C) nonmetals.
    (D) gases.

13. What is the mass of 1 mole of NaCl?

    (A) 58.44
    (B) 59.25
    (C) 58.60
    (D) 57.60

14. Properties of ionic bonding include

    (A) the transfer of one or more electrons from one atom or group of atoms to another.
    (B) molten compounds conducting electricity.
    (C) solids with high melting points.
    (D) all of the above

15. Balance the following chemical equation: $Mg + P_4 \rightarrow Mg_3P_2$.

    (A) $Mg_3 + P_4 \rightarrow Mg_3P_4$
    (B) $Mg + P_4 \rightarrow 2Mg_3P_2$
    (C) $6Mg + P_4 \rightarrow 2Mg_3P_2$
    (D) $P_4 + Mg_3 \rightarrow 2Mg_3P_2$

Answers and Explanations

1. **D.** All of the answers are true regarding the Periodic Table.

2. **C.** Bases have a bitter taste. Answers A, B, and D are all properties of acids.

3. **A.** This is also known as Avogadro's number.

4. **B.** An ion is an atom that has an electrical charge due to the addition or subtraction of electrons.

5. **A.** Weight is a measure of gravitational attraction of the Earth for the body and varies with distance from the center of the Earth. A meter is a standard unit of length.

6. **D.** All of the answer choices describe a reaction in a chemical change.

7. **B.** An element is a substance that cannot be decomposed into simpler substances by chemical changes. A mixture is a combination of two or more pure substances in which each substance retains its own composition and properties. A substance is something that cannot be further broken down by physical means.

8. **A.** Molecular mass is the sum of the atomic weights of the elements in the formula each taken the number of times the element occurs.

9. **B.** Neutralization is the combination of hydrogen ions (H^+) with hydroxide ions (OH^-) in aqueous solution. A base is a substance that contains the OH group and produces hydroxide ions (OH^-) in aqueous solution. A base is a proton acceptor.

10. **A.** A nonelectrolyte is a water-soluble substance whose aqueous solutions do not conduct electricity. Dissociation is a process in which a solid ionic compound separates into its ions in solution. Ionization is the process in which a molecular compound separates to form ions in solution.

11. **A.** Ca is in Column 2 on the Periodic Table and has a +2 charge.

12. **C.** They are all nonmetals.

13. **A.** Add the atomic weight of Na (sodium) and Cl (chloride). Na is 22.99 and Cl is 35.45.

14. **D.** All of the answers are properties of ionic bonding.

15. **C.** This shows the reaction between magnesium and phosphorus to form phosphide. Because you can't decrease the numbers on either side of the equation, you have to increase. Start with phosphorus. There are 4 on the left and 2 on the right. Add a 2 coefficient to the molecule to the right of the arrow: $2Mg_3P_2$. Next, balance the magnesium. Because we just added a coefficient of 2 to the molecule on the products side, we have 6 Mg atoms on that side. Now, to balance Mg atoms on the reactant side, add a coefficient of 6 before Mg. The chemical equation is now balanced.

Let's Get Physical

This final science review chapter is all about physics, which rounds out the entire battery of science topics on which nursing school entrance exams tend to test candidates. Where chemistry and the biological sciences focus on what makes up things in our universe, physics is all about how they move and the energy associated with them.

This chapter reviews common principles you encounter in high school physical science classes. We walk you through mass and energy concepts, speed, movement, wavelengths, electricity, and more. Then we give you some practice questions to test just how much you know. So, let's get to it!

What to Expect

More than any other science section you may encounter on a nursing school entrance exam, the physics sections ask you to *apply* the principles more than asking you questions about them. So, when you prepare for this section, make sure that you do lots of practice questions that have you calculating velocity, ohms, and amplitude. (If you don't know what those are, you will soon.)

ⒶⒷⒸⒹ
ⒶⒷⒸⒹ
ⒶⒷⒸⒹ
ⒶⒷⒸⒹ
ⒶⒷⒸⒹ
ⒶⒷⒸⒹ

Before we jump into our discussion of various concepts in physics, familiarize yourself with some basic vocabulary that you'll be using throughout this chapter.

Physics Vocabulary

Term	Definition
Energy	The amount of work a force can exert. Measured in joules.
Force	Something that changes the motion of an object.
Mass	The amount of matter an object has. Measured in kilograms.
Matter	Anything that occupies space and has mass.
Motion	The change in position of an object over a period of time.
Speed	How fast an object is moving.
Work	Transfer of energy through force over a distance.

Weight and Mass

People often get mass and weight confused. Mass is the amount of matter an object has. This amount doesn't change in relation to the environment. Weight, however, measures the amount of gravitational force exerted on an object. The weight of an object changes when the gravitational force on an object changes.

If you took a trip to the moon, where there is much less gravity than here on Earth, you would weigh less because the force of gravity being exerted on your body is less. Your mass, however, would stay the same.

Determining the mass of an object is an important calculation in physics.

Formula: Multiply the object's volume (V) measured in cubic meters by its density (d) measured in kilograms per cubic meter (explained in Chapter 12) to find mass (mass = dv).

Example: What is the mass of a solid cube that has a volume of 25 m³ and a density of 4 kg/m³?

Answer: Mass = 4 × 25 = 100 kg

In science, you will quite often be working with measurements of mass. There's a good reason for this: science is universal, so universal measurements are used. Here in the United States, we're used to foot, mile, and pound. Science follows the International System of Units (SI System), which means that as a nurse, you will follow it, too.

The SI System is very similar to the metric system, but it is not the same. For example, the metric measure of temperature is Celsius and the SI measure is Kelvin. The following are SI measurements for length, mass, and volume:

Measures of length:

1 millimeter (mm) = .01 centimeter

1 centimeter (cm) = 10 millimeters

1 meter (m) = 100 centimeters

1 kilometer (km) = 1,000 meters

Measures of mass:

1 milligram (mg) = .001 grams

1 gram (g) = 1,000 milligrams

1 kilogram (kg) = 1,000 grams

Measures of volume:

1 milliliter (mL^3) = .001 liter

1 centiliter (cL^3) = .01 liter

1 deciliter (dL^3) = .1 liter

1 liter (L^3) = 1,000 milliliters

1 kiloliter (kL^3) = 1,000 liters

Measures of area:

1 square millimeter (mm^2) = .01 centimeter^2

1 square centimeter (cm^2) = 100 millimeters^2

1 square meter (m^2) = 10,000 centimeters^2

1 square kilometer (km^2) = 1,000,000 meters^2

Here are some additional units and the quantities they measure that you will see in this chapter:

Ampere (A) = Electric current

Hertz (Hz) = Frequency

Joule (J) = Energy, work, quantity of heat

Kelvin (K) = Temperature

Newton (N) = Force

Ohm (O or Ω) = Resistance

Pascal (Pa) = Pressure

Volt (V) = Voltage

Watt (W) = Power

Energy and Work

Energy is the amount of work a force can exert. Work is the transfer of energy through force over a distance. These two concepts are two peas in a pod, which is why we discuss them in the same section.

Energy comes in lots of different forms. In Chapter 10, we talked about energy in the form of ATP. In Chapter 12, we talked about energy in the form of heat. In this chapter, we look at kinetic energy and potential energy.

Potential Energy

When we talk about potential energy (*PE*), we're referring to energy that is stored in an object to be released later. The presence of potential energy means that the piece of matter has the potential to do work or convert that potential energy into kinetic energy (discussed in the next section).

The water behind a dam has *tons* of potential energy. Take the Hoover Dam, for instance. It holds back an estimated 10 trillion gallons of water. As we learned in Chapter 12, within the molecular structure of matter, atoms are constantly banging into each other and creating energy. This is particularly true with liquids.

Now think of all the molecules in 10 trillion gallons of water held back by the Hoover

Dam and the energy they produce simply by being held back. This is an example of potential energy. Because the dam holds the water back, the only energy it produces is whatever it has at rest (simply existing in its natural environment). Now take that dam away and you've released that stored-up energy, with devastating consequences.

Any piece of matter that exists within a force field—such as the Earth's gravitational force—has potential energy. Here is how you would calculate the potential energy of an object:

Formula: Multiply the object's mass (m) by the gravitational force (g) exerted on it and its height (h) above Earth's surface: $PE = mgh$.

Example: What is the potential energy of a ball that has a mass of 0.46 kg when it is on the 102nd floor of the Empire State Building, 381 meters high?

Answer: Remember that gravitational force is 9.8 meters per second squared, or 9.8 m/s².

$PE = .46 \times 9.8 \times 381 = 1,717.548$ joules

Kinetic Energy

Kinetic energy (KE) is the energy generated by motion. When you throw a ball, you release energy. When a plate falls off the table and crashes to the floor, energy is released. These are all forms of kinetic energy.

Going back to the Hoover Dam example, the potential energy of the water is converted into kinetic energy to generate electricity. Power stations close to the dam funnel carefully controlled amounts of water into turbines. As the water moves the turbines, the potential energy is released as kinetic energy. The turbines then harness that kinetic energy and turn it into electricity. This is called hydroelectric power.

Your job on a nursing school entrance exam will be to calculate the amount of kinetic energy that is released through motion.

Formula: Multiply the object's mass (m) by the square of its *velocity* (v), and then multiply that value by half: $KE = \frac{1}{2}mv^2$.

Example: If a kettle bell weighing 64 kg is tossed out a window at a velocity of 6 m/s, what would be the amount of kinetic energy being released?

Answer: $KE = \frac{1}{2} \times 64 \times 6^2$

$KE = \frac{1}{2} \times 64 \times 36$

$KE = 32 \times 36$

$KE = 1,152$ joules

Work, Work, Work

Now that you know a little about different types of energy, let's talk about work. We defined it previously as a transfer of energy through force over distance.

If you've ever push-started a manual transmission car or kicked a ball, you've performed work. The energy in your body was transferred to the car or ball, which then turned its potential energy into kinetic energy. And all of this can be measured:

Formula: Multiply force (measured in Newtons) by distance: $W = fd$.

Example: If you push an IV stand 4.5 meters across a parking lot with a force of 5 N, how much work have you done?

Answer: $W = 5 \times 4.5 = 22.5$ joules

Motion

If you're looking for explanations about motion—which is simply any kind of movement—Sir Isaac Newton is your man. We talked about astronomer Johannes Kepler in our discussion of planetary movement in Chapter 9. Newton was a Kepler fan and followed in his footsteps, studying all kinds of motion. Among his many discoveries, Newton developed three laws that serve as the basis for mechanical theory.

Newton's First Law

Newton's First Law is also known as *the law of inertia*. It states that objects tend to resist changes in motion. An object in motion tends to stay in motion, and an object at rest tends to stay at rest, unless a force is exerted upon it.

For example, a rock will never move unless a force, say a stream of water, comes along with enough force to make it move. Conversely, if you're riding in a car and that car hits a wall, your body will keep moving forward unless it is held back with a seatbelt. Even with a seatbelt, you are still jerked forward with the same amount of force with which you were traveling. Anyone who has had whiplash or bruising from a seatbelt can

tell you that the force is considerable—and painful.

Newton's Second Law

This law is all about how a force influences the motion of an object: the acceleration of an object is directly proportional to the net force acting on the object. It also states that an object accelerates in the direction of the net force acting on it. Essentially, this tells you how to calculate force, which we used in the previous section to calculate work.

Formula: To calculate force, multiply the mass (m) of the object by its acceleration (a): $F = ma$.

Example: To push-start your car, you have to push hard enough to accelerate it at a rate of .10 m/s². If you do this with a car that weighs 1,500 kg, how much force do you have to exert to get to this speed?

Answer: $F = 1,500 \times .10 \rightarrow 150$ Newtons

TEST TIP

Newtons are always used to measure force. One Newton is equal to the force required to accelerate a mass of 1 kg by 1m/s².

Newton's Third Law

This is the one that states, "For every action, there is an equal and opposite reaction." It means that every motion results in the creation of another motion that runs in the opposite direction.

For example, when you jump up and down, you are exerting force on the ground in order to push yourself up. But the ground is also pushing back at you, which you can feel in your feet. Similarly, if you threw a ball at a wall, the action of the ball hitting the surface of the wall will propel it away—the opposite reaction.

Speed

You now know a few things about motion, so you're ready to measure it, beginning with speed. This is the rate at which an object moves.

Formula: $\text{Speed} = \frac{\text{Distance}}{\text{Time}}$

Example: You live 25 kilometers away from work. How fast would you have to drive from your house to make it to work in 20 minutes?

Answer: Speed $= \frac{25}{20}$ or 1.25 km/minute

> **NURSING NOTES**
>
> The formula for speed is also the formula for calculating velocity. The difference between speed and velocity is that velocity takes direction into consideration. So the velocity of the previous example would be 1.25 km/minute traveling west, or some similar directional qualifier. As long as both speed and direction remain constant, velocity is said to be constant.

Acceleration

Acceleration expresses a rate of change in velocity. This can mean an increase (which most of us think of when we consider acceleration), decrease, or a change in direction (even if your speed remains the same). You can use the following formula to calculate positive acceleration (increase in velocity) and negative acceleration (decrease in velocity).

Formula: Subtract the initial rate of velocity (vi) from the final rate of velocity (vf), and divide that value by the length of time (t) in which the change occurs: $A = \dfrac{vf - vi}{t}$

Example: You're driving to work at a velocity of 85 km/hour when you get a call from your boss saying there's an emergency and you need to get in as soon as possible. It takes you 25 seconds to increase your velocity to 100 km/hour. What is your rate of acceleration in m/s²?

Answer: First, you want to convert your velocity into meters per second by dividing the number of total seconds in an hour by the number of meters in a kilometer (this works out to be 3.6): $85 \div 3.6 = 23.61$; $100 \div 3.6 = 27.78$. Then subtract $27.78 - 23.61$ to get 4.17. Finally, divide that by the amount of time it took to increase velocity: $4.17 \div 25 = .1668$ m/s².

Another acceleration concept you should familiarize yourself with is gravitational acceleration. What this basically says is that objects that have no other force acting on them besides gravity fall at the same rate of acceleration (9.8 m/s²) regardless of mass. This means that, in theory, a car and a paper clip dropped in an environment with no air friction (essentially a vacuum) would both hit the ground at the same time; the ratio of weight to mass is the same for both the heavy object and the light object.

> **TEST TIP**
>
> Acceleration is always expressed in units of distance per squared time.

Thermodynamics

Thermodynamics deals with the compression of gases and temperatures. We talked a little about this in our discussion of matter in Chapter 12, particularly when we explained states of matter and how they are converted from one state to another.

Thermodynamics is a very complex branch of science, but luckily, should it pop up on your exam, there are only a few main concepts that you should be familiar with.

Pressure

Let's revisit our definition of gases: Atoms in this state are very loosely bonded and will fill the entirety of any container that holds it (think of helium inside a balloon). Gases do not take on any form of their own, nor do they have a fixed volume.

Because of these loose bonds, the molecules in gases are constantly banging into each other. The same is true for liquids, even though the bonds between liquid molecules are stronger (like elastic bands). When gas and liquid molecules are contained, they also bang into their container, which in turn creates pressure.

> **TEST TIP**
>
> Pressure is measured in Pascals (Pa) or pounds per square inch (PSI).

Familiarize yourself with a few laws that deal with gases and pressure:

- **Boyle's Law.** This law deals with pressure and volume. It states that as the pressure of gas increases, the volume of a fixed amount of gas decreases and vice versa. When you pop a balloon, you are applying Boyle's Law. As you push down on the outside of the balloon, you're decreasing the volume of gas inside. This increases the pressure, and when it becomes too much for the bonds holding the balloon molecules to withstand, the balloon bursts.

- **Charles' Law.** This law deals with gas volume and temperature. It states that as the temperature increases, so does the volume of gas. As it decreases, so does the volume. Have you ever taken a helium-filled balloon outside on a cold day? What happens? It seems like the balloon deflates some. When you go back inside, it fills out again. This is Charles' Law at work.

Temperature

We discussed in Chapter 12 that temperature is a measure of average kinetic energy. When the atoms in an object move fast, the object feels hot. When they move slowly, the object feels cold.

Three main scales are used to measure temperature:

- **Fahrenheit.** This is the scale that we commonly use in the United States. Some important Fahrenheit temperatures you should know:
- Boiling point of water: 212°F
- Freezing point of water: 32°F
- *Absolute zero: –459.67°F*
- **Celsius.** This is the metric scale for temperature. Most of the world uses this scale, but most sciences use the SI scale, which is Kelvin. Important Celsius temps you should know:
- Boiling point of water: 100°C
- Freezing point of water: 0°C
- Absolute zero: –273.15°C
- **Kelvin.** This is the SI scale and the one you'll see most in physics and chemistry in particular. Important Kelvin temps you should know:
- Boiling point of water: 373.15 K
- Freezing point of water: 273.15 K
- Absolute zero: 0 K

Term	Definition
Current (I)	Flow of electricity through a conductor, measured in amperes
Insulator	Something through which electricity passes poorly or not at all
Ohm (Ω)	Measure of resistance
Power (P)	Amount of energy transferred during a specified time; measured in watts
Resistance	Slows down the flow of electricity
Volt (V)	Measure of voltage
Voltage	Strength with which current flows through a conductor; measured in volts
Watt (W)	Measure of electric power

What do you do if you have a Fahrenheit temperature and need it in Celsius or Kelvin to complete a question? There are easy conversion equations that you can use to do this. You may also find these helpful on the math section of your test. (We snuck a few into the practice tests at the back of the book to get you started.):

Fahrenheit to Celsius: $\frac{5}{9} \times$ (Fahrenheit – 32)

Fahrenheit to Kelvin: ($\frac{5}{9} \times$ [Fahrenheit – 32] + 273)

Celsius to Fahrenheit: ($\frac{9}{5} \times$ Celsius) + 32

Celsius to Kelvin: Celsius + 273

Kelvin to Celsius: Kelvin – 273

Kelvin to Fahrenheit: ([Kelvin – 273] $\times \frac{9}{5}$) + 32

It's Electric!

The following are some terms to familiarize yourself with before we continue with our discussion of electricity.

Electricity Vocabulary

Term	Definition
Ampere (A)	Measure of current
Conductor	A material through which electricity can pass easily

Electricity is the flow of electrons through a conductor. In Chapter 12, we talked about electrons and how they are the only subatomic particles that get passed from atom to atom. When this passage occurs, you have an electrical charge because the balance of protons and electrons is now disrupted. When an atom accepts an electron (or more), it has a negative charge. When an atom gives away an electron, it has a positive charge.

Continuous movement of electrons results in an electric current, which we measure in amperes (amps). To make electricity useful for human purposes, we capture the flow of negative electrons using a conductor—and all of this usually happens in some kind of circuit (discussed later in this chapter).

Voltage and Ohm's Law

Voltage measures how much electrical force a power source applies. Think of this as the amount of force pushing the current through a conductor at a certain rate. When there is resistance added to the conductor, this slows down the rate the current travels and increases the voltage needed to push the current through to the end of the conductor.

For example, say you add a dimmer switch to your bedside lamp. As the current flows from the wall outlet through the wires leading to the lamp, it hits the dimmer switch, which adds resistance to the wire. If the resistance is high, only some of the electricity makes it to the lamp, and you have dimmer light. If the resistance is low, more electricity makes it to the lamp and you have brighter light.

All of this discussion about currents, voltage, and resistance leads us to Ohm's Law. Ohm's Law is used to define the proportional relationship among currents, voltage, and resistance within a circuit.

Ohm's Law states that electric current is directly proportional to voltage. So the more voltage you have, the greater the current is. Ohm's Law also states that electric current is inversely proportional to resistance—the higher the resistance, the lower the current.

These laws result in several equations that you will need to know for electricity-related questions on your exam.

Ohm's Law Equations

Value Sought	Equation	Translation
Ampere (A)	$A = \frac{V}{\Omega}$	amps = $\frac{volts}{resistance}$
Ohms (Ω)	$\Omega = \frac{V}{A}$	ohms = $\frac{volts}{amps}$
Voltage (V)	$V = A \times \Omega$	volts = amps × ohms
Watts (W)	$W = V \times A$	watts = volts × amps

Circuits

A circuit is a system of connected conductors that direct the path of electricity. As long as electrons are able to move along their desired paths, the circuit is complete. A complete circuit may also be referred to as closed. When the electrons stop moving, the circuit is called open.

Simple Circuit

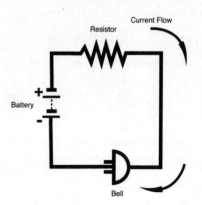

A basic circuit, such as the one shown, starts with a power source (a battery in this case) that generates an electric current, which then flows through a conductor and back to the power source, completing the circuit. Along the way, it can meet resistors or other components that can change the path and properties of the electricity.

The two types of circuits you should be familiar with for your nursing school entrance exam are:

▶ **Series.** A circuit that provides a single-flow path. Think about strings of lights in which, if one bulb goes out, the whole string does.

Series Circuit

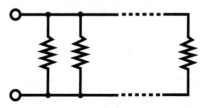

▶ **Parallel.** A circuit that provides several flow paths. These are the strings of lights that, when a single bulb goes out, the rest stay lit.

Parallel Circuit

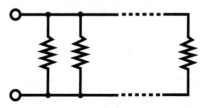

Waves

A wave is a rhythmic movement of energy through a medium that does not cause the medium to permanently change. Think of the ringing of a bell. The energy you apply to hit the bell causes the molecules that make it up to vibrate the air so much that a sound wave is produced—energy that you can't see, but can hear. When that sound wave comes into contact with another form of matter, it displaces the molecules in that matter, but

only for as long as the wave affects it. When the wave is gone, so is the energy to move the molecules.

Waves come in a variety of shapes and forms. The following diagram shows characteristics that are common to all waves:

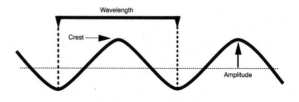

The midline (the dotted line that runs through the middle of the wave in the diagram) represents what the medium looks like when the wave is not passing through it. This series of crests and valleys (formally called a *trough*) is the general shape of a wave, or the shape that the medium takes as the wave moves through it.

Based on a wave diagram, you can calculate several measures:

▶ **Wavelength.** This is a measure of any two corresponding points on a wave. Wavelength can also be measured by the distance from one crest to the next, between troughs, or the distance from the beginning of a *cycle* to the end of a cycle.

▶ **Wave speed.** This is a measure of how fast the wave is travelling. Multiply the wavelength by the frequency (see below).

▶ **Amplitude.** This measures the height of a wave. It's calculated by slicing a line down the middle of a crest and measuring the height from crest top to the midline. If you measure from the midline to the bottom of a trough, this is called negative amplitude.

Frequency

Frequency is the measure of any periodic event expressed as the number of complete cycles per second. In terms of waves, frequency tells us how many complete waves have occurred in a selected time frame.

Formula: To measure frequency, divide the number of times a complete wave is made during a given time: $\frac{\text{Times Event Takes Place}}{\text{Amount of Time Elapsed}}$

Example: During the course of five minutes, a sound wave crests 150 times. What is its frequency?

Answer: You need to break this down into cycles per second, so multiply 5×60 to figure out the seconds (300). Now divide: $\frac{150}{300} = \frac{1}{2} = .5$. Your answer is .5 Hz.

Types of Waves

There are lots of types of waves. Light waves, for example, are made up of photons (light energy). But radio waves, x-rays, and gamma rays are also forms of light—you just can't see them. All of these waves are sorted into the spectrum (the electromagnetic spectrum to be precise) based on their wavelengths.

Generally, waves with the highest and lowest energy can't be seen, but the ones in the middle can be seen.

In addition to light waves, you should know a few things about sound waves, which are mechanical as opposed to electromagnetic. The frequency of the wave determines its pitch. Sound waves with high frequencies hurt our ears because they can't withstand the amount of energy that the sound waves deliver. Ultrahigh and ultralow frequencies are so far beyond our capacity for hearing that they are impossible for us to hear.

The volume of a sound wave depends on its amplitude. The lower the amplitude, the lower the intensity of the sound. The higher the amplitude, the higher the intensity of sound.

How Waves Move

You know that waves follow the up-and-down pattern shown in the earlier diagram. But did you know that that pattern can take on a pattern of its own? The two main wave patterns to know for your test are the following:

▶ **Transverse.** This pattern causes particles in the wave to move perpendicular to the direction of the wave. For example, if a wave is moving forward, the pattern of the wave would be to move up and down. Electromagnetic waves are transverse.

▶ **Longitudinal.** This pattern moves parallel to the direction the wave is travelling. So if the wave is moving straight ahead, its pattern is straight ahead, too. Sound is a longitudinal wave.

In addition to following these patterns, waves behave in different ways when they come in contact with different forms of matter. The results are:

▶ **Reflection.** This happens when waves bounce back after colliding with a surface. You can see this effect with light (mirrors) and sound (echoes).

▶ **Refraction.** Have you ever heard of bending light through prisms? This is refraction. When a wave's direction changes as a result of passing through a new medium, refraction takes place.

▶ **Diffraction.** This is where waves bend to go around obstacles in their way. An example of this is the U.S. Capitol Building's whispering spot. There is a place you can stand under the rotunda that joins the Senate and House of Representatives' respective sides of the building. If you speak softly there, the sound waves are diffracted off of the inside of the rotunda and travel down to the other side of the room. If you're standing on that side, you can hear exactly what's being whispered several yards away.

▶ **Interference.** This is what happens when two waves collide. Static on your cellphone or tuning to one radio station and having the programming from another interrupt your signal are both examples of interference.

▶ **Dispersion.** This occurs when a wave is split up by frequency. In a rainbow, white light is broken up into colors—the visual representation of the varying wavelengths of that light—and you have dispersion.

Nuclear Physics

Our final discussion in this chapter has to do with the physics of atoms. In the early twentieth century, scientists discovered that atoms could be split, which up until that time had been thought to be an impossibility. The effects of this discovery are with us today in the form of atomic energy formed by nuclear reactions.

> **NURSING NOTES**
>
> The discovery that atoms can be split is ironic because the word atom comes from the Greek word for "indivisible."

This is an extremely complex area of physics, so we're just going to boil this down to three main concepts:

▶ **Radiation.** When the nucleus of an atom begins to break down or enter a transformational process, it gives off radioactive energy in the form of alpha particles (large, made up of two protons and two neutrons), beta particles (similar to electrons, but originate in the nucleus), or gamma rays (electromagnetic energy in the form of photons). This process is called radioactive decay. Radioactive isotopes are the atoms most vulnerable to this type of reaction. When they go through radioactive decay, they transform from one type of atom to another (alpha to beta, beta to gamma, etc.).

▶ **Fission.** This takes a nucleus and splits it apart. The result is that a large amount of energy is produced.

▸ **Fusion.** This is a nuclear reaction that joins the nuclei of at least two atoms, resulting in one big nucleus and the creation of an enormous amount of energy.

▸ The processes of nuclear fission and fusion take place every day in nuclear power plants, which harness the energy created by the reactions and turn them into forms of energy that you can use.

Practice Questions

For each of the following questions, choose the best answer.

1. How much force does it take to accelerate a 5 kg box across the floor at a rate of .5 m/s²?

    (A) 2.5 N
    (B) 5.2 N
    (C) 10 N
    (D) 20 N

2. How much current can 25 volts push through 8 ohms of resistance?

    (A) 3.125 amps
    (B) 13.25 amps
    (C) 31.25 amps
    (D) 311.25 amps

3. −273.15°C =

    (A) 373.15 K
    (B) 32°F
    (C) 0 K
    (D) 212°F

4. You're riding the bumper cars at the carnival. The jerking action of the cars hitting each other is an example of

    (A) Newton's First Law.
    (B) Newton's Second Law.
    (C) Newton's Third Law.
    (D) Charles' Law.

5. During the course of an hour, a light wave completes 4,500 cycles. What is its frequency?

    (A) 1.25 Hz
    (B) 12.5 Hz
    (C) 25.2 Hz
    (D) 125 Hz

6. According to Charles' Law, if you have a beaker full of carbon dioxide gas and you heat it up, what will happen to the gas?

    (A) It will increase in volume.
    (B) It will increase in pressure.
    (C) It will decrease in volume.
    (D) It will decrease in pressure.

7. You break a bulb on a string of lights, and they all go out. What type of circuit do these lights operate on?

    (A) parallel
    (B) reactive
    (C) inverse
    (D) series

8. Energy is measured in

    (A) grams.
    (B) Newtons.
    (C) joules.
    (D) watts.

9. How much work do you do by pushing a stroller 25.6 m with a force of 12 N?

   (A) 2.32 joules
   (B) 23.2 joules
   (C) 236.2 joules
   (D) 307.2 joules

10. Resistance is measured in units of

    (A) volts.
    (B) amps.
    (C) watts.
    (D) ohms.

11. The law of thermodynamics that deals with pressure and gases is

    (A) Charles' Law.
    (B) Kepler's Law.
    (C) Boyle's Law.
    (D) Newton's Law.

12. A rainbow is an example of

    (A) refraction.
    (B) dispersion.
    (C) diffraction.
    (D) interference.

13. What is the potential energy of a kettle bell that has a mass of 6 kg when it is 68 m above the ground?

    (A) 122.4 joules
    (B) 256.28 joules
    (C) 399.4 joules
    (D) 3,998.4 joules

14. ATP, heat, and electricity are all forms of

    (A) mass.
    (B) reaction.
    (C) energy.
    (D) power.

15. If you have 12 ohms of resistance, through which you need to conduct 6 amps of electricity, how many volts are necessary to accomplish this?

    (A) 2
    (B) 18
    (C) 60
    (D) 72

Answers and Explanations

1. **A.** To calculate force, you multiply the mass (m) of the object by its acceleration (a): $F = ma$. F = 5 kg x 0.5 m/s^2 = 2.5 N

2. **A.** Your formula is $\text{amps} = \frac{\text{volts}}{\text{resistance}}$:
$A = \frac{25}{8} = 3\frac{1}{8} = 3.125$

3. **C.** Answer A is Kelvin's boiling point. B and D are Fahrenheit's freezing and boiling point, respectively.

4. **C.** This is the "for every action there is an equal and opposite reaction." Car A hits Car B, and Car B hits back.

5. **A.** We need to break this down into cycles per second, so multiply 60×60 to figure out the seconds (3600). Now divide: $\frac{4500}{3600} = 1\frac{1}{4} = 1.25$. Your answer is 1.25 Hz.

6. **A.** Charles' Law states that as the temperature of a gas increases, so does the volume of gas.

7. **D.** Series circuits only have one path through which current can flow.

8. **C.** Mass is measured in grams. Force is measured in newtons. Power is measured in watts.

9. **D.** The formula for work is $W = fd$: $12 \times 25.6 = 307.2$ joules.

10. **D.** Resistance is measured in ohms. Volts measure voltage. Amps measure current. Watts measure power.

11. **C.** Boyle's Law states that as the pressure of gas increases, the volume of a fixed amount of gas decreases and vice versa. Kepler's and Newton's Laws have to do with motion. Charles' Law has to do with gases and temperature.

12. **B.** Dispersion is when a wave is split up by frequency, which is what happens when you see a rainbow.

13. **D.** Your formula is $PE = mgh$: $6 \times 9.8 \times 68 = 3,998.4$ joules.

14. **C.** These are all forms of energy.

15. **D.** Your equation is $V = A \times \Omega$: $6 \times 12 = 72$ volts.

Strength Training: Test Your Skills

Trial and error, plus answers and detailed explanations for every question, can be even more of an effective learning tool than straight studying—which is what this part is all about. Because this book covers several types of tests, we've developed two practice exams that cover all the subject areas.

Something to keep in mind: the questions in this part were written based on our experience with the exam, subject matter, and test design. They are not official test questions from any of the exams. Our intent is to give you more familiarity with the test structure and types of content known to be given on the test so that you can better prepare yourself.

Practice Test 1

Word Knowledge

Time: 40 minutes

Questions: 40

Directions: For each of the following questions, choose the best answer out of the choices given.

1. After hearing the news of the CEO's resignation, the board decided to <u>table</u> the decision about selling the company until the next meeting.

   The underlined word in the previous sentence most nearly means

   (A) set up.
   (B) put off.
   (C) celebrate.
   (D) vote on.

2. The job fair was a <u>virtual</u> meat market of employers and prospective employees.

   The underlined word in the previous sentence most nearly means

   (A) something that is almost the real thing.
   (B) something that is exactly the real thing.
   (C) something that is not the real thing.
   (D) something that is the opposite of something else.

3. Truncate most nearly means

   (A) elongate.
   (B) freshen up.
   (C) cut off.
   (D) envelope.

4. exacerbate : aggravate ::

   (A) sick : ill
   (B) inform : violate
   (C) admire : envy
   (D) lost : found

5. Believing everything everyone tells you is not a(n) _____ way to collect information.

   (A) forgivable
   (B) efficient
   (C) discerning
   (D) pardonable

6. A cadre of civilian resistors formed when the government's constitution was thrown out and a new regime took power.

   The underlined word in the previous sentence most nearly means

   (A) organized group.
   (B) boon.
   (C) treaty.
   (D) quagmire.

7. Xenophobe describes someone who is afraid of

   (A) spiders.
   (B) things that are foreign.
   (C) enclosed spaces.
   (D) flying.

8. transdermal : skin ::

   (A) hand : foot
   (B) intravenous : vein
   (C) today : tomorrow
   (D) move : rent

9. Though the teacher told her student that if he did not improve his home-work grades he would not pass the course, he still took a(n) _____ attitude to her comments and to completing his assignments.

   (A) studious
   (B) blasé
   (C) slight
   (D) average

10. Apropos most nearly means

    (A) breezy.
    (B) flip.
    (C) outrageous.
    (D) fitting.

11. Jay was capricious in his baseball team preference; he supported the Mets when the team was having a good year, but switched to the Yankees if they took the lead.

    The underlined word in the previous sentence most nearly means

    (A) staunchly loyal.
    (B) uncertain.
    (C) static.
    (D) erratic.

12. <u>Spartan</u> most nearly means the opposite of

   (A) austere.
   (B) elaborate.
   (C) outdated.
   (D) generous.

13. prescribe : betray ::

   (A) delirious : ranting
   (B) offbeat : strange
   (C) subscribe : disagree
   (D) offend : insult

14. Dave did not want to serve on a jury, so he did not register to vote in hopes that he could _____ being added to the list of county residents that makes up the jury pool.

   (A) volunteer
   (B) facilitate
   (C) celebrate
   (D) circumvent

15. The handsome man walked with a confident <u>gait</u> when he entered the room, which disappeared when he tripped over a waiter and smeared hors d'oeuvres all over his expensive suit.

   The underlined word in the previous sentence most nearly means

   (A) tray.
   (B) bearing.
   (C) grade.
   (D) smile.

16. <u>Egregious</u> most nearly means the opposite of

   (A) averse.
   (B) extroverted.
   (C) wonderful.
   (D) slow.

17. The anesthetic from my dental work earlier in the day was still in effect, thus making me _____ my words in the meeting.

   (A) garble
   (B) jumble
   (C) plait
   (D) berate

18. contract : obligation ::

   (A) correction : mistake
   (B) memoir : life
   (C) formidable : substantial
   (D) acute : severe

19. <u>Maverick</u> most nearly means

   (A) nonconformist.
   (B) famous.
   (C) pleased with oneself.
   (D) conventional.

20. The cake icing tasted bad; the butter they used to make it probably was <u>rancid</u>.

   The underlined word in the previous sentence most nearly means

   (A) new.
   (B) fresh.
   (C) spoiled.
   (D) improved.

21. Mucus that you cough up from your lungs is called

    (A) gross.
    (B) sputum.
    (C) asthma.
    (D) drainage.

22. A precocious two-year-old recited all of the lyrics to the "Star-Spangled Banner" for his preschool class.

    The underlined word in the previous sentence most nearly means

    (A) tiresome.
    (B) energetic.
    (C) advanced.
    (D) annoyed.

23. masochist : pain ::

    (A) anterior : posterior
    (B) seated : entrenched
    (C) hedonist : pleasure
    (D) expensive : opulent

24. After my mother's funeral, I thanked her friends for being so _____ in their kind offer to help with the preparations.

    (A) grateful
    (B) false
    (C) active
    (D) solicitous

25. cranium : skull ::

    (A) radius : ulna
    (B) mandible : masticate
    (C) patella : kneecap
    (D) sternum : ribs

26. Complacent most nearly means

    (A) vivacious.
    (B) haggard.
    (C) perky.
    (D) content.

27. Even though the newspapers were all predicting a landslide win for the other candidate, the mayor was _____ in his belief that he would win the election.

    (A) steadfast
    (B) depressed
    (C) anxious
    (D) appreciative

28. endogenous : exogenous ::

    (A) forage : look
    (B) native : alien
    (C) khat : plant
    (D) bellow : speak

29. Misogynistic describes someone who

    (A) loves animals.
    (B) is afraid of water.
    (C) doesn't like women.
    (D) doesn't like sports.

30. I am going to specialize in triage because I am good at assessment and determining priorities.

    The underlined word in the previous sentence most nearly means

    (A) treating patients.
    (B) taking blood.
    (C) prioritizing patients.
    (D) administering medication.

31. <u>Sabotage</u> most nearly means the opposite of

    (A) create.
    (B) wreck.
    (C) sink.
    (D) enflame.

32. hypothermia : cold ::

    (A) enraged : angry
    (B) borrow : belong
    (C) fading : ending
    (D) sorry : contrite

33. When Paige received an expensive new sports car for her 16th birthday, her brother was _____, because he'd only gotten a new game system for his.

    (A) indignant
    (B) healthy
    (C) average
    (D) pacified

34. Despite the haunted house's <u>foreboding</u> exterior, the show inside was pretty funny.

    The underlined word in the previous sentence most nearly means

    (A) cheerful.
    (B) intricate.
    (C) new.
    (D) apprehensive.

35. constrict : dilate ::

    (A) lost : forgotten
    (B) beautiful : pretty
    (C) spoken : directed
    (D) facilitate : stall

36. <u>Emollient</u> most nearly means

    (A) bomb.
    (B) balm.
    (C) razor.
    (D) right.

37. The mother gave the boy in the movie an <u>admonitory</u> look when he took a cookie from the table after she told him he was not allowed to have dessert.

    The underlined word in the previous sentence most nearly means

    (A) scolding.
    (B) sinister.
    (C) sly.
    (D) arch.

38. If someone is <u>febrile</u>, they are

    (A) frozen.
    (B) uptight.
    (C) inconsolable.
    (D) feverish.

39. extension cord : power ::

    (A) train : people
    (B) hate : detest
    (C) introvert : extrovert
    (D) florid : reticent

40. <u>Patrician</u> most nearly means

    (A) male.
    (B) blue-blooded.
    (C) pious.
    (D) forgiven.

Grammar

Time: 40 minutes

Questions: 40

Directions: For each of the following questions, choose the best answer out of the choices given.

1. Which of the answer choices is grammatically correct?

    (A) I want you to go to the store I got the bread from.
    (B) Where is the store at?
    (C) The store is just down the street.
    (D) Is it easy to get inside?

2. How many prepositional phrases are in the following sentence?

    Despite all of the years of study I already completed to become a psychologist, I recently decided to change my major to nursing.

    (A) 1
    (B) 2
    (C) 3
    (D) 4

3. What punctuation is needed to correct this sentence?

    I have just one thing to say, vote for me!

    (A) a colon instead of a comma
    (B) a semicolon instead of a comma
    (C) a dash instead of a comma
    (D) no change

4. Which of the answer choices is grammatically correct?

    (A) At the end of the day; there was a going away party for Laura.
    (B) I never had a doubt that you would pass the course: it was just a matter of time.
    (C) We need a few things from the baby boutique: booties, sleepers, blankets, and washcloths.
    (D) Amy ran up the hill; and she quickly picked up the bag she left there.

5. What punctuation is needed to correct this sentence?

    Where do you think you're going!

    (A) a question mark instead of an exclamation point
    (B) a period instead of an exclamation point
    (C) a comma after "Where"
    (D) no change

6. Which of the answer choices is grammatically correct?

    (A) After working a 12-hour shift, Carly was wary and looking forward to a good long nap.
    (B) The company issued a statement in which they announced the sale of the U.S. division.
    (C) The waiting room was filled with patients who were getting restless.
    (D) There was little that could be done because there were fewer then three people available to help.

7. What punctuation is needed to correct this sentence?

    The peoples response to the election was overwhelming.

    (A) an apostrophe before the s in "peoples"
    (B) an apostrophe after the s in "peoples"
    (C) a question mark instead of a period
    (D) no change

8. How many prepositions are in the following sentence?

    Over the river and through the woods to grandmother's house we go.

    (A) 1
    (B) 2
    (C) 3
    (D) 4

9. Which form of the verb "to be" would make this sentence grammatically correct?

    We _____ going to leave in the morning.

    (A) are
    (B) am
    (C) be
    (D) is

10. What punctuation is needed to correct this sentence?

    We were greeted with a Spartan stage which was dressed only with four bar stools, a projection screen, and a computer.

    (A) a comma after "We"
    (B) a comma after "stage"
    (C) a colon after "with"
    (D) no change

11. Which form of the verb "to be" would make this sentence grammatically correct?

    Either Forman or Archer _____ coming to bring my keys.

    (A) are
    (B) am
    (C) be
    (D) is

12. Which word best completes this sentence?

    I've been a fan of both _____ music for many years.

    (A) artists
    (B) artists'
    (C) artist's
    (D) woman's

13. What punctuation is needed to correct this sentence?

Before you jump to conclusions let me explain what happened.

    (A) a comma after "Before"
    (B) a comma after "you"
    (C) a comma after "conclusions"
    (D) no change

14. Which verb would make this sentence grammatically correct?

We _____ on the ice when we were driving up the hill yesterday.

    (A) backslided
    (B) backslid
    (C) backslode
    (D) backslidden

15. Which form of the verb "to be" would make this sentence grammatically correct?

Both of our parents _____ thinking we need to go to college.

    (A) are
    (B) am
    (C) be
    (D) is

16. What is the possessive noun in the following sentence?

Barry's saving grace was that he quickly fixed his mistakes.

    (A) Barry's
    (B) grace
    (C) his
    (D) mistakes

17. What punctuation is needed to correct this sentence?

Jake began writing his memoir about five years ago; not long after his daughter was born.

    (A) a comma instead of a semicolon
    (B) a colon instead of a semicolon
    (C) a period instead of a semicolon
    (D) no change

18. Which word would make this sentence grammatically correct?

Fortunately, it turned out to be a(n) _____, sunny day.

    (A) bright
    (B) invitingly
    (C) beautifully
    (D) lavishly

19. If a subject has more than one element, it is called a _____ subject.

    (A) fractured
    (B) singular
    (C) compound
    (D) plural

20. What kind of error is present in the following sentence?

Like the sands of time.

    (A) run-on sentence
    (B) sentence fragment
    (C) subject/verb agreement
    (D) ambiguous pronoun

21. Which of the following statements is true?

    (A) There are more adjectives than adverbs.
    (B) Adjectives end in -ly.
    (C) Adjectives only modify nouns or pronouns.
    (D) Adverbs only modify nouns or pronouns.

22. What kind of grammatical error is present in the following sentence?

    Blake am a college graduate.

    (A) run-on sentence
    (B) sentence fragment
    (C) ambiguous pronoun
    (D) subject/verb agreement

23. What word(s) make(s) up the predicate in the following sentence?

    I stayed up late on Monday night and ordered pizza.

    (A) stayed up
    (B) stayed up late
    (C) ordered
    (D) stayed up and ordered

24. Which of the answer choices is grammatically correct?

    (A) The speech, which was very eloquently presented, was just the right length for the occasion.
    (B) My dad is a great baseball player, and has played every Sunday afternoon since he was in high school at the local park.
    (C) The CEO, after accepting his lifetime achievement award for leading his industry, joined their team at the table where they all sat.
    (D) The panel speakers prepared its presentations for the conference.

25. What punctuation is needed to correct this sentence?

    Running and other cardiovascular exercises are good for your heart: you should get some in every day.

    (A) a comma instead of a colon
    (B) a semicolon instead of a colon
    (C) an exclamation point instead of a period
    (D) no change

26. Which word best completes this sentence?

    In general, the people of the town were pretty accepting of the news that the community park would be _____.

    (A) broken
    (B) crushed
    (C) blanketed
    (D) renovated

27. Which word would make this sentence grammatically correct?

I wish I _____ a millionaire.

(A) can be
(B) was
(C) were
(D) is

28. A group of words that has a subject and a verb is a

(A) clause.
(B) phrase.
(C) prepositional phrase.
(D) declarative sentence.

29. Which word best completes this sentence?

The concert _____ with a surprise guest performance.

(A) closed
(B) bellowed
(C) reeked
(D) prepared

30. What punctuation is used when you are joining two independent clauses and you want to emphasize the second of the two?

(A) colon
(B) period
(C) comma
(D) semicolon

31. Which word would make this sentence grammatically correct?

If I don't have to go to work tomorrow, we _____ go visit Grandma.

(A) can't
(B) can
(C) promised
(D) didn't

32. What punctuation is needed to correct this sentence?

One of the best things about this time of year is back to school shopping.

(A) a colon after "is"
(B) hyphenate "best things"
(C) hyphenate "back to school"
(D) no change

33. A general type of noun is called a

(A) common noun.
(B) collective noun.
(C) proper noun.
(D) possessive noun.

34. What shows to whom or for what the action in a sentence is performed?

(A) compound subject
(B) preposition
(C) indirect object
(D) direct object

35. Which word in the following sentence is used incorrectly?

I could care less if you got caught smoking on campus.

(A) could
(B) less
(C) caught
(D) campus

36. If the speaker is detached from the subject in a sentence, the sentence is written in

(A) first person perspective.
(B) second person perspective.
(C) third person perspective.
(D) the past.

37. Which word in the following sentence is used incorrectly?

For all intensive purposes, I already have the job.

(A) For
(B) intensive
(C) have
(D) job

38. Which word best completes this sentence?

The singer also performed newer songs that were less familiar, but certainly _____.

(A) generous
(B) memorable
(C) treatable
(D) proud

39. Which word in the following sentence is used incorrectly?

When Lynn said she was going to the movies, she inferred that she would bring a date.

(A) going
(B) inferred
(C) bring
(D) date

40. Adjectives are

(A) groups of words that don't have a subject and verb, but act as a unit.
(B) used to modify verbs, other adjectives, and adverbs.
(C) used to describe or modify a noun or pronoun.
(D) indirect objects.

Spelling

Time: 40 minutes

Questions: 40

Directions: For each of the following examples, choose the letter that shows the correctly spelled word.

1. (A) anbulatory (B) amblatory
(C) ambulatory

2. (A) latteral (B) lateral (C) latarel

3. (A) infectious (B) infectcious
(C) infecious

4. (A) horomone (B) hormone
(C) hoormone

5. (A) basal (B) basel (C) baceal

6. (A) metebolic (B) metobolic
(C) metabolic

7. (A) cuntagion (B) contageon
(C) contagion

8. (A) Eustacean (B) Eustachian
(C) Eustacoan

9. (A) sepsis (B) sepsus (C) sepsess

10. (A) distanded (B) distended
(C) destended

11. (A) akute (B) accute (C) acute

12. (A) benine (B) benign (C) binine

13. (A) febrile (B) febral (C) feberile

14. (A) variant (B) varient (C) variunt

15. (A) subtol (B) subtel (C) subtle

16. (A) address (B) adress (C) addres

17. (A) persperation (B) perspiration
(C) persparation

18. (A) analisis (B) analysis (C) analisys

19. (A) ommited (B) omited (C) omitted

20. (A) dependent (B) dependant
(C) dependint

21. (A) absess (B) abcess (C) abscess

22. (A) superficial (B) superficiel
(C) superfishal

23. (A) circlatory (B) circulatory
(C) circleatory

24. (A) nuetron (B) nutron (C) neutron

25. (A) naturally (B) naturaly
(C) natrually

26. (A) publiclly (B) publically
(C) publicly

27. (A) completely (B) compleetly
(C) completlee

28. (A) accommadate (B) accomodate
(C) accommodate

29. (A) abdomenal (B) abdominal
(C) abdomunal

30. (A) abrasion (B) abbrasion
(C) abrashion

31. (A) referal (B) referral (C) referrall

32. (A) beggar (B) begger (C) begar

33. (A) firey (B) fiery (C) fierie

34. (A) amature (B) ameteur (C) amateur

35. (A) parallel (B) parralel (C) paralell

36. (A) liklihood (B) likelyhood
(C) likelihood

37. (A) resevoir (B) reservoir (C) reservior

38. (A) obedience (B) obediance
(C) obediunce

39. (A) sensury (B) sensery (C) sensory

40. (A) percipcion (B) preception
(C) perception

Reading Comprehension

Time: 40 minutes

Questions: 30

Directions: Read each of the following passages and choose the best answer for each of the questions that follow it.

Use the following passage to answer questions 1 through 7:

Five-year-old Emma Zeilnhofer of West Milford, New Jersey, grew nervous when she saw her mom, Sue, arguing with her partner, Millie, over the color of an umbrella. Millie insisted it was pink; Sue scoffed, rolled her eyes, and called it purple. Upset by this exchange, Emma ran between the couple and shouted, "Mommy, be nice to Millie! Now say you're sorry."

Though Sue and Millie were only engaging in a little playful banter, Emma saw their trivial debate as a full-on fight. How do you explain the subtleties of friendly sarcasm to a kid?

"It's important that you don't deny your child's sense of reality by insisting that 'we weren't fighting,'" says Virginia Shiller, Ph.D., a clinical psychologist with the Yale Child Study Center in New Haven, Connecticut. A good reaction might be: "Sometimes I sound angry when I'm not. I don't want to hurt anyone's feelings. I'm really just teasing." That's a concept she can understand.

Role-playing with your child can also help her distinguish between a fun discussion and a serious argument. Try two games: First, start a quarrel about something unimportant to your child, something she'll find silly. She'll giggle, for example, when you insist that the sky is green, not blue. Then pretend you're fighting over a topic that hits closer to home—say, taking turns with a toy. "You've been playing with it all day!" you could complain vehemently and then explain, "See, in this case, I'm really mad."

Now is also a good time to point out that teasing can go too far and that she should speak up if someone's ribbing is rubbing her the wrong way. That way, you'll help her learn that it's better to use good humor than bullying banter with her friends.

1. The author would most likely agree with which of the following statements?

    (A) You should always correct a child when she thinks you are arguing but you are only kidding around with someone else.

    (B) Role-playing might help a child understand playful banter.

    (C) A child should stay quiet if others' joking behavior is bothering him.

    (D) You should explain playful sarcasm to a child in a logical manner.

2. In the fifth paragraph, the word "ribbing" most nearly means

    (A) bullying.

    (B) praise.

    (C) complaining.

    (D) teasing.

3. In the first paragraph, what were the two women arguing over?

    (A) the color of an umbrella

    (B) rolling of eyes in response to something

    (C) whether or not the daughter should run in the house

    (D) how to say sorry

4. Which of the following statements from the passage is an opinion?

    (A) "Emma ran between the couple and shouted ..."

    (B) "Sometimes I sound angry when I'm not."

    (C) "Role-playing with your child can also help her distinguish between a fun discussion and a serious argument."

    (D) "... she should speak up if someone's ribbing is rubbing her the wrong way."

5. The purpose of this passage is to

    (A) correct the behavior of children.

    (B) present a common situation and offer advice about how to handle it.

    (C) present hard-and-fast rules for parenting.

    (D) point out the negative consequences of parenting.

6. Based on information in the passage, it can be inferred that

    (A) parents shouldn't be sarcastic in front of their children.

    (B) when a child's upset as a result of playful teasing among adults, it can turn into a teachable moment.

    (C) children should be seen and not heard.

    (D) parents need to discipline their children.

7. According to the passage, a role-playing game that would help a child understand playful teasing would be

   (A) a card game where the child has to lie about what cards she has.
   (B) to put on a puppet show that re-enacts a teasing situation.
   (C) to pretend you really think the sky is green, prompting the child to counter with the fact that it's blue.
   (D) none of the above

Use the following passage to answer questions 8 through 14:

It may seem like getting a cold or coming down with food poisoning is easy to do, given the number of times you've likely experienced both throughout your life. But what most people don't realize is that a "perfect storm" of conditions must be present for a person to become infected with the microorganisms that cause these ailments.

First, an infectious agent or pathogen must be present and strong enough to make it through the entire chain of infection. This is entirely dependent on the strength of the agent's ability to multiply (virulence), move and enter the body through tissues (invasiveness), and cause illness (pathogenicity). Infectious agents that are strong in all these areas, such as *Escherichia coli* (*E. coli*) or *Clostridium botulinum* (*C. botulinum*), have a greater chance of being transmitted.

The second factor needed in the chain of infection is a reservoir or place where the agent can live and grow. This can be anything from the soil in your garden to the lining of your digestive tract to your computer keyboard. The conditions must be right for an infectious agent to live in a reservoir for any period of time, and changes in condition can quickly lead to death for the agent.

Next, there must be some way for the infectious agent to leave the reservoir and enter a person's body. These are known as the portal of exit, mode of transmission, and portal of entry. For example, a portal of exit for a digestive pathogen may be fecal matter. If a person uses a bathroom where infected fecal matter has been and does not wash their hands properly, those hands can pick up the pathogens and act as the mode of transmission if they make contact with the mouth, eyes, or blood—all points of entry.

Even with exposure to an infectious agent, though, it does not guarantee transmission. The person who is exposed must be susceptible to the invasion of the microorganism. This means that he or she must not have adequate physical or immunological resistance to the infectious agent, giving it enough time and the right environment to live and multiply.

All of these conditions must be present for an infection to occur.

8. According to the passage, a "microorganism" is

    (A) something that cures illness.

    (B) an infection.

    (C) something that causes infection.

    (D) a degree of strength.

9. According to the passage, a "reservoir" that could hold infectious agents

    (A) could be anything.

    (B) is confined to only a few types of objects.

    (C) is difficult to find.

    (D) would be expensive to buy.

10. Based on what is stated in the passage, which of the following is an opinion?

    (A) All links in the chain of infection must be in place for transmission to occur.

    (B) Hands can act as a portal of entry for a pathogen.

    (C) Not everyone who is exposed to a pathogen gets ill as a result.

    (D) Everyone needs to protect themselves against pathogen transmission.

11. According to the passage, the ability to move and enter the body through tissues is called

    (A) "virulence."

    (B) "E. coli."

    (C) "invasiveness."

    (D) "pathogenicity."

12. In the second sentence of the fifth paragraph, the word "susceptible" most nearly means

    (A) alive.

    (B) vulnerable.

    (C) agreeable.

    (D) averse to.

13. Based on the information from the passage, it can be inferred that

    (A) pathogens can be deadly.

    (B) washing your hands properly can disrupt the chain of infection.

    (C) avoiding infection is an easy process.

    (D) avoiding infection is harder than most people may think.

14. A good title for this passage would be

    (A) The Making of a Pathogen.

    (B) How to Avoid Infections.

    (C) E. Coli and Other Bacteria: How They Work.

    (D) The Chain of Infection Explained.

Use the following passage to answer questions 15 through 21:

Simple, handmade soap is the product of a chemical reaction when fat and lye are combined in precise proportion. The acids in the oil and the bases in lye react the moment they come into contact with each other; this is usually done in a pot or some other type of tall, sturdy, metallic container.

It takes time for all of the molecules in both the oil and the lye to come into contact with each other and saponify or turn into soap. What begins as a heterogeneous mixture becomes a homogeneous one that is creamy in color after many minutes or sometimes hours of stirring. To test if saponification has occurred, dribble some of the mixture from a spoon onto the surface of the rest of the solution in the pot. If the dribbles remain visible on the surface instead of sinking down, you know that your solution has become soap.

Your next step is to pour it into molds and let it slowly cool over a few days. This allows the acids and bases to continue their reactions and for the mixture to solidify. When cooled, you can cut the soap into bars and allow it to cure for about six to eight weeks. This is an important step because even though your soap is solidified after cooling, it is still too harsh to use on skin. During the weeks of curing, the acids and bases in the soap continue to neutralize each other. The bars themselves will also harden.

Handmade soap is becoming increasingly popular because soap makers often use vegetable oils, such as olive oil or coconut oil, as the base for their products. This produces a naturally moisturizing soap that is gentle on the skin, whereas the additives in commercial soap can irritate and dry out skin.

15. The author would most likely agree with which of the following statements?

   (A) Commercial soap is the best you can buy.
   (B) Selling commercial soap is more profitable than selling hand-made soap.
   (C) Handmade soap smells better than commercial soap.
   (D) Handmade soap is better for sensitive skin than commercial soap.

16. According to the passage,

   (A) fat and lye must be combined in precise proportion to make soap.
   (B) animal fat cannot be used to make soap.
   (C) vegetable oils are unpopular ingredients among soap makers.
   (D) lavender is a main ingredient for making soap.

17. *Saponification* is

    (A) the name for the practice of making soap in pots.
    (B) the point where a soap mixture takes on a creamy color.
    (C) the chemical reaction between soap and lye.
    (D) the point where an oil/lye solution can become soap.

18. In the third paragraph, the word "cure" most nearly means

    (A) ridding the body of disease.
    (B) using animal fat to make soap.
    (C) the hardening and neutralization of soap.
    (D) adding herbs to soap.

19. The tone of the passage is

    (A) informative.
    (B) skeptical.
    (C) bossy.
    (D) gloomy.

20. What kind of fat would be good for making a vegetable-based soap?

    (A) beef tallow
    (B) lard
    (C) coconut oil
    (D) chicken fat

21. Which of the following statements about the passage is not a fact?

    (A) It takes weeks for soap to harden into usable bars.
    (B) Handmade soap is better than commercial-made soap.
    (C) Acid and base molecules in a solution react to create soap.
    (D) The acids and bases in a soap solution neutralize each other.

Use the following passage to answer questions 22 through 25:

Is capital punishment a just punishment for murder? This is one of the most debated topics in American society, and it exemplifies the type of argument that asks one of the essential questions of our existence: what is justice? Because laws are created by people, one could say that justice is what is deemed to be moral and right by the majority.

But what of those who do not agree with these ideas? Are their impressions of justice more or less valid within the scope of the universe? Is there any such thing as a universal right or wrong?

Certainly, most cultures find killing to be wrong, yet every culture kills, whether it is deemed to be right or wrong. Does this mean that killing is a universal right, even though large numbers of people believe it to be wrong?

Questions such as these will likely never be answered, because for every definitive opinion given, there will also be a counteropinion that is just as persuasive. Therefore, arguing for or against capital punishment is a futile task.

22. The speaker in this passage is

    (A) addressing a text.

    (B) arguing with someone else.

    (C) debating with himself.

    (D) responding to a comment.

23. This passage consists of

    (A) a series of questions, answers, and speculation.

    (B) incontrovertible facts.

    (C) academic research.

    (D) biased opinion.

24. In the end, the speaker decides that

    (A) debating the topic is essential.

    (B) every academic should debate this topic.

    (C) there will be only one answer to this debate.

    (D) debating the topic is useless.

25. The purpose of this passage is to

    (A) reason out different perspectives on a social issue.

    (B) persuade the reader to support capital punishment.

    (C) persuade the reader to oppose capital punishment.

    (D) present facts to the reader.

Use the following passage to answer questions 26 through 30:

Owning a pet can result in several health benefits. Studies have shown that cat and dog owners tend to suffer fewer cardiovascular ailments, such as high blood pressure or high cholesterol. They have also found that pet owners who have had heart attacks tend to survive longer, and the presence of a pet in the house is given credit for this phenomenon.

Children who are born into and raised in homes with dogs and other furry companions have shown increased immune system function and decreased risk of developing allergies and asthma. Interacting with pets can also result in increased brain activity and has a calming effect on the body, which is a great help when hormones during puberty cause stress levels in children to rise.

The reason for this is that interacting with a pet can cause your brain to release pleasurable hormones, such as serotonin and dopamine. These chemicals can help stave off depression and increase your general sense of well-being.

26. According to the passage,

    (A) serotonin produces feelings of well-being.

    (B) puberty can be stressful.

    (C) the presence of pets in a house can affect a child's immune system.

    (D) all of the above

27. Based on the passage, it can be inferred that

    (A) having a dog around a baby will make the baby sick.
    (B) common beliefs about cats causing allergies in children are likely untrue.
    (C) a child raised with pets will most likely develop asthma.
    (D) playing with pets can make children hyperactive.

28. The main idea of the passage is

    (A) pets can cause the brain to release pleasurable hormones, such as serotonin and dopamine.
    (B) interacting with pets can result in increased brain activity and have a calming effect on the body.
    (C) owning a pet can result in several health benefits.
    (D) pet owners who have had heart attacks tend to survive longer.

29. Based on information in the passage, buying a pet would be a good gift idea for someone who has

    (A) a brain tumor.
    (B) surgical scars.
    (C) heart palpitations.
    (D) dry skin.

30. According to the passage, dopamine is

    (A) a chemical.
    (B) a hormone.
    (C) both A and B.
    (D) none of the above

Math

Time: 40 minutes

Questions: 40

Directions: Carefully read each question and choose the answer choice that best answers the question.

1. If 1 foot equals 30.48 cm, how many centimeters are in a yard?

    (A) 85.67
    (B) 91.44
    (C) 98.52
    (D) 102.98

2. $2\frac{5}{6}$

    (A) $\frac{9}{6}$
    (B) $\frac{10}{6}$
    (C) $\frac{13}{6}$
    (D) $\frac{17}{6}$

3. At what rate would you have to drive in order to travel 75 miles in 20 minutes?

    (A) 3.75 mph
    (B) 22.55 mph
    (C) 150 mph
    (D) 225 mph

4. Find the LCM of 16 and 12.

    (A) 6
    (B) 26
    (C) 36
    (D) 48

5. $\frac{5}{9} \div \frac{3}{9} =$

    (A) $\frac{5}{27}$
    (B) $1\frac{2}{3}$
    (C) $\frac{3}{5}$
    (D) $2\frac{3}{5}$

6. You have two complementary angles. One of the angles is 45°. The value of the missing angle is

    (A) 45°
    (B) 90°
    (C) 130°
    (D) 180°

7. If $8x + 6 > 6x - 4$, then $x >$

    (A) –2
    (B) 2
    (C) –5
    (D) 5

8. All four sides are congruent, and angles are right angles in a

    (A) pentagon.
    (B) hexagon.
    (C) triangle.
    (D) square.

9. The total surface area of a cylindrical solid that has a radius of 5 feet and a height of 12 feet is

   (A) 60 ft.^{2}

   (B) 112 ft.^{2}

   (C) 533.8 ft.^{2}

   (D) 635.6 ft.^{2}

10. A lecture hall has 266 people attending a speech about biology. Of these people, 60 are history majors, 144 are biology majors, and the rest are undeclared. What is the ratio of history majors to biology majors?

    (A) 5:12

    (B) 30:31

    (C) 12:5

    (D) 31:30

11. $k^2 + 2k + 6$ is a

    (A) coefficient.

    (B) constant.

    (C) quadratic expression.

    (D) variable.

12. $\frac{a^2d}{cd} \times \frac{4y}{2a} =$

    (A) $\frac{2c}{a}$

    (B) $\frac{2ay}{c}$

    (C) $\frac{4a}{c}$

    (D) $\frac{4c}{a}$

13. $3 + 2[1 + 2(1 + 2)]^2$

    (A) 36

    (B) 49

    (C) 98

    (D) 101

14. $(x^3)^3 =$

    (A) x^{-4}

    (B) x^6

    (C) x^9

    (D) x^{-9}

15. Factor: $a^2 - 49$

    (A) $(a - 7)(a - 7)$

    (B) $(a + 7)(a + 7)$

    (C) $(a + 7)(a - 7)$

    (D) none of the above

16. 1 pound = how many grams?

    (A) 28.35

    (B) 283.5

    (C) 453.6

    (D) 464.3

17. You're used to getting up at 8 A.M. To get to your new job on time, you have to get up at 4:30 A.M. Assuming you go to bed at the same time every night, how much less sleep will you get during the course of one full week?

    (A) about $\frac{1}{4}$ of the day

    (B) about $\frac{1}{2}$ of the day

    (C) about $\frac{2}{4}$ of the day

    (D) about 1 day

18. A concert hall can hold 1,253 people. If tonight's show sold out only 82% of the hall, about how many tickets were sold?

    (A) 226

    (B) 568

    (C) 1,027

    (D) 1,171

19. How would you write .36 as a fraction?

   (A) $\frac{2}{15}$

   (B) $\frac{3}{15}$

   (C) $\frac{25}{9}$

   (D) $\frac{9}{25}$

20. If $a = 6$, $b = \sqrt{4}$, and $c = \frac{2}{4}$, then $b^2 + 6ac - b^2c =$

   (A) 18

   (B) 20

   (C) 22

   (D) 24

21. $36.245 + 103.62 =$

   (A) 138.685

   (B) 138.586

   (C) 139.865

   (D) 1,398.65

22.

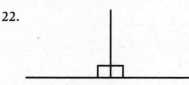

These angles are

   (A) supplementary.

   (B) complementary.

   (C) acute.

   (D) parallel.

23. Your car thermometer says it's 42°F at your house when you leave to run some errands. When you get to the store, it reads 38°F. About how much of a drop in temperature is this measured in degrees Celsius?

   (A) 2°

   (B) 3°

   (C) 4°

   (D) 5°

24. What is 36% of 148?

   (A) 35.82

   (B) 53.28

   (C) 54.28

   (D) 65.36

25. .0257 divided by 32.48 is about

   (A) .00791.

   (B) .00791.

   (C) .000791.

   (D) .0000791.

26. Which of these answers is a whole number?

   (A) $\sqrt{122}$

   (B) $\sqrt{265}$

   (C) $\sqrt{361}$

   (D) $\sqrt{402}$

27. What is the sum of a series of seven consecutive numbers with a median of 4?

   (A) 7

   (B) 16

   (C) 22

   (D) 28

28. The following diagram is an example of a

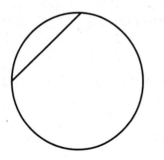

    (A) circumference.

    (B) chord.

    (C) radius.

    (D) diameter.

29. Music lessons for your child will cost $1,265 per year. If you get a part-time job that pays $6.05 per hour, how many hours will you have to work in a year to pay for the music lessons?

    (A) 209.09

    (B) 290.90

    (C) 2,090.90

    (D) 2,909.90

30. What is 6.59843 rounded to the nearest tenth?

    (A) 6.5

    (B) 6.6

    (C) 6.61

    (D) 6.62

31. 62 mi/hr = about how many km/hr?

    (A) 1.61

    (B) 99.8

    (C) 122.9

    (D) 265.2

32. Solve for y: $4y = 128$.

    (A) 32

    (B) 36

    (C) 38

    (D) 42

33. Find the area of a trapezoid with the following values: $h = 8$, $b_1 = 11$, and $b_2 = 14$.

    (A) 10

    (B) 20

    (C) 50

    (D) 100

34. What is the mode of the following set of numbers: 22, 13, 24, 22, 13, 64, 24, 64, 22, 13, 64, 13, 24?

    (A) 13

    (B) 22

    (C) 24

    (D) 64

35. Solve for x: $62°C = x°F$

    (A) 72.6°F

    (B) 94.2°F

    (C) 143.6°F

    (D) 154.2°F

36. The simplest form of $\sqrt{80}$ is

    (A) $2\sqrt{4}$

    (B) $3\sqrt{6}$

    (C) $4\sqrt{5}$

    (D) $6\sqrt{4}$

37. A mathematical statement that combines terms and operations is a(n)

    (A) expression.
    (B) variable.
    (C) constant.
    (D) equation.

Use the following chart to answer questions 38 through 40.

January Sales

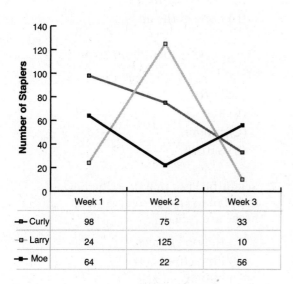

	Week 1	Week 2	Week 3
—◻— Curly	98	75	33
--◻-- Larry	24	125	10
—◼— Moe	64	22	56

38. Larry, Moe, and Curly are competing to be named salesman of the month. To earn this title, one of them would have to sell 250 staplers within a 4-week window. How many staplers would Curly have to sell in week 4 to hit the goal?

    (A) 24
    (B) 44
    (C) 156
    (D) 206

39. Larry loses a key customer who cancels his last two orders of staplers. The first order for 15 staplers was placed in week 1. The second order for 57 staplers was placed in week 2. Given this reduction in Larry's sales record, how many staplers does he have to sell in week 4 to make his 250-stapler goal?

    (A) 63
    (B) 96
    (C) 163
    (D) 206

40. If Moe, Larry, and Curly's sales manager wants his team to reach a sales goal of 1,000 staplers for the month of January, how many more staplers would each of the three men have to sell to reach that target?

    (A) 125
    (B) 156
    (C) 165
    (D) 493

Life Science

Time: 35 minutes

Questions: 30

Directions: For each of the following questions, choose the best answer.

1. The highest layer of the atmosphere is the

   (A) stratosphere.
   (B) exosphere.
   (C) mesosphere.
   (D) troposphere.

2. About 85 percent of Earth's total volume is located in the

   (A) asthenosphere.
   (B) lithosphere.
   (C) outer core.
   (D) mantle.

3. Photosynthesis takes place in

   (A) leaves.
   (B) chloroplasts.
   (C) both A and B.
   (D) neither A nor B.

4. Physical characteristics of an organism, such as having a spine or a shell, are one factor that determines their classification into which taxon?

   (A) kingdom
   (B) phylum
   (C) class
   (D) order

5. Eukaryotic cells are found primarily in

   (A) more complex organisms.
   (B) simple organisms.
   (C) dead organisms.
   (D) none of the above

6. The largest planet in our solar system is

   (A) Earth.
   (B) Mars.
   (C) Jupiter.
   (D) Saturn.

7. Scientific laws that describe how the planets in our solar system move are called

   (A) Newton's Laws.
   (B) Einstein's Laws.
   (C) Voltaire's Laws.
   (D) Kepler's Laws.

8. Sedimentary rock is

   (A) a result of cooling lava.
   (B) a result of erosion of igneous rock.
   (C) transformed in the Earth's interior.
   (D) not where fossils are found.

9. You buy an apple from the local grocer and eat it. The apple is

   (A) a producer.
   (B) a consumer.
   (C) a decomposer.
   (D) a food web.

10. Which kind of biome is characterized by heavy vegetation in the form of trees and plants?

    (A) marine
    (B) tundra
    (C) forest
    (D) grasslands

11. Some earthquakes happen as a result of

    (A) the gravitational pull of the moon.
    (B) the shifting of Earth's tectonic plates.
    (C) an increase in the volume of liquid rock in the outer core of the Earth.
    (D) global warming.

12. The planets orbit the sun in

    (A) circles.
    (B) triangles.
    (C) stars.
    (D) ellipses.

13. The only planet that rotates on its side is

    (A) Mars.
    (B) Venus.
    (C) Uranus.
    (D) Mercury.

14. A pistil is the part of a plant that

    (A) holds the plant's ovaries and ovules.
    (B) keeps the plant rooted to the ground.
    (C) delivers water and nutrients to the plant.
    (D) contains the plant's pollen.

15. ATP, NADPH, and oxygen are used to convert carbon dioxide and water into carbohydrates and oxygen during which phase of photosynthesis?

    (A) light-dependent reactions
    (B) light-independent reactions
    (C) photon capture
    (D) none of the above

16. Aerobic respiration needs what gas to take place?

    (A) carbon dioxide
    (B) hydrogen
    (C) nitrogen
    (D) oxygen

17. Cytosol is

    (A) the whole of a cell's internal components.
    (B) the outer structure or a cell that holds everything else inside.
    (C) the fluid that makes up the majority of a cell.
    (D) subcellular structures that perform a specific function in the lifecycle of a cell.

18. *Canis familiaris* are names that identify a dog in terms of which two taxa?

     (A) genus and species
     (B) family and genus
     (C) order and family
     (D) class and order

19. The portion of a plant that is above ground and provides structure for the plant and its appendages is called the

     (A) root system.
     (B) shoot.
     (C) flower.
     (D) stamen.

20. Aquatic biomes that are characterized by a lack of salt in the water are called

     (A) terrestrial.
     (B) marine.
     (C) freshwater.
     (D) tundra.

21. A system that takes into consideration all of the different food chains within an environment and looks at how they all affect each other is called a

     (A) food web.
     (B) food chain.
     (C) biome.
     (D) ecosystem.

22. What happens when the moon passes behind the Earth?

     (A) The moon is cast in shadow.
     (B) The Earth is cast in shadow.
     (C) The moon casts a shadow on the Earth.
     (D) The sun is blocked from the Earth.

23. Which planet do scientists suspect is made up of mostly hydrogen, with no real surface to speak of?

     (A) Uranus
     (B) Saturn
     (C) Neptune
     (D) all of the above

24. If the sky looks like a blanket of clouds has been rolled out across it, you're looking at

     (A) cumulus clouds.
     (B) cirrus clouds.
     (C) cumulonimbus clouds.
     (D) stratus clouds.

25. Ozone is made in the

     (A) stratosphere.
     (B) exosphere.
     (C) mesosphere.
     (D) troposphere.

26. The inner core of the Earth is made up of

     (A) solid iron and nickel.
     (B) liquid iron and nickel.
     (C) solid ferromagnesium silicates.
     (D) liquid ferromagnesium silicates.

27. Which planet(s) make one complete revolution around the sun in less time than Mars?

     (A) Mercury
     (B) Venus
     (C) Earth
     (D) all of the above

28. Bacteria are often made up of what kind of cell?

    (A) eukaryotic

    (B) plant cell

    (C) prokaryotic

    (D) animal

29. The groove where tectonic plates meet is called a

    (A) mountain.

    (B) fault line.

    (C) volcano.

    (D) tsunami.

30. Molten rock is called what when underground?

    (A) lava

    (B) igneous

    (C) metamorphic

    (D) magma

Biology

Time: 35 minutes

Questions: 30

Directions: For each of the following questions, choose the best answer.

1. Using the Punnett square, what would the blood type of an offspring be if both parents are AO blood type?

   (A) type A only
   (B) type O only
   (C) type A or O
   (D) all ABO types are possible

2. How do enzymes help in cellular metabolism?

   (A) They are proteins that provide chemical reactions in a cell by lowering the amount of energy needed to start these reactions.
   (B) Only small quantities are needed because they do not change or get used up in the reaction.
   (C) Only one enzyme is needed to control all the reactions.
   (D) A and B.

3. Organelles that make or synthesize proteins for use in the cell are

   (A) lysosomes.
   (B) vacuoles.
   (C) ribosomes.
   (D) centrioles.

4. Long chains of amino acids joined by peptide bonds are

   (A) lipids.
   (B) proteins.
   (C) inorganic compounds.
   (D) NADH.

5. The first step in cellular respiration is

   (A) the electron transport chain.
   (B) fermentation.
   (C) Krebs cycle.
   (D) glycolysis.

6. Spindles finish elongating in which phase of mitosis?

   (A) prophase
   (B) metaphase
   (C) anaphase
   (D) telophase

7. Adenine pairs with

   (A) thymine.
   (B) cytosine.
   (C) guanine.
   (D) A and C.

8. DNA unwinds in the

   (A) ribosomes.
   (B) golgi.
   (C) chromatin.
   (D) centrioles.

9. When Mendel conducted his pea plant experiments, he noticed that the ratio of tall plants to short plants was

   (A) 3:1
   (B) 1:3
   (C) 4:1
   (D) 1:4

10. Which of the following types of cells does not go through mitosis?

    (A) skin cells
    (B) heart cells
    (C) liver cells
    (D) sperm

11. Redox is the process by which

    (A) cells replicate.
    (B) atoms lose and gain electrons.
    (C) DNA replicates.
    (D) sugar is turned into ATP.

12. Chloroplasts are found in the cells of

    (A) cats.
    (B) dogs.
    (C) plants.
    (D) monkeys.

13. What gives a cell its structure?

    (A) centrioles
    (B) cytoplasm
    (C) cytoskeleton
    (D) cilia

14. Messenger RNA

    (A) pairs up free nucleotides in the chromatin with their partner nucleotides.
    (B) coils new strands into separate double helixes.
    (C) unzips the DNA strand.
    (D) copies the DNA's sequence in a process called transcription.

15. ADP turns into

    (A) $FADH_2$
    (B) ATP
    (C) NADH
    (D) lipids

Use the following diagram for questions 16 through 18. "T" indicates an allele for tallness. "t" indicates an allele for shortness.

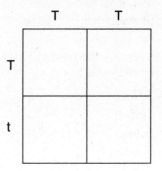

16. What is the probability of these two people having a child that carries a recessive gene for height?

    (A) 1:4
    (B) 2:4
    (C) 3:4
    (D) 4:4

17. The alleles shown at the top of the diagram are

    (A) homozygous.
    (B) heterozygous.
    (C) phenotypical.
    (D) none of the above

18. Based on the data in the square, if this couple had four children, how many would most likely be tall?

    (A) 1
    (B) 2
    (C) 3
    (D) 4

19. Polysaccharides are types of

    (A) enzymes.
    (B) nucleic acids.
    (C) carbohydrates.
    (D) proteins.

20. Oxygen enters the blood in alveoli capillaries through

    (A) diffusion.
    (B) osmosis.
    (C) redox.
    (D) synthesis.

21. Glycolysis takes place in

    (A) chromatin.
    (B) mitochondria.
    (C) endoplasmic reticula.
    (D) cytoplasm.

22. Cellular respiration converts one molecule of glucose into

    (A) 34 ATP.
    (B) 36 ATP.
    (C) 38 ATP.
    (D) 40 ATP.

23. A cell creates all the carbs, lipids, proteins, and enzymes needed to reproduce at some stage during

    (A) S stage.
    (B) G1 stage.
    (C) G2 stage.
    (D) mitosis.

24. A person is homozygous recessive for a particular trait if the person has

    (A) two dominant alleles for the trait.
    (B) two recessive alleles for the trait.
    (C) one dominant and one recessive allele for the trait.
    (D) more than two alleles for the trait.

25. Gametes have how many chromosomes?

    (A) 23
    (B) 32
    (C) 46
    (D) 92

26. Pyrimidines are

    (A) nucleotides.
    (B) cytosine.
    (C) thymine.
    (D) all of the above

27. A carrier of a gene

    (A) does not have the gene in his
        genetic code and does not
        express it physically.
    (B) has the gene in his genetic
        code but does not express it
        physically.
    (C) has the gene in his genetic code
        and expresses it physically.
    (D) none of the above

28. Enzymes are

    (A) chemicals that act as catalysts to
        speed up a reaction by lowering
        a reaction's activation energy.
    (B) redox molecules.
    (C) information carriers.
    (D) molecules that store energy.

29. The anaerobic phase of cellular
    respiration

    (A) takes place in the mitochondria.
    (B) occurs in the absence of oxygen.
    (C) produces a large amount of
        energy of ATP molecules.
    (D) converts pyruvic acid to
        acetyl-coenzyme A and enters
        the citric acid cycle.

30. A diploid cell has how many
    chromosomes?

    (A) 23
    (B) 32
    (C) 46
    (D) 92

Anatomy and Physiology

Time: 35 minutes

Questions: 30

Directions: For each of the following questions, choose the best answer.

1. Which type of muscle is found in the walls of organs such as the stomach and intestines?

    (A) smooth visceral muscle
    (B) skeletal muscle
    (C) multiunit smooth muscle
    (D) cardiac muscle

2. A bone that is part of the upper limbs is

    (A) metatarsal.
    (B) metacarpal.
    (C) tibia.
    (D) fibula.

3. Major events in inspiration include which of the following?

    (A) As the diaphragm moves downward, the size of the thoracic cavity is increased.
    (B) Atmospheric pressure, greater on the outside, forces air into the respiratory tract through air passages.
    (C) Tissue recoiling around the lungs causes the air pressure within the lungs to increase.
    (D) A and B

4. What structure is responsible for making enzymes that detoxify substances we ingest?

    (A) pancreas
    (B) liver
    (C) gallbladder
    (D) small intestine

5. What element of the blood is a factor in phagocytosis?

    (A) red blood cells
    (B) white blood cells
    (C) platelet cells
    (D) plasma cells

6. The normal amount of urine produced in a 24-hour period is approximately

    (A) 300–600 mL.
    (B) less than 300 mL.
    (C) 1,500–2,000 mL.
    (D) more than 3,000 mL.

7. Which hormone helps stimulate the thickening of the endometrium during menstruation?

    (A) testosterone
    (B) progesterone
    (C) FSH (follicle-stimulating hormone)
    (D) corpus leuteum

8. Which of the following is not part of the axial skeleton?

    (A) vertebral column
    (B) skull
    (C) thoracic cage
    (D) upper limbs

9. Which part of the autonomic nervous system is concerned primarily with preparing the body for energy-expending, stressful, or emergency situations?

    (A) sympathetic
    (B) parasympathetic
    (C) somatic
    (D) visceral

10. The root "hypo" means

    (A) brain.
    (B) neck.
    (C) extreme beyond.
    (D) extreme below.

11. Which of the following is a major event of muscle contraction?

    (A) Stimulation occurs when acetylcholine is released from the end of a motor neuron.
    (B) Muscle fibers lengthen.
    (C) Cross bridges between actin and myosin filaments are broken.
    (D) Cholinesterase causes acetylcholine to decompose.

12. A ventral wound is found

    (A) in the abdomen.
    (B) on the side of something.
    (C) below something.
    (D) above something.

13. Which of the following would be considered nonrespiratory air movements?

    (A) inspiration
    (B) expiration
    (C) inspiratory reserve volume
    (D) yawning

14. If neurons are classified by their structural or functional differences, which of the following neurons would be considered functional?

    (A) sensory neurons
    (B) motor neurons
    (C) bipolar neurons
    (D) A and B

15. Blood is made up of all the following except

    (A) erythrocytes.
    (B) bile.
    (C) platelets.
    (D) leukocytes.

16. The upper GI tract consists of

    (A) salivary glands.
    (B) the stomach.
    (C) the esophagus.
    (D) all of the above

17. The pancreas secretes hormones that

    (A) activate the sympathetic nervous system.
    (B) activate the parasympathetic nervous system.
    (C) regulate glucose in the blood.
    (D) regulate the release of female sexual hormones.

18. The opening of the uterus, located at the bottom of the organ and that leads to the vagina, is the

    (A) cervix.
    (B) ovary.
    (C) egg.
    (D) zygote.

19. You are in a car accident. Which part of your nervous system kicks in and floods your body with adrenaline?

    (A) parasympathetic
    (B) sympathetic
    (C) central
    (D) somatic

20. Which of the following is a function of bones?

    (A) They provide shape and support for body structures.
    (B) They produce blood cells.
    (C) They act as levers to aid in body movement.
    (D) all of the above

21. An axon

    (A) travels from neuron to neuron.
    (B) extends off all sides of the rounded cell body like branches from a tree.
    (C) is a long fiber that extends from a cell body to the muscle that receives the impulse.
    (D) receives impulses from the brain or other neurons.

22. Thin fingerlike projections that line part of the duodenum and all of the jejunum and ileum are called

    (A) villi.
    (B) cilia.
    (C) axons.
    (D) chyme.

23. How many bones are in the cervical vertebrae?

    (A) 5
    (B) 7
    (C) 12
    (D) 15

24. The latissimus dorsi are found in the

    (A) chest.
    (B) thighs.
    (C) shoulders.
    (D) abdomen.

25. Striated muscles attach to

    (A) organs.
    (B) bones.
    (C) cartilage.
    (D) tissue.

26. What secretes fluid that makes up semen through the ejaculatory duct?

    (A) seminal vesicle
    (B) prostate gland
    (C) both A and B
    (D) vas deferens

27. The pea-shaped gland located near the bottom of the hypothalamus that can be accessed surgically through the nasal cavity or the roof of the mouth is the

   (A) pineal gland.
   (B) thyroid.
   (C) parathyroid.
   (D) pituitary gland.

28. What kind of neuron takes information from the central nervous system (CNS) to muscles and glands that perform some kind of action?

   (A) sensory
   (B) motor
   (C) somatic
   (D) autonomic

29. When air enters the bronchi, it travels to the

   (A) trachea.
   (B) bronchioles.
   (C) larynx.
   (D) pharynx.

30. Bones are classified according to

   (A) their shape.
   (B) the number of osteoclasts present.
   (C) the joint that the bone articulates with.
   (D) the ligaments and tendons that are connected to the bone.

Chemistry

Time: 35 minutes

Questions: 30

Directions: For each of the following questions, choose the best answer.

1. Five moles of Al equal how many grams?

   (A) 27
   (B) 54
   (C) 124
   (D) 135

2. A bowl of jellybeans in assorted colors is an example of a(n)

   (A) homogeneous mixture.
   (B) heterogeneous mixture.
   (C) solution.
   (D) electrolyte.

3. ^{12}C has how many neutrons?

   (A) 6
   (B) 8
   (C) 12
   (D) 16

4. NaCl is the chemical formula for

   (A) butane.
   (B) propane.
   (C) salt.
   (D) lye.

5. A solution with a pH of 8 is

   (A) slightly acidic.
   (B) slightly basic.
   (C) very acidic.
   (D) very basic.

6. Elements in columns 3–12 on the Periodic Table are

   (A) transition metals.
   (B) nitrogens.
   (C) noble gases.
   (D) alkaline Earth metals.

7. Nonmetals are

   (A) bad conductors of heat.
   (B) dull.
   (C) unable to be shaped or thinned through physical means.
   (D) all of the above

8. Balance the following equation: $Al + CuO \rightarrow Al_2O_3 + Cu$

   (A) $Al + 3CuO \rightarrow Al_2O_3 + 3Cu$
   (B) $2Al + CuO \rightarrow Al_2O_3 + Cu$
   (C) $2Al + 3CuO \rightarrow Al_2O_3 + 3Cu$
   (D) $2Al + 3CuO \rightarrow Al_2O_3 + Cu$

9. Which of the following is not a noble gas?

   (A) helium
   (B) calcium
   (C) argon
   (D) radon

10. The only substance that naturally exists in all three states of matter is

   (A) water.
   (B) nitrogen.
   (C) aluminum.
   (D) magnesium.

11. How many moles of H_2SO_4 would you need to produce 375 grams of sulfuric acid?

   (A) 2.34 moles
   (B) 3.82 moles
   (C) 12.23 moles
   (D) 98 moles

12. Avogadro's number is

   (A) 23.24.
   (B) 6.202×10^{23}.
   (C) 6.022×10^{23}.
   (D) 42.13.

13. Which of the following is a compound?

   (A) Ti
   (B) Li
   (C) H
   (D) C6H12O6

14. A substance that is made up of a single atom with specific properties that can't be chemically broken down into simpler parts is a(n)

   (A) compound.
   (B) element.
   (C) tincture.
   (D) solution.

15. The scientist who defined the four main concepts upon which modern atomic theory is based is

   (A) Einstein.
   (B) Kepler.
   (C) Dalton.
   (D) Galileo.

16. O^+ indicates a(n)

   (A) anion.
   (B) cation.
   (C) isotope.
   (D) neutron.

17. Balance the following equation:
    $(NH_4)_2CO_3 \rightarrow NH_3 + CO_2 + H_2O$

   (A) $(NH_4)2CO_3 \rightarrow 2NH_3 + CO_2 + H_2O$
   (B) $(NH_4)2CO_3 \rightarrow 2NH_3 + 4CO_2 + H_2O$
   (C) $(NH_4)2CO_3 \rightarrow 2NH_3 + 2CO_2 + H_2O$
   (D) $(NH_4)2CO_3 \rightarrow 2NH_3 + 3CO_2 + H_2O$

18. An element in the fifth row of the Periodic Table has how many electron orbitals?

   (A) 2
   (B) 3
   (C) 4
   (D) 5

19. In $3N_2H_6O_4$, the coefficient is

   (A) 2.
   (B) 3.
   (C) 6.
   (D) 4.

20. The chemical symbol for gold is

    (A) Au.
    (B) As.
    (C) Ru.
    (D) Hg.

21. Bonds that are formed when an atom loses electrons that are then picked up by another atom are called

    (A) covalent.
    (B) ionic.
    (C) synthetic.
    (D) displaced.

22. $2Al(s) + Fe_2O_3(aq) \rightarrow Al_2O_3(aq) + 2Fe(s)$ is a

    (A) single displacement reaction.
    (B) decomposition reaction.
    (C) synthesis reaction.
    (D) double displacement reaction.

23. To dilute a solution where water is the solvent and magnesium is the solute, you would

    (A) add more magnesium to the solution.
    (B) add calcium to the solution.
    (C) add water to the solution.
    (D) run an electric current through the solution.

24. If you were to taste a solution that was basic (which you should never do), it would taste

    (A) sweet.
    (B) sour.
    (C) like nothing.
    (D) bitter.

25. How many grams of $Na_2S_2O_3$ would you need to use up 22 g of I_2 using this reaction: $I_2 + 2Na_2S_2O_3 \rightarrow 2NaI + Na_2S_4O_6$?

    (A) 8.12 g
    (B) 11.55 g
    (C) 27.37 g
    (D) 53.16 g

26. What is the molarity (M) of the solute in a solution made up of 22 liters of water and 12 moles of sugar?

    (A) .55 M
    (B) .59 M
    (C) 1.59 M
    (D) 1.89 M

27. Express the following number in scientific notation: 0.0000628

    (A) 6.28×10^5
    (B) 6.28×10^{-5}
    (C) 62.8×10^6
    (D) 62.8×10^{-6}

28. Which of the following could you add to a reaction to reduce the amount of activation energy needed for a reaction to occur?

    (A) solute
    (B) heat
    (C) catalyst
    (D) ions

29. A gas-to-liquid change of matter is an

  (A) endothermic change called
  sublimation.
  (B) exothermic change called
  condensation.
  (C) endothermic change called
  vaporization.
  (D) exothermic change called
  deposition.

30. Nucleons are the

  (A) number of isotopes an element
  has.
  (B) number of valence electrons an
  atom has.
  (C) number of protons the atom
  has and can be found on the
  Periodic Table of Elements.
  (D) total number of protons and
  neutrons in an atom.

Physics

Time: 35 minutes

Questions: 30

Directions: For each of the following questions, choose the best answer.

1. Potential energy is

    (A) the energy an object possesses because of its position or composition.
    (B) the capacity for doing work directly.
    (C) any burning reaction.
    (D) the amount of energy absorbed from an object's surroundings.

2. You multiply an object's volume by its density to find its

    (A) mass.
    (B) kinetic energy.
    (C) potential energy.
    (D) force.

3. What is the kinetic energy of a 2,600-kg pickup truck that is traveling at a velocity of 34 m/s on a highway?

    (A) 1,300 joules
    (B) 14,884 joules
    (C) 1,502,800 joules
    (D) 10,502,800 joules

4. A nuclear reaction that joins the nuclei of at least two atoms is

    (A) radiation.
    (B) fission.
    (C) fusion.
    (D) none of the above

5. How much voltage do you need to push 120 amps of current through 15 ohms of resistance?

    (A) 1,800 volts
    (B) 2,300 volts
    (C) 2,400 volts
    (D) 2,800 volts

6. What law of physics explains why your body moves forward into the seatbelt when you suddenly slam on the brakes of your car?

    (A) Kepler's Law of Planetary Motion
    (B) Newton's First Law
    (C) Newton's Second Law
    (D) Newton's Third Law

7. Suppose it takes you 800 joules of work to move a distance of 50 meters against a force. If you cut your distance in half, what happens to your workload?

    (A) It stays the same.
    (B) It doubles.
    (C) It gets halved.
    (D) No way to tell.

8. The mass of an object that has a volume of 53 m^3 and a density of 24 kg/m^3 is

    (A) 1,072 kg.
    (B) 1,172 kg.
    (C) 1,272 kg.
    (D) 1,372 kg.

9. The type of radiation that emits helium ions and contains two protons and two neutrons is known as

   (A) alpha radiation.
   (B) beta radiation.
   (C) gamma radiation.
   (D) radioisotopes.

10. What is the momentum of a 1,000-kg car that is traveling west on a highway at 65 m/s?

    (A) 28,000 kg/m/s
    (B) 37,000 kg/m/s
    (C) 46,000 kg/m/s
    (D) 65,000 kg/m/s

11. The force of gravity on Earth is always equal to

    (A) 6.8 m/s^2.
    (B) 8.6 m/s^2.
    (C) 8.9 m/s^2.
    (D) 9.8 m/s^2.

12. A cube has a mass of .25 kg. What is its mass in milligrams?

    (A) 250 mg
    (B) 2,500 mg
    (C) 25,000 mg
    (D) 250,000 mg

13. Light travels through a prism and changes its direction. This is an example of

    (A) fission.
    (B) refraction.
    (C) reflection.
    (D) dispersion.

14. A sound wave completes 215 cycles in 65 seconds. What is the frequency of the wave?

    (A) .30 Hz
    (B) .62 Hz
    (C) 3.31 Hz
    (D) 3.33 Hz

15. A light bulb is connected to a series circuit. The bulb will only light up when the circuit

    (A) is closed.
    (B) is open.
    (C) is parallel.
    (D) has resistance.

16. 152.65 K =

    (A) 120.35°C
    (B) 120.35°F
    (C) –120.35°C
    (D) –120.35°F

17. The fizz in your soda decreases when you go outside on a cold day. This is because

    (A) a decrease in temperature causes gas volume to decrease.
    (B) an increase in temperature causes gas volume to increase.
    (C) as the pressure of gas increases, the volume of a fixed amount of gas decreases.
    (D) as the pressure of gas decreases, the volume of a fixed amount of gas increases.

18. Which of the following is not an SI measurement?

    (A) newton
    (B) ohm
    (C) ounce
    (D) watt

19. What is the potential energy of a chair that has a mass of 42 kg when it hangs 1,126 meters above ground?

    (A) 36,461.6 newtons
    (B) 36,461.6 joules
    (C) 436,461.6 kg
    (D) 463,461.6 joules

20. What is the wave speed of a radio wave that has a frequency of 62 Hz and a wavelength of 15 m?

    (A) 320 m/s
    (B) 560 m/s
    (C) 930 m/s
    (D) 1,022 m/s

21. You push your bike 15.29 meters with a force of 10 N. How much work have you done?

    (A) 52.9 joules
    (B) 152.9 joules
    (C) 1,529 joules
    (D) 1,852.9 joules

22. Pressure is measured in

    (A) pascals.
    (B) newtons.
    (C) hertz.
    (D) watts.

23. You know the value of volts. What other value do you need to calculate wattage?

    (A) ohms
    (B) amps
    (C) current
    (D) insulators

24. Liquid molecules have bonds like

    (A) straws.
    (B) metal bands.
    (C) tight string.
    (D) elastic bands.

25. You travel 423 km in 6 hours. What is your average speed?

    (A) 65.5 km/hr
    (B) 68.5 km/hr
    (C) 70.5 km/hr
    (D) 73.5 km/hr

26. What is your rate of acceleration if you decrease your driving speed from 45 m/s to 32 m/s in 65 seconds?

    (A) $-.2$ m/s^2
    (B) .2 m/s^2
    (C) -123 km/s^2
    (D) 123 km/s^2

27. Transfer of energy through force over a distance is

    (A) force.
    (B) speed.
    (C) motion.
    (D) work.

28. Something through which electricity can't pass easily is

    (A) resistance.

    (B) a conductor.

    (C) an insulator.

    (D) voltage.

29. Transverse waves

    (A) reflect off of soft surfaces.

    (B) move parallel to the direction the wave is travelling.

    (C) have high frequencies.

    (D) cause particles in the wave to move perpendicular to the direction of the wave.

30. If you pop a bubble, you are applying

    (A) Boyle's Law.

    (B) Newton's First Law.

    (C) Charles' Law.

    (D) Newton's Second Law.

Practice Test 1: Answers and Explanations

Word Knowledge

1. **B.** "Table" makes the most sense because it means to put off until another time. None of the other answers make sense.

2. **A.** "Virtual" refers to something that is like another thing. In this case, the sentence is comparing a job fair to a meat market.

3. **C.** *Truncate* means "to clip or cut off." *Elongate* means "to make longer." *Envelope* means "to surround."

4. **A.** *Exacerbate* is another word for "aggravate." *Sick* is another word for "ill." You may be tempted to choose C, but "admire" and "envy," though related, are not synonyms. Envy implies wanting something someone else has, which is not necessarily true when you admire something. B has no relationship, and D shows opposites.

5. **C.** When you take all information to be fact, you're simply collecting it, not evaluating it at all. The context clues tell us that the underlined word is the opposite of what the sentence is talking about. Therefore, "discerning" (evaluative) is the correct answer.

6. **A.** A *cadre* is a group that leads a new organization, often associated with political, military, or religious interests. The other answers don't fit: a *boon* is a blessing or something good that happens. A *treaty* is a formal agreement. A *quagmire* is something that's difficult to get out of.

7. **B.** Roots will help you here. *Phobe* means "fear," so the secret to getting this one correct is identifying the roots for the answer choices. *Arachne* is a Greek root meaning "spider"; *xenos* is a Greek root meaning "stranger"; *claustrum* is a Latin root that means "a shut-in place"; and *aero* means "to fly." This makes B the best choice.

8. **B.** Something that is "transdermal" transfers substances through the skin. Something that is "intravenous" transfers substances through a vein.

9. **B.** Context clues in the sentence indicate that the answer we're looking for shows the student did not change his attitude or did not think the teacher's advice was important. The only answer choice that reflects this is B. *Studious* means "interested in or engaging in study." The other answer choices don't really make sense.

10. **D.** As you can infer from the sound of the word, *apropos* refers to something that's appropriate or fitting.

11. **D.** *Capricious* means "to be unstable or going back and forth." Answers A and C are the opposite of this. Answer B is not supported by the sentence, because Jay's loyalties align with whoever is winning.

12. **B.** *Spartan* refers to something that is disciplined, strict, or simply utilitarian, like the warriors of ancient Sparta. Answer B is the opposite of this; Answers C and D don't make sense. Answer A describes strictness and discipline.

13. **C.** In this case, *prescribe* means "to advise in good faith." "Betray" is the opposite of this. When you "subscribe" to something you agree with it; "disagree" is the opposite of

this. The rest of the answer choices are synonyms to one degree or another.

14. **D.** It's obvious from the context of the sentence that Dave is trying to avoid jury duty. *Circumvent* means "to avoid."

15. **B.** "Gait" refers to how someone walks. "Bearing" is the only answer choice that has any association with how a person moves, as it describes posture or the way a person carries him or herself.

16. **C.** "Egregious" is an extreme negative, so your answer choice needs to be an extreme negative as well. *Averse* is not extreme; it just means "opposed to something." *Extroverted* means "outgoing," which is neutral, as is *slow*. C, *wonderful*, is your best bet.

17. **A.** Anyone who has had their mouth numbed in the dentist's chair knows that the anesthetic impairs one's ability to speak. Using context clues, you can figure out that to *garble* is "to make something unintelligible." *Jumble* means "to mix up." *Plait* means "to braid." *Berate* means "to scold."

18. **B.** A *contract* details information about an obligation. A *memoir* details information about a life. Answer A shows an opposite relationship. C and D are "same as" relationships.

19. **A.** A *maverick* goes against the grain and does the unexpected. D is the opposite of this, and although B and C may apply to a maverick, they don't define the word.

20. **C.** *Rancid* means "spoiled."

21. **B.** Yes, the mucus you cough up from your lungs may be gross and it may also be a sign of drainage, but it is

called *sputum*. Asthma is a disease of the lungs involving inflammation and constriction of airways.

22. **C.** *Precocious* refers to a child who is advanced for his or her age. This answer makes the most sense.

23. **C.** A *masochist* is someone who seeks pain. A *hedonist* is a person who seeks pleasure. Answer A shows opposites (front and back). B and D show similarities.

24. **D.** You can infer from the sentence that the "kind offer" was most likely out of concern for the aggrieved daughter. The other answer choices don't make sense in this context.

25. **C.** *Cranium* is another word for "skull." *Patella* is another word for "kneecap." None of the other choices show this relationship: the radius is located next to the ulna; the mandible is used to masticate food; and the sternum connects to the ribs.

26. **D.** *Complacent* means "to be satisfied or content." *Vivacious* and *perky* are synonyms that mean "upbeat" or "full of energy." *Haggard* describes something that is worn or tired.

27. **A.** The sentence talks about someone who believes against the odds. The mayor is determined to keep hope alive. *Steadfast* means "to stay firm in a belief." Answers B and D don't make sense with the context clues in the sentence, which tell us the underlined word would mean the opposite of what the beginning of the sentence implies. Answer D just doesn't make sense.

28. **B.** Even if you don't know that *endogenous* means "originating from within" and *exogenous* means "originating from outside," the prefixes tell you there is an opposite relationship here. *Endo* means "internal;" *exo* means "external." Answer A shows a synonymous relationship. *Khat* is a type of plant, so C doesn't fit. *Bellow* is an extreme form of speaking.

29. **C.** The prefix *mis* means "to be against something." The root *gyn* means "woman or female." Answer C is your best choice.

30. **C.** When you "triage" a situation, you determine what is most urgent and what needs to be attended to after that. The sentence doesn't indicate any of the other answers.

31. **A.** When you "sabotage" something, you purposely cause it harm or to not work. This means Answer A is your best bet because this is the opposite.

32. **A.** "Hypothermia" is a severe form of being cold. "Enraged" is a severe form of being angry. You "borrow" something that belongs to someone else. C and D show similarities between the words, but not extremes.

33. **A.** The sentence implies that the brother is upset at the unfairness of the situation. "Healthy" and "average" are simply not strong enough to match a starved appetite. "Pacified" has to do with calming, which is the opposite of what we need. Your answer is *indignant*, which means "angry."

34. **D.** Haunted houses are designed to be sinister and scary. This is the type of word we're looking for in the blank. None of the other answers have this connotation. To be *apprehensive* means "to have anxiety or fear."

35. **D.** "Constrict" is the opposite of "dilate." *Facilitate* means "to begin something," while *stall* means "to hold back or prevent from moving forward." These are opposites. Answer A shows related words, but with no definite information about what that relationship is. B shows a relationship of degree. C has no relationship.

36. **B.** An *emollient* is something that soothes or relaxes, especially when applied to the skin. Think "lip balm."

37. **A.** Based on the context of the sentence, you're looking for a word that means "reprimanding." A sinister look implies evil intent on the part of the mom, which is not represented in the sentence. *Sly* and *arch* mean "calculating or mischievous." *Scolding*, however, means "reprimanding."

38. **D.** "Febrile" refers to fever (nice alliteration to help you remember there). Answer A is the opposite of what you're looking for, and B and C don't fit.

39. **A.** An extension cord brings power from one place to another. A train brings people from one place to another. B shows similarities. C and D show opposites.

40. **B.** Someone who is "patrician" comes from the upper class. Though the other answers may apply to someone who is patrician, they do not define the word.

Grammar

1. **C.** All of the other answer choices have prepositions as the last word, which is not grammatically correct.

2. **D.** They are "Despite all of the years," "of study," "to become a psychologist," and "to nursing."

3. **A.** A colon is used after an independent clause to indicate to your reader that you will be starting a list, a quote, an example, or another related idea of emphasis.

4. **C.** This is the only answer choice that uses the correct punctuation. Answers A and D should have a comma, not a semicolon. Answer B should have a semicolon, not a colon.

5. **A.** This sentence starts with a question word, making it a question that needs a question mark.

6. **C.** "Who" modifies "patients," which is correct. In Answer A, "wary" should be "weary." Answer B uses "they" to replace "the company," which is an inanimate object and takes the pronoun "it." Answer D uses "then" instead of "than."

7. **A.** People is a plural noun that does not take an "s" to make it plural. So when you make it possessive, you add "'s."

8. **C.** The prepositions in this sentence are "over," "through," and "to."

9. **A.** Plural subject, plural verb.

10. **B.** The clause beginning with "which" is dependent and needs to be separated by a comma.

11. **D.** Because there is "either," the subject is singular and takes the singular verb, "is."

12. **B.** You need a plural possessive noun there. D is not grammatically correct, because "both" is plural. Answer A is incorrect because that is simply the plural form of "artist." Answer C is the singular possessive form of "artist."

13. **C.** You need a comma after this dependent clause in order to set it off from the independent clause that follows it.

14. **B.** "Backslid" is the simple past form of "backslide."

15. **A.** "Both our parents" takes a plural verb.

16. **A.** You may be tempted to say Answer C is correct, too, but this is a possessive pronoun, not noun.

17. **A.** "Not long after his daughter was born" is a dependent clause that needs to be separated from the sentence with a comma.

18. **A.** You're looking for an adjective here, and Answer A is the only adjective. The rest are all adverbs.

19. **C.** There is no such thing as a fractured subject. A singular subject refers to one noun performing an action, while a plural subject refers to more than one noun performing an action.

20. **B.** There is no verb in this sentence, which makes it a fragment.

21. **C.** Adjectives modify nouns and pronouns; adverbs modify everything else.

22. **D.** The subject and verb do not match up. "Blake" is a third-person singular subject. "Am" is a first-person singular form of "to be." This sentence needs the third-person singular form, which is "is."

23. **D.** This is a compound predicate. The subject did not do one or the other, she did both.

24. **A.** Answer B has a misplaced modifier situation. "At the park" modifies "in high school," when it is clearly meant to modify "every Sunday afternoon." There's a pronoun disagreement with Answer C; "their" should be "his." In Answer D, the subject, "the panel speakers," is plural but the verb, "its," is singular.

25. **B.** A semicolon connects two related independent clauses.

26. **D.** A park can't be broken or crushed. It can be blanketed with snow or leaves. But that's not the case here. D makes the most sense.

27. **C.** This sentence is in the subjunctive case, which means that it is stating a hypothetical or desire. You use "were" in this case in conjunction with "wish." You could also use "could" or "would" in the subjunctive case, but they wouldn't work in this sentence.

28. **A.** Phrases are groups of words that don't have a subject and verb but act as a unit. A prepositional phrase has a preposition, a noun/pronoun as the direct object, and sometimes a modifier. A declarative sentence is a statement and ends with a period.

29. **A.** A concert can't bellow, reek, or prepare. It can open and it can close, making A the best choice.

30. **A.** A period ends a declarative sentence. A comma separates two independent clauses when a conjunction is used and both clauses are equal. A semicolon connects two related independent clauses when no conjunction is used (or separates items in a list that contains commas within an item or items).

31. **B.** A and C don't make sense with the beginning of the sentence. D doesn't work because it talks about the past in a part of the sentence that refers to the future.

32. **C.** "Back-to-school" is being used as a compound modifier for "shopping." It needs to be hyphenated so that the words act as a single adjective.

33. **A.** Collective nouns name a group. Proper nouns identify specific people, places, things, or ideas. Possessive nouns show ownership of something.

34. **C.** A compound subject has more than one subject for one verb. A preposition links nouns, pronouns, and phrases to other words in a sentence by describing some kind of relationship. A direct object shows who or what receives the action in the sentence.

35. **A.** This should be "I couldn't care less." Saying you "could care less" doesn't make sense.

36. **C.** In first person perspective, the speaker is the subject. In second person perspective, the speaker is addressing someone specific (you). Perspective has nothing to do with tense.

37. **B.** This should be "intents and purposes."

38. **B.** Songs can't really be generous, treatable, or proud. They can be memorable and the mention of "less familiar" makes this the best choice.

39. **B.** When you infer, you use information you take in to come to a conclusion. This doesn't make sense for this sentence. You want "imply" instead, because that means to hint at something.

40. **C.** Phrases are groups of words that don't have a subject and verb, but act as a unit. Adverbs modify verbs, adjectives, and other adverbs. Indirect objects show to what or whom an action is performed.

Spelling

1. C		31. B	
2. B		32. A	
3. A		33. B	
4. B		34. C	
5. A		35. A	
6. C		36. C	
7. C		37. B	
8. B		38. A	
9. A		39. C	
10. B		40. C	
11. C			
12. B			
13. A			
14. A			
15. C			
16. A			
17. B			
18. B			
19. C			
20. A			
21. C			
22. A			
23. B			
24. C			
25. A			
26. C			
27. B			
28. C			
29. B			
30. A			

Reading Comprehension

1. **B.** The fourth paragraph says: "Role-playing with your child can also help her distinguish between a fun discussion and a serious argument." All of the other answer choices go against information in the passage.

2. **D.** Context clues early in the sentence point to "teasing."

3. **A.** The first sentence says: "Five-year-old Emma Zeilnhofer of West Milford, New Jersey, grew nervous when she saw her mom, Sue, arguing with her partner, Millie, over the color of an umbrella."

4. **D.** This statement is the one that is most clearly an opinion. The inclusion of "should" implies that this is advice that is given, and in the context of the rest of the passage, it makes sense.

5. **B.** This answer makes the most sense.

6. **B.** All of the other answer choices are contradicted by the passage.

7. **C.** This game is described in the fourth paragraph.

8. **C.** The last sentence of the first paragraph states that "the microorganisms that cause these ailments." From this you can infer that microorganisms cause infection.

9. **A.** The third paragraph states that a reservoir "can be anything from the soil in your garden to the lining of your digestive tract to your computer keyboard."

10. **D.** Each of the other answer choices is directly supported by statements in the passage.

11. **C.** The second paragraph defines invasiveness as how a pathogen can "move and enter the body through tissues."

12. **B.** The sentence where the word is found reads: "The person who is exposed must be susceptible to the invasion of the microorganism." The word is further explained in the following sentence, which points to B as your answer: "This means that he or she must not have adequate physical or immunological resistance to the infectious agent."

13. **B.** The passage specifically discusses washing hands: "If a person uses a bathroom where infected fecal matter has been and does not wash his or her hands properly, those hands can pick up the pathogens and act as the mode of transmission if they make contact with the mouth, eyes, or blood—all points of entry." Answer A may be right, but it's not supported by the passage. Answers C and D are not supported by the passage.

14. **D.** The passage does not address any of the topics listed in the other answer choices. It does, however, thoroughly explain the chain of infection.

15. **D.** This is stated in the final paragraph, where it says: "This produces a naturally moisturizing soap that is gentle on the skin, whereas the additives in commercial soap can irritate and dry out skin."

16. **A.** This is stated in the first line of the passage.

17. **D.** The last sentence in the second paragraph says saponification is "when your solution has reached a point where it will become soap."

18. **C.** The third paragraph says: "During the weeks of curing, the acids and bases in the soap continue to neutralize each other. The bars themselves will also harden."

19. **A.** This passage is providing information in a neutral tone. Answer A is the best choice.

20. **C.** This is the only vegetable-based oil listed.

21. **B.** All of the other statements are based on facts from the passage. By saying something is better than something else, the speaker of the statement is stating an opinion.

22. **C.** Because no other source of information is being presented to us, it can be assumed that all the debate is coming from the speaker.

23. **A.** Answer B is too extreme and inaccurate. Answer C is incorrect since there is no academic information in the passage. There is no indication of bias one way or another in the speaker's words, which eliminates Answer D.

24. **D.** The final sentence reads, "Therefore, arguing for or against capital punishment is a futile task."

25. **A.** There are no actual facts presented in the passage, just suppositions from the speaker. There is also no clear-cut persuasion going on here, because the speaker concludes that no decision can be made either way on the topic. Answer A makes the most sense.

26. **D.** Each of these statements is supported by the passage.

27. **B.** The passage states that studies show "children who are born into and raised in homes with dogs and other furry companions have shown increased immune system function and decreased risk of developing allergies and asthma." None of the other choices are supported by the passage.

28. **C.** The rest of the answer choices are details presented in the passage.

29. **C.** The passage specifically says, "Studies have shown that cat and dog owners tend to suffer fewer cardiovascular ailments, such as high blood pressure or high cholesterol." The heart is a key part of the cardiovascular system. No mention of the other areas of health were made in the passage.

30. **C.** The passage states: "The reason for this is that interacting with a pet can cause your brain to release pleasurable hormones, such as serotonin and dopamine. These chemicals can help stave off depression and increase your general sense of well-being."

Math

1. **B.** There are 3 feet in a yard, so multiply 30.48 times 3 to get 91.44.

2. **D.** Multiply the denominator by the whole number and then add the numerator: $6 \times 2 + 5 = 17$. Place the 17 over the denominator for your final improper fraction.

3. **D.** Use the Distance = Rate × Time formula here: $75 = r \times 20$. Divide 75 by 20 to get 3.75 minutes. Now multiply this by 60, because your answers show miles per *hour*, not miles per minute. Final answer is 225 mph.

4. **D.** $16 = 2 \times 2 \times 2 \times 2$, and $12 = 2 \times 2 \times 3$. Our factors are 2 and 3. The most times 2 appears in one factorization is four, while 3 only appears once. Multiply $2 \times 2 \times 2 \times 2 \times 3 = 48$.

5. **B.** Because we're dividing fractions, flip the second fraction and multiply across to get your answer. Then reduce.

6. **A.** Complementary angles are two angles that share a common side and whose combined value equals 90°.

7. **C.** Solve like any other equation, keeping track of the direction of the inequality.

$8x + 6 > 6x - 4$

$8x - 6x + 6 > \underline{6x - 6x} - 4$

$2x + 6 > -4$

$2x + 6 - 6 > -4 - 6$

$2x > -10$

$\frac{2x}{2} > \frac{-10}{2}$

$x > -5$

8. **D.** Pentagons have five sides. Hexagons have six sides. Triangles have three sides.

9. **C.** To calculate total surface area, use the formula $TSA = 2\pi r(r + h)$. Plug in your values and solve:

$TSA = 2 \times 3.14 \times 5 \times (5 + 12)$

$TSA = 2 \times 3.14 \times 5 \times 17$

$TSA = 2 \times 3.14 \times 5 \times (17)$

$TSA = 6.28 \times 5 \times 17$

$TSA = 31.4 \times 17$

$TSA = 533.8$

10. **A.** The ratio is 60:144. Both of these numbers have 12 as a common factor. If you divide both by 12, you have 5:12, which is your final answer.

11. **C.** This is an example of a quadratic expression: $ax^2 + bx + c$.

12. **B.** Multiply straight across and then take out lowest terms:

$\frac{a^2 d}{cd} \times \frac{y}{2a} = \frac{4a^2 dy}{2acd} = \frac{4a\,\cancel{ad}\,y}{2\,\cancel{acd}} = \frac{4y}{2c} = \frac{2y}{c}$

13. **D.** Start with the inner expression in parentheses (not the brackets, which indicate that all processes within must be addressed first) and calculate the answer, 3. The parentheses around the 3 indicate that you must multiply. Within the brackets, multiply 2×3 first and then add $1 + 6$. Next, apply the exponent to the 7 to get 49. Next, multiply 2×49 to get 98; finally, add the 3. Your work should look like this: $3 + 2\,[1 + 2(3)]^2 = 3 + 2\,[1 + 6]^2 = 3 + 2\,[7]^2 = 3 + 2 \times 49 = 3 + 98 = 101$.

14. **C.** When you apply an exponent to terms in parentheses that have powers, you multiply exponents to simplify the expression:

$(x^3)^3 = x^{3 \times 3} = x^9$.

15. **C.** This involves simple factoring, because you have a binomial made up of squares. Break it into two binomial expressions that have the roots of the squares. In this case, *a* and 7. Because the original expression has a negative, at least one of your signs is going to be a negative as well. If you FOIL the binomials, the two middle terms will have to cancel each other out in order to give you your original expression. This means one sign will be negative and one positive. In this case, it doesn't matter which. The correct answer is $(a + 7)(a - 7)$.

16. **C.** 1 ounce = 28.35 grams. 16 ounces makes 1 pound. Multiply 16×28.35 to find that 1 pound is equal to about 453.6 grams.

17. **D.** You lose 3.5 hours of sleep per day. Multiply this over a 7-day week, and you end up losing 24.5 hours total. This equals about a whole day.

18. **C.** This question is all about percents. Calculate 82 percent of 1,253: $.82 \times 1,253 = 1,027$.

19. **D.** .36 is the same as $\frac{36}{100}$. However, this is not the simplest form of the fraction. Reduce by 4, the GCF for these two numbers. Your final fraction should be $\frac{9}{25}$.

20. **B.** Start by simplifying the variables:

$a = 6$

$b = \sqrt{4} = 2$

$c = \frac{2}{4} = \frac{1}{2}$

Now replace the variables with their values in the expression:

$2^2 + 6 \times 6 \times \frac{1}{2} - 2^2 \times \frac{1}{2}$

Finally, work the order of operations, starting with exponents:

1. $4 + 6 \times 6 \times \frac{1}{2} - 4 \times \frac{1}{2}$

2. $4 + 18 - 2$

3. $22 - 2 = 20$

21. **C.** 103.620
    +36.245
    139.865

22. **A.** Supplementary angles together make a straight line. The sum of the angles equals 180°. Complementary angles make a right angle. Acute angles have a degree value of less than 90. Parallel refers not to angles, but to lines that run next to each other but never meet.

23. **A.** To solve this problem, you need to convert your original temperatures from Fahrenheit to Celsius using the following formula: $(F - 32) \times \frac{5}{9} = C$:

$(42 - 32) \times \frac{5}{9} = 10 \times \frac{5}{9} = \frac{10}{1} \times \frac{5}{9} = \frac{50}{9} = 5.56 \text{ C}$

$(38 - 32) \times \frac{5}{9} = 6 \times \frac{5}{9} = \frac{6}{1} \times \frac{5}{9} = \frac{30}{9} = 3.33 \text{ C}$

Now find the difference between the temperature when you left your house and the temperature at the store: $5.56 - 3.33 = 2.23$. Round down to 2 because the question is asking "about how much of a change" this is.

24. **B.** $.36 \times 148 = 53.28$

25. **C.** You don't have to divide this problem out completely to get to the answer; only enough to tell you how many zeros come after the decimal point:

$$32.48\overline{)\,.0257}$$

$$3248\overline{)\,025700}^{\,.0007}$$

As you can see, you move the decimal place to the right two places in both the divisor and the dividend. 3248 does not go into 25, 257, or 2570. It does go into 25700, which means three zeroes go after the decimal point before you can show how many times the divisor goes into the dividend.

26. **C.** $\sqrt{361} = 19$

27. **D.** If the median of a set of seven numbers is 4, your numbers are 1, 2, 3, 4, 5, 6, 7. Add them all together to get 28.

28. **B.** A chord is a segment in a circle that touches any two points of the edge. A diameter is a type of chord, but it has to go directly through the center of the circle. The line in this diagram does not.

29. **A.** Divide the amount of money needed by the hourly rate to get the number of hours that you will have to work:

$$6.05\overline{)\,1265.00}$$

$$605\overline{)\,126500.00}^{\,209.09}$$
$$\underline{-\,1210}$$
$$550$$
$$\underline{-\,000}$$
$$5500$$
$$\underline{-\,5445}$$
$$550$$
$$\underline{-\,000}$$
$$5500$$
$$\underline{-\,5445}$$
$$55$$

30. **B.** The first place after the decimal point is the tenths place. The number is 5, so you look to the number next to it to see if you should round up or down. The number in the hundredths place is 9, which means you round up to 6.6.

31. **B.** One mile = 1.609344 kilometers. Multiply 1.609344 by 62 and you get 99.779328 kilometers.

32. **A.** This is a simple equation. Isolate the y by dividing each side by 4. This gives you 32 as your answer.

33. **D.** Use the formula for calculating the area of a trapezoid here:

$$A = \tfrac{1}{2}h(b_1 + b_2) = \tfrac{1}{2}8(11+14) = 4 \times 25 = 100$$

34. **A.** Mode describes the number within a set of numbers that appears the most times. In this case, 13 appears four times, while all the others only appear three times.

35. **C.** Convert Celsius to Fahrenheit using the following formula: $°C \times \frac{9}{5} + 32 = F$. Plug in your numbers and solve.

36. **C.** Roots can be simplified if the number under the radical sign has a factor that is a perfect square. In this case,

    you have: $\sqrt{80} = \sqrt{16 \times 5} = \sqrt{4 \times 4 \times 5}$.

    Factor out the square and place it outside as a coefficient. The remaining factor stays inside the radical

    sign: $4\sqrt{5}$.

37. **A.** A variable is a letter in an equation or expression that stands in place of an unknown quantity. A constant is a number that stands by itself in an expression or equation. An equation is a mathematical statement that shows two equal expressions.

38. **B.** The chart tells you that so far, Curly has already sold 206 staplers. He needs to sell at least 44 more to reach his goal.

39. **C.** Overall, Larry has sold 159 staplers. Subtract the cancelled order from this amount (159 – 72), and you'll find his adjusted total is 87. Now subtract that amount from the goal, which is 250, and you have the number of staplers Larry would have to sell to meet his goal: 163.

40. **C.** During week 1, 186 staplers were sold. During week 2, 222 were sold. During week 3, 99 were sold. The total is 507. Subtract that from 1,000 and find that Moe, Larry, and Curly would have to sell 493 staplers collectively. Divide that amount by 3 and get 164.33, or 165 whole staplers, because they wouldn't be able to sell part of a stapler.

Life Science

1. **B.** Answers A and C make up the middle atmosphere. D makes up the lower atmosphere.

2. **D.** Answers A and B make up part of the mantle, but it's the mantle itself that makes up about 85 percent of the Earth's volume.

3. **C.** Photosynthesis takes place in the leaves of a plant, specifically in the chloroplasts of the cells.

4. **B.** The other factor is the degree of evolution relation to others within a population.

5. **A.** Simple organisms have prokaryotic cells. Dead organisms can have either, since the answer doesn't specify what type of organism.

6. **C.** All of the other planets are smaller than Jupiter.

7. **D.** It was Kepler who discovered the fixed elliptical movements of the planets.

8. **B.** Answer A describes igneous rock. C describes metamorphic rock. D is not true.

9. **A.** You, a consumer, eat the apple. The apple is the fruit of a plant, which are producers.

10. **C.** Marine biomes are saltwater bodies. Tundra is like frozen desert in Arctic areas and at the tops of high mountains. Grasslands are plains that don't have many trees at all.

11. **B.** The Earth's tectonic plates kind of float on top of the asthenosphere, which is made up of semiliquid rock. Because of this, tectonic plates shift, which results in earthquakes, volcanic eruptions, tsunamis, and the occasional sinking or creation of an island. The increasing use of fossil fuels has imbalanced the carbon cycle. Carbon dioxide is being released into the atmosphere faster than it is being used. This is causing the Earth to warm.

12. **D.** Kepler's first law establishes this.

13. **C.** Uranus rotates on a horizontal axis. All of the other planets revolve on a vertical axis.

14. **A.** Pistils are a plant's female reproductive organ.

15. **B.** These reactions take place in the second part of photosynthesis and do not require light to happen.

16. **D.** Aerobic respiration needs oxygen for ATP production. Anaerobic respiration does not need oxygen for ATP production.

17. **C.** Answer A describes cytoplasm. B describes a plasma membrane. D describes organelles.

18. **A.** *Canis* is the genus and *familiaris* is the species.

19. **B.** The root system is underground. The flower and stamen are parts of a plant's reproductive system.

20. **C.** Freshwater biomes are defined by their lack of salt, whereas marine biomes have a high concentration of salt in the water. The other types of biomes in the answer choices are land based, not aquatic.

21. **A.** This is the definition of a food web.

22. **A.** This describes a lunar eclipse. The Earth blocks sunlight from reaching the moon.

23. **C.** Neptune is one of 4 gas giants, which is a large planet that is not made up of mostly solid matter. Scientists speculate that Neptune is mostly made up of hydrogen with no real surface to speak of.

24. **D.** Stratus clouds blanket the sky and are uniform in color.

25. **A.** The higher up in the stratosphere you get, the higher the temperature rises, which results in the formation of ozone. This helps deflect solar radiation from reaching the lower atmosphere.

26. **A.** The inner core is about 750 miles thick and made of solid iron and nickel. The outer core is made entirely of molten rock, mostly iron and nickel.

27. **D.** Kepler's third law of planetary motion states that the amount of time it takes a planet to orbit the sun one time depends on its distance from the sun. This means that the farther a planet is from the sun, the longer it takes to orbit it. Because A, B, and C are all closer to the sun, they all make the trip in less time. Specifically, in Earth days, Mercury = 88, Venus = 225, Earth = 365, and Mars = 685.

28. **C.** Bacteria are simple organisms, mostly prokaryotes.

29. **B.** A mountain is a mass of land that is much higher than the other landforms around it. A volcano is a vent in the Earth's surface that allows heat, gas, and magma to travel from the interior of the planet to the surface. A tsunami is a huge series of waves that are generated as a result of a seismic activity that disturbs a large volume of water.

30. **D.** Underground, it's magma. When it reaches the surface, it's lava.

Biology

1. **C.** The possibilities are AA, AO, and OO.

2. **D.** Each reaction is controlled by a specific enzyme.

3. **C.** Lysosomes hold enzymes that the cell creates. Vacuoles act as storage containers within a cell. Centrioles are little tube-like structures whose only purpose is to assist in cell division, whether through asexual or sexual reproduction.

4. **B.** Lipids are fats. Inorganic compounds don't have carbon in their make-up. NADH stands for nicotinamide adenine dinucleotide. It is a coenzyme used in cellular respiration.

5. **D.** The order is glycolysis, Krebs cycle, and electron transport chain.

6. **B.** During metaphase, the spindles finish elongating, and the chromosomes attach themselves along the length of the spindle apparatus.

7. **A.** Adenine can only pair with thymine. Guanine can only pair with cytosine.

8. **C.** DNA replication takes place in chromatin. All of the other answer choices are organelles.

9. **A.** Mendel observed that for every breeding of purely tall plants with purely short plants (no hybrids), three tall plants and one short plant would be reduced.

10. **D.** Mitosis happens with all types of cells except those used in sexual reproduction.

11. **B.** *Oxidation* refers to the process by which atoms lose electrons. This is always coupled with a process called *reduction*, which is the gain of electrons by an atom. Together, they are called *redox*.

12. **C.** Chloroplasts are specialized organelles within which photosynthesis takes place.

13. **C.** Cytoskeletons are made of strands of protein that help give a cell structure and also anchor the structures inside the cell. Centrioles are little tube-like structures whose only purpose is to assist in cell division. Cytoplasm holds all of the internal structures inside a cell. Cilia are hair-like structures that wiggle in order to make a cell move.

14. **D.** Enzymes perform the functions in A and C.

15. **B.** ADP is turned into ATP during the electron transfer chain process of cellular respiration.

16. **B.** The top two boxes combine to make "TT" and the bottom two boxes combine to make "Tt." This is a 2:4 split.

17. **A.** Homozygous gene pairs are made up of two of the same alleles. Heterozygous gene pairs are made up of two different alleles. *Phenotypical* refers to phenotype, which is the physical expression of genes.

18. **D.** The tallness gene is dominant. Each of the four boxes has a dominant allele for tallness in it, which means that it is most likely to be the one expressed. The recessive allele would be carried, not expressed.

19. **C.** Polysaccharides are a type of sugar, which is a carbohydrate.

20. **A.** Diffusion is simply the passing of molecules across a plasma membrane. This happens in the lungs when oxygen-poor blood is pumped from the heart.

21. **D.** DNA replication takes place in chromatin. The Krebs cycle takes place in mitochondria. Endoplasmic reticula assist ribosomes in creating proteins and act as a storage center for ions and steroids.

22. **C.** If you add together the 2 ATP from glycolysis, the 2 ATP from the Krebs cycle, and the 34 from the electron transport chain, you have a total of 38 ATP produced from one molecule of glucose.

23. **B.** G_1 is a growth stage and can last years in slow-growing cells. New organelles that will be passed on to the daughter cells created at the end of mitosis are also formed and stored.

24. **B.** Homozygous for a trait means that the person has two of the same alleles.

25. **A.** A gamete only has 23 single chromosomes (not paired ones like in mitosis), as opposed to the 46 present in other cells. This is so that when a gamete mixes with another gamete, the resulting cell has the 46 chromosomes it should instead of 92.

26. **D.** Deoxyribonucleic acid (DNA) is a nucleic acid made up of sequenced pairs of two types of nucleotides: purines (adenine and guanine) and pyridimines (cytosine and thymine).

27. **B.** This means that the information that causes this condition is written in their genetic code but does not affect the person who carries that code. Because the gene is not expressed, it is said to be "carried."

28. **A.** B describes $FADH_2$. C describes nucleic acids. D describes lipids.

29. **B.** A, C, and D all occur in aerobic respiration.

30. **C.** When a gamete is by itself, with its 23 chromosomes, it's called a *haploid*. When the number of its chromosomes doubles after fertilization, the resulting cell (zygote) is called a *diploid*.

Anatomy and Physiology

1. **A.** Skeletal muscle allows for movement of bones at joints and maintenance of posture. Multiunit smooth muscle occurs as separate fibers and is found in irises of eyes and walls of blood vessels. Cardiac muscle is found only in the heart.

2. **B.** Answers A, C, and D are bones of the lower limbs.

3. **D.** Tissue recoiling around the lungs causes the air pressure within the lungs to increase and is a major event in expiration.

4. **B.** The liver is a filter for the blood that removes wastes, toxins, and bacteria that are transferred into the bloodstream from the intestine.

5. **B.** White blood cells protect the body against infection by attacking invading parasites, viruses, bacteria, and sometimes allergens, in addition to helping dispose of dead or damaged cells. They do this through phagocytosis, a process of surrounding another cell and breaking it down. The red blood cells carry oxygen. Platelets are fragments in the blood. Plasma is the liquid portion of the blood.

6. **C.** Adults produce around 1.5 to 2 liters of urine daily. This converts to 1,500 to 2,000 milliliters. Both A and B may be related to kidney problems. D can be related to excessive fluid intake or a problem with antidiuretic hormone production.

7. **B.** Progesterone maintains the lining of the uterus (endometrium) for pregnancy and regulates menstruation. Follicle-stimulating hormone (FSH) secreted by the pituitary gland helps to produce sperm cells in males and stimulate the ovaries to enlarge in females at puberty. Testosterone stimulates the development of secondary sex characteristics and helps sperm cells to mature. During ovulation, the corpus luteum is formed, which helps thicken the uterine wall.

8. **D.** Upper limbs are part of the appendicular skeleton.

9. **A.** Answer B, the parasympathetic part of the autonomic nervous system, is active under ordinary, restful conditions and counterbalances the effects of the sympathetic section and restores the body to a restful state. Answer C is not a part of the autonomic nervous system, and Answer D does not name a part of the nervous system.

10. **D.** Answer A is "crani." B is "cervic." C is "hyper."

11. **A.** Answers B, C, and D are major events in muscle relaxation.

12. **A.** Answer B is "lateral." C is "inferior." D is "superior."

13. **D.** With yawning, not all alveoli are ventilated, and some blood may pass through the lungs without being oxygenated; the low oxygen level triggers the yawn reflex.

14. **D.** Bipolar neurons are classified as structural.

15. **B.** Bile is secreted by the liver and stored in the gallbladder.

16. **D.** Each of these answer choices names a part of the upper GI tract.

17. **C.** The adrenal glands do A and B. Ovaries control female sexual hormones.

18. **A.** Ovaries hold eggs. A zygote is a fertilized egg.

19. **B.** The sympathetic nervous system provides a response to stress, often referred to as "fight or flight." When a stressor, such as a scare or sexual arousal, affects the body, the nerves in this system react by generating more energy, hormones, and efficient blood flow to vital organs to prepare your body to handle the stress. In a sympathetic response, adrenaline flows, your heart rate increases, your temperature goes up, and your respiration increases.

20. **D.** All of the answers are functions of bone.

21. **C.** Answers B and D describe dendrites. Answer A describes impulses.

22. **A.** Cilia are fine hairs in the nose and trachea. Axons are part of neurons. Chyme is a mixture of stomach juices and food.

23. **B.** Thoracic vertebrae have 12; lumbar vertebrae have 5.

24. **C.** *Latissimus dorsi* literally means "broadest muscle in the back" in Latin.

25. **B.** Striated muscles are also known as *skeletal muscles* because they are attached to the bones of the skeleton.

26. **C.** The vas deferens connects the testes to the seminal vesicle and prostate gland.

27. **D.** The pineal gland is a tiny gland at the top of the brain stem. The thyroid and parathyroid glands are located together around the outside of the throat.

28. **B.** Sensory neurons bring information about a stimulus to the CNS. Somatic and autonomic describe subsystems within the peripheral nervous system.

29. **B.** Air travels through the parts named in all of the other answer choices before it gets to the bronchioles.

30. **A.** Bones can be classified according to their osseous tissue type (compact or spongy) and their shape (long, short, flat, or irregular).

1. **D.** The atomic weight of aluminum is 27. Multiply that by 5 to get 135 grams.

2. **B.** Heterogeneous mixtures are those that contain two or more substances that retain all of their distinct physical and chemical properties. Because jellybeans are made up of two or more substances, each with specific physical and chemical properties, this is a heterogeneous mixture. An electrolyte is a substance that conducts [...] when in a sol[...] homogeneou[s...] more substan[...] solutions tha[...] concentratio[n...]

3. **A.** Carbon ha[s...] 6 and a mass [...] the atomic n[...] number and [...] neutrons, w[...]

4. **C.** The chem[...] sodium chl[oride...]

5. **B.** On the p[...] higher up t[...] basic the so[...] you go, the [...]

6. **A.** Nitrogen [...] gases are i[...] Earth met[...]

7. **D.** All of th[...] nonmetal[...]

8. **C.** To brin[g...] the same proportion as the Al on the right, you add 2 as a coefficient. Now balance the oxygens by adding a 3 to the CuO compound on the left. This also raises the number of Cu on the left, so to balance it out, add 3 as a coefficient to the Cu on the right.

9. **B.** Calcium is an alkaline metal.

10. **A.** Water is the only substance on Earth that naturally exists in all three states of matter.

11. **B.** This is the formula for sulfuric acid. You need to use stoichiometry for this. We first figure out the atomic weight of the H_2SO_4:

$$H = 1 \times 2 = 2$$

4

mass: $2 + 32 + 64 = 98$

[...] that 1 mole of H_2SO_4 is [...] divide this number into 375 [...] s Number $= 6.022 \times 10^{23}$, [...] uch more compact way [...] 2,200,000,000,000,000,00 [...] ium. B is lithium. H is [...] is the chemical formula [...] which is a compound. [...] und is when two or more [...] re chemically bonded [...] tincture is a solution that [...] l as the solvent. A solution [...] re of a solute with a solvent. [...] , Jonathan Dalton published [...] ystem of Chemical [...] y, which presented four [...] t atomic relationships that nas served as the basis of modern atomic theory.

16. **B.** A cation is an atom with a positive charge. An anion is an atom with a negative charge. An isotope is when there are two atoms of the same element that contain different numbers of neutrons. A neutron is a subatomic particle that carries no charge.

17. **A.** The only thing you have to do here is add a 2 as a coefficient to the NH_3 on the right side of the equation.

18. **D.** Each of the elements in a row has the same number of orbitals as the row's number.

19. **B.** A coefficient comes before the element and is not a subscript.

20. **A.** B is arsenic, C is ruthenium, and D is mercury.

21. **B.** The result of this loss of electrons is that one atom takes on a negative charge, while the other takes on a positive charge. The atoms are then attracted to each other because they are now ions of opposing charges. A covalent bond occurs when one or more electron pairs are shared between two atoms. The others do not apply to bonds.

22. **A.** A single displacement reaction is one where an element reacts with a compound and replaces an element in the compound. A synthesis reaction combines two reactants that break the existing chemical bonds and form new ones. A decomposition reaction is the opposite of a synthesis reaction. A double displacement reaction happens when ionic compounds are added to an aqueous solution—each pair of elements in the compounds separate to become cations and anions. Within the solution, new ionic bonds are formed between ions of opposite charge, resulting in a swap of ion partners.

23. **C.** When you add volume to the solvent in a solution, you reduce the molarity of a solution, thereby diluting it.

24. **D.** Bases taste bitter.

25. **C.** For every diatomic molecule of iodine, you need two molecules of $Na_2S_2O_3$, so your ratio is 1:2. Now find out how many moles of I_2 are in 22 g of I. The atomic weight of iodine is 127; multiply by 2 to get 254 amu. This tells us that 1 mole of I_2 is equal to 254 g. Divide the number of grams in your equation by the number of grams that equals 1 mole of I_2: 22 ÷ 254 = .0866. This means that 22 g is equal to .0866 moles of I_2.

   Since we have a 1:2 ratio between I_2 and $Na_2S_2O_3$, you now multiply .0866 by 2 to find out how many moles of $Na_2S_2O_3$ you need for this reaction: .0866 × 2 = .1732 moles of $Na_2S_2O_3$ to use up 22 g of I_2. Now multiply this by the atomic mass of $Na_2S_2O_3$ and get 27.37 g:

   Na = 23 × 2 = 46

   S = 32 × 2 = 64

   O = 16 × 3 = 48

   46 + 64 + 48 = 158 × .1732 = 27.37 g

26. **A.** Divide 12 by 22 to get .55.

27. **B.** When you have a number that is less than 1, you move the decimal point after the first nonzero number after the decimal's original position and express the number of places moved with a negative exponent.

28. **C.** This is the definition of a catalyst. In a solution, one substance is called a *solute* and one substance is called a *solvent*. Heat is usually used to accelerate a chemical reaction. An ion is an atom that carries an electrical charge.

29. **B.** A (sublimation) describes a solid-to-gas change. C (vaporization) describes a liquid-to-gas change. D (deposition) describes a gas-to-solid change.

30. **D.** Nucleons represent the total number of protons and neutrons for an element; this is also the mass number for the element.

Physics

1. **A.** Kinetic is the energy of motion. Exothermia is any emission of energy into the environment. Endothermia is the absorption of energy from the surrounding environment.

2. **A.** This is the formula for mass.

3. **C.** The formula for kinetic energy is $\frac{1}{2}mv^2$: $\frac{1}{2} \times 2{,}600 \times 34^2 = \frac{1}{2} \times 2{,}600 \times 1{,}156 = 1{,}300 \times 1{,}156 = 1{,}502{,}800$ joules.

4. **C.** Radiation is when the nucleus of an atom begins to break down or enter a transformation process. Fission takes an atom and splits it apart.

5. **A.** Your formula is Volts = Amps × Ohms: $120 \times 15 = 1{,}800$ volts.

6. **B.** Kepler's Law has to do with how the planets move in ellipses. Newton's Second Law has to do with calculating force; his third law is "For every action, there is an equal and opposite reaction."

7. **C.** Work is directly proportionate to distance traveled.

8. **C.** Your formula is mass = dv: $24 \times 53 = 1{,}272$ kg.

9. **A.** Beta radiation is composed of high-energy, high-speed electrons and is negatively charged. Gamma radiation is composed of high-energy, electromagnetic radiation that has no charge.

10. **D.** Momentum is calculated by multiplying velocity times mass: $1{,}000 \times 65 = 65{,}000$. It's expressed in kilogram meters per second.

11. **D.** On Earth, the force of gravity is always equal to 9.8 m/s² or 32.2 f/s².

12. **D.** One kilogram = 1,000,000 milligrams. If you divide 1,000,000 by 4 and then find what one quarter (.25) of your kilograms is in milligrams, you find that .25 kg = 250,000 mg.

13. **B.** Fission has to do with splitting atoms. Reflection is the bouncing of waves off a surface. Dispersion is when a wave is split up by frequency.

14. **C.** To measure frequency, divide the number of times a complete wave is made during a given time: $215 \div 65 = 3.308$. Round up to 3.31 and you have your answer.

15. **A.** A circuit needs to be closed to be complete. This ensures the current makes it from the power source to the light bulb.

16. **C.** To go from Kelvin to Celsius, subtract 273 from the Kelvin value: $152.65 - 273 = -120.35$.

17. **A.** This is an example of Charles' Law. The temperature goes down when going into a cold environment, so the gas volume decreases.

18. **C.** Ounce is a measure of volume in the American system of measures.

19. **D.** First, potential energy (any energy, actually) is measured in joules, so A and C are out. Your formula is $PE = mgh$: $42 \times 9.8 \times 1{,}126 = 463{,}461.6$ joules.

20. **C.** Wave speed is a measure of how fast the wave is travelling. Multiply the wavelength measure by the frequency: $15 \times 62 = 930$ m/s.

21. **B.** Your formula is $W = fd$: $10 \times 15.29 = 152.9$ joules.

22. **A.** Newtons measure force. Hertz measures frequency. Watts measure power.

23. **B.** Watts = volts × amps.

24. **D.** Liquids have loose bonds but not as loose as those in gases.

25. **C.** Divide distance by time here: $423 \div 6 = 70.5$ km/hr.

26. **A.** To calculate deceleration, subtract final speed from your initial speed and then divide the difference by the time it took to go from one speed to the other: $32 - 45 = -13$; $-13 \div 65 = -0.2$ m/s^2.

27. **D.** Force is something that changes the motion of an object. Speed is how fast an object is moving. Motion describes any object that changes distance over a period of time.

28. **C.** Resistance is something that slows down the flow of electricity. Conductors are materials through which electricity can pass easily. Voltage is the strength with which current flows through a conductor.

29. **D.** Transverse wave patterns cause particles in the wave to move perpendicular to the direction of the wave. For example, if a wave is moving forward, the pattern of the wave would be to move up and down.

30. **A.** Boyle's Law deals with pressure and volume. It states that as the pressure of gas increases, the volume of a fixed amount of gas decreases and vice versa. When you pop a bubble, you apply pressure to the outside of the bubble, which increases the pressure of the gas inside. The bubble bursts when the amount of pressure breaks the bonds of the bubble.

Practice Test 2

Word Knowledge

Time: 40 minutes

Questions: 40

Directions: For each of the following questions, choose the best answer out of the choices given.

1. Seattle's _____ climate makes it ideal for those who are not overly fond of extremely cold or hot weather.

    (A) lacking
    (B) excessive
    (C) seasonal
    (D) temperate

2. <u>Myriad</u> most nearly means

    (A) mild.
    (B) many.
    (C) mindful.
    (D) myopic.

3. After conducting tests to see if the infection spread further into the tissue, the doctor concluded that it was confined to the epidermis of the hand.

   The underlined word in the previous sentence most nearly means

   (A) muscle.
   (B) bone structure.
   (C) inner layer of skin.
   (D) outer layer of skin.

4. Belligerent most nearly means

   (A) welcoming.
   (B) abusive.
   (C) smelly.
   (D) active.

5. Barry goaded me to finally get rid of my old analog TV and get a flat-screen TV.

   The underlined word in the previous sentence most nearly means

   (A) promised.
   (B) prompted.
   (C) forgave.
   (D) teased.

6. The increasing length of the war quickly _____ the country's finances and manpower.

   (A) infused
   (B) depleted
   (C) sustained
   (D) marginalized

7. Swank most nearly means

   (A) blistering.
   (B) famous.
   (C) svelte.
   (D) grand.

8. We need someone who can picture the overall campaign as well as design the minutia needed to lead us to our goal.

   The underlined word in the previous sentence most nearly means

   (A) details.
   (B) big picture.
   (C) time frame.
   (D) appeal.

9. Vivacious most nearly means

   (A) staid.
   (B) brisk.
   (C) reticent.
   (D) living.

10. penitent : regret ::

    (A) valued : disregard
    (B) awed : reverence
    (C) overwhelmed : sedate
    (D) fanciful : logical

11. Because of my dyslexia, I often _____ p and b when I write the word plumber; it ends up looking like blumper.

    (A) impress
    (B) transpose
    (C) ruin
    (D) berate

12. When the IV bag had drained off all its contents, it hung <u>flaccid</u> on the stand.

The underlined word in the previous sentence most nearly means

(A) limp.

(B) strong.

(C) contained.

(D) taut.

13. A <u>perforation</u> is a(n)

(A) disease.

(B) syndrome.

(C) tear.

(D) emergency.

14. capitol : laws ::

(A) foreign : unfamiliar

(B) original : trite

(C) torrent : downpour

(D) bakery : pastries

15. Although Jimmy was _____ about being away from home for the first time, it helped that he had his best friend with him as he took the bus to camp.

(A) apprehensive

(B) fantastical

(C) courteous

(D) reluctant

16. The Halloween block party was a spooky affair with lots of <u>costumery</u> on people young and old.

The underlined word in the previous sentence most nearly means

(A) people dancing.

(B) people talking.

(C) people in costumes.

(D) people fighting.

17. <u>Oblique</u> most nearly means

(A) indirect.

(B) nimble.

(C) straightforward.

(D) easy.

18. cog : grandfather clock ::

(A) delve : get into

(B) hatchback : car

(C) strawberry : jam

(D) microchip : computer

19. <u>Intrepid</u> most nearly means

(A) nautical.

(B) warm.

(C) daring.

(D) boring.

20. The weather went from a light drizzle to a fierce downpour that <u>pelted</u> me with raindrops.

The underlined word in the previous sentence most nearly means

(A) repeatedly hit.

(B) hardly felt.

(C) overcome.

(D) dressed in furs.

21. murder : crows ::

    (A) crime : shame
    (B) harass : bother
    (C) pod : dolphins
    (D) listen : absorb

22. The ankle joint is located at the <u>distal</u> end of the tibia or shin bone.

    The underlined word in the previous sentence most nearly means

    (A) hardest.
    (B) broken.
    (C) farthest.
    (D) top.

23. <u>Introvert</u> describes someone who is

    (A) excited.
    (B) optimistic.
    (C) pessimistic.
    (D) shy.

24. After a(n) _____ search effort that encompassed hundreds of miles, the man was not able to locate a source of water for the village.

    (A) heroic
    (B) fortuitous
    (C) intimate
    (D) immense

25. annual : year ::

    (A) decennial : decade
    (B) slow : progress
    (C) filtered : distilled
    (D) treatment : synopsis

26. If you have an arterial <u>occlusion</u>, that means one of your arteries is

    (A) blocked.
    (B) hardened.
    (C) transforming.
    (D) buried.

27. A <u>laceration</u> is a(n)

    (A) disease.
    (B) syndrome.
    (C) cut.
    (D) emergency.

28. When the patient complained of pain on the right side of his chest, the doctor considered causes of <u>unilateral</u> distress in this area of the body.

    The underlined word in the previous sentence most nearly means

    (A) one sided.
    (B) two sided.
    (C) same side.
    (D) no sides.

29. Because the lesion was changing in shape over time, the dermatologist felt it necessary to <u>excise</u> it.

    The underlined word in the previous sentence most nearly means

    (A) add on.
    (B) cut off.
    (C) burn.
    (D) freeze.

30. <u>Corrosive</u> most nearly means

    (A) challenging.
    (B) strengthening.
    (C) basic.
    (D) eroding.

31. <u>Inexorable</u> most nearly means

    (A) beautiful.
    (B) revered.
    (C) balanced.
    (D) unrelenting.

32. attrition : gain ::

    (A) over : above
    (B) pass : fail
    (C) forever : infinity
    (D) oblivion : nothing

33. forge : metal ::

    (A) castle : home
    (B) arsenal : armory
    (C) plateau : landform
    (D) stove : food

34. <u>Distended</u> most nearly means

    (A) angry.
    (B) red.
    (C) torn.
    (D) swollen.

35. The <u>gratuitous</u> praise John was giving me made me question his motives.

The underlined word in the previous sentence most nearly means

    (A) welcome.
    (B) generous.
    (C) unwarranted.
    (D) creative.

36. Though the years had taken their toll on Olivia's 100-year-old body, you could still see a <u>vestige</u> of her younger self when you looked at her.

The underlined word in the previous sentence most nearly means

    (A) picture.
    (B) shred.
    (C) frame.
    (D) parody.

37. Her smile and optimistic words of encouragement in even the toughest circumstances made Jane the ideal candidate to be a(n) _____ team leader.

    (A) darkening
    (B) threatening
    (C) sanguine
    (D) unconscious

38. Persnickety most nearly means

    (A) unintelligible.
    (B) particular.
    (C) cranky.
    (D) fluid.

39. The move from working the intake desk in the emergency room to working the intake desk in the maternity ward was a <u>lateral</u> move.

The underlined word in the previous sentence most nearly means

    (A) a step up.
    (B) a step down.
    (C) a demotion.
    (D) at the same level.

40. Laconic most nearly means
    (A) florid.
    (B) angry.
    (C) pithy.
    (D) lazy.

Grammar

Time: 40 minutes

Questions: 40

Directions: For each of the following questions, choose the best answer out of the choices given.

1. Collective nouns

   (A) indicate tense.
   (B) are plural.
   (C) name a person.
   (D) name a group.

2. Which word best completes this sentence?

   Why _____ there no more potato chips left?

   (A) is
   (B) are
   (C) would
   (D) could

3. Which word in the following sentence is used incorrectly?

   The hotel is just a little further down the expressway.

   (A) is
   (B) just
   (C) further
   (D) expressway

4. Which word best completes this sentence?

   Ben saw no alternative but to take matters into _____ own hands.

   (A) its
   (B) their
   (C) his
   (D) her

5. Which of the answer choices is grammatically correct?

   (A) Jennie questioned her teacher, Miss Jones, when she gave her test back.
   (B) The man walked to the doctor's office when they could have taken the bus.
   (C) Her mom was angry when she came home with a scrape in the car's bumper.
   (D) Anyone who paid attention to the lecture doesn't have to worry about his or her performance on the test.

6. Which verb would make this sentence grammatically correct?

   My girlfriend and I _____ to the movies last week.

   (A) stayed out
   (B) going out
   (C) go out
   (D) went out

7. Which word in the following sentence is used incorrectly?

   Ross just could not except that his girlfriend was breaking up with him.

   (A) just
   (B) except
   (C) was
   (D) up

8. Which word best completes this sentence?

Vicky _____ to take a walk in the evening.

(A) likes
(B) complains
(C) eats
(D) sings

9. What word(s) make(s) up the predicate in the following sentence?

Listen to the rain fall outside.

(A) Listen
(B) to the rain
(C) fall
(D) outside

10. Many adverbs end with the suffix

(A) -ly.
(B) -ed.
(C) -ing.
(D) -s.

11. Which word best completes this sentence?

There used to be a _____ of trees in this neighborhood.

(A) markedly
(B) fortunate
(C) graceful
(D) host

12. Which word in the following sentence is used incorrectly?

My grandfather emigrated to the United States after World War II.

(A) My
(B) emigrated
(C) after
(D) II

13. What is the adjective in the following sentence?

My previous anatomy professor was much easier to understand.

(A) My
(B) previous
(C) professor
(D) easier

14. Which pronoun would make this sentence grammatically correct?

Jordan made the picture _____.

(A) herself
(B) itself
(C) themself
(D) themselves

15. What punctuation is needed to correct this sentence?

The mail carrier rang the doorbell, and he handed me the package.

(A) no comma after "doorbell"
(B) a semicolon after "doorbell"
(C) a colon after "doorbell"
(D) no change

16. Which word in the following sentence is used incorrectly?

I object to wearing fur and leather on principal.

(A) object
(B) wearing
(C) leather
(D) principal

17. What is the indirect object in the following sentence?

On her blog, Beverly listed all of the things she wanted to do this summer.

(A) On her blog
(B) all of the things she wanted to do this summer
(C) this summer
(D) the things

18. The verb *to be* is

(A) only used in first person.
(B) regular.
(C) irregular.
(D) only used in third person.

19. Which word would make this sentence grammatically correct?

Neither my mom _____ my sister knows anything about my missing skirt.

(A) or
(B) were
(C) nor
(D) are

20. What is the prepositional phrase in the following sentence?

Our new house is just over the river.

(A) Our new house
(B) over the river
(C) the river
(D) just over

21. Which word best completes this sentence?

The night was full of memories from those who have been touched by the legendary actor's _____.

(A) outbursts
(B) toys
(C) life
(D) motorcycles

22. Which word in the following sentence is used incorrectly?

There's no use trying to illicit information out of me; I don't know anything.

(A) There's
(B) trying
(C) illicit
(D) anything

23. Possessive pronouns show

(A) ownership.
(B) description.
(C) action.
(D) who receives action.

24. What shows the action the subject of a sentence is performing?

  (A) preposition
  (B) predicate
  (C) direct object
  (D) indirect object

25. Words that link nouns, pronouns, and phrases to other words in a sentence by describing some kind of relationship are

  (A) pronouns.
  (B) adverbs.
  (C) adjectives.
  (D) prepositions.

26. What shows who or what is performing the action in a sentence?

  (A) regular verbs
  (B) relative pronouns
  (C) predicate
  (D) subject

27. Which word best completes this sentence?

  When the entire _____ was released on DVD, I was excited to finally be able to catch up on all that I'd missed.

  (A) series
  (B) serious
  (C) seals
  (D) sears

28. Which word in the following sentence is used incorrectly?

  Set yourself down right here and take a load off your feet.

  (A) Set
  (B) right
  (C) load
  (D) off

29. Which verb would make this sentence grammatically correct?

  When we were kids, we _____ this silly nursery rhyme over and over.

  (A) sing
  (B) sang
  (C) sung
  (D) have sung

30. What is the adverb in the following sentence?

  The test was amazingly easy.

  (A) test
  (B) was
  (C) amazingly
  (D) easy

31. Which word in the following sentence is used incorrectly?

  That is a capitol idea!

  (A) That
  (B) is
  (C) capitol
  (D) idea

32. What is/are the pronoun(s) in the following sentence?

    That has to be the hardest question anyone has ever asked me.

    (A) That
    (B) That and anyone
    (C) anyone and me
    (D) That, anyone, and me

33. Which of the answer choices is grammatically correct?

    (A) The cars and the vans was expected to arrive by 3 p.m.
    (B) The gas tank and nozzle need to be repaired.
    (C) I remember either the rides or the cotton candy stand were at the end of the aisle.
    (D) I have no doubt the neither Greg nor his brother's cousins is going to come to the concert.

34. What punctuation is needed to correct this sentence?

    Though we are more educated about mental illness than we were in previous decades, we're still battling stigmas that are continually inflamed by the media.

    (A) a comma after "Though"
    (B) a semicolon instead of a comma after "decades"
    (C) no apostrophe in "we're"
    (D) no change

35. What is the subject in the following sentence?

    The elegant woman took her time looking through the rack of designer dresses.

    (A) the rack of designer dresses
    (B) The elegant woman
    (C) took her time
    (D) looking through

36. Which word would make this sentence grammatically correct?

    The church group boarded the bus and greeted _____ driver.

    (A) their
    (B) its
    (C) there
    (D) it's

37. Which of the answer choices is grammatically correct?

    (A) Their is very little that I don't know about that topic.
    (B) The smell in the lab was assaulting they're senses.
    (C) Is there anything better than a warm spring afternoon?
    (D) That is neither here nor their.

38. Which word in the following sentence is used incorrectly?

    There saying that it will only be a few more minutes until we're seated.

    (A) There
    (B) saying
    (C) until
    (D) we're

39. Which of the answer choices is grammatically correct?

   (A) To whom would you like to speak?
   (B) Who are you going to call?
   (C) Who should I ask about my check?
   (D) Who do you want to talk to?

40. Which word best completes this sentence?

   It seems there are a million ideas and plans out there to help people lose _____.

   (A) time
   (B) change
   (C) wait
   (D) weight

Spelling

Time: 40 minutes

Questions: 40

Directions: For each of the following examples, choose the letter that shows the correctly spelled word.

1. (A) resparation (B) respiration (C) resperation
2. (A) edeema (B) adema (C) edema
3. (A) palpitation (B) palpatation (C) palpetation
4. (A) dialation (B) dilation (C) dielation
5. (A) disstension (B) distenshun (C) distension
6. (A) cyst (B) syst (C) cysst
7. (A) epedemic (B) epademic (C) epidemic
8. (A) obstruction (B) obastruction (C) obstructcion
9. (A) posterior (B) postearior (C) postirior
10. (A) reumatic (B) rheumatic (C) rumatic
11. (A) sty (B) stie (C) stei
12. (A) anelgesic (B) analgesic (C) anilgesic
13. (A) antecoagulant (B) anticagulant (C) anticoagulant
14. (A) tranquillizer (B) tranquiliser (C) tranquilliser
15. (A) surgeon (B) surgon (C) surgoen
16. (A) phisician (B) physician (C) physican
17. (A) quarentine (B) quarantine (C) quarintine
18. (A) peacable (B) piecable (C) peaceable
19. (A) dominent (B) domanant (C) dominant
20. (A) recessive (B) reccessive (C) reccesive
21. (A) begnining (B) beggining (C) beginning
22. (A) acomplish (B) accomplish (C) akomplish
23. (A) hemmorhage (B) hemmorage (C) hemorrhage
24. (A) concieve (B) conceive (C) conceve
25. (A) buiscit (B) biscit (C) biscuit
26. (A) irresisteble (B) irresistible (C) irresistable
27. (A) ireversible (B) irreversible (C) irreversable
28. (A) femoral (B) femeral (C) femerol
29. (A) recead (B) receed (C) recede
30. (A) mussle (B) muscle (C) muscel
31. (A) yield (B) yeild (C) yeald
32. (A) undowtedly (B) undoutedly (C) undoubtedly
33. (A) theries (B) theorys (C) theories
34. (A) secede (B) cecede (C) cesede
35. (A) personel (B) personnel (C) personnell
36. (A) psycholigy (B) psycology (C) psychology

37. (A) questionnaire (B) questionnare
    (C) questionaire

38. (A) restaraunt (B) restraunt
    (C) restaurant

39. (A) privilege (B) privledge
    (C) privalege

40. (A) permissable (B) permissible
    (C) permisible

Reading Comprehension

Time: 40 minutes

Questions: 30

Directions: Read each of the following passages, and choose the best answer for each of the questions that follow.

Use the following passage to answer questions 1 through 6:

Wind farms are one of the leading sources of sustainable energy growth in the United States. Such farms contain one or more turbines with giant blades that are turned by the wind. This action converts the kinetic energy of the wind into mechanical energy through the rotation of the blades. The mechanical energy is then routed to a generator within the turbine, which converts that energy into yet another form: electricity.

Winds of between 16 and 50 km/hr are needed to start a wind turbine's blades turning and get it up to speed for the best possible energy production. This means that establishing wind farms in areas that experience a steady flow of high-energy wind are a good idea. Strips of land facing the ocean are a great option. Winds from the sea are constantly blowing because of the lack of interference from buildings or landforms. With electronic settings that will automatically shut down the blades should high-force winds, such as those in a hurricane, gust and possibly damage the turbine, the risk of damage to an investment in this area is low.

1. A good title for this passage would be

   (A) Wind Farms Produce the Most Electricity in the Nation
   (B) Sustainable Energy Now!
   (C) Wind Farms: A Sustainable Energy Source Based on Science
   (D) The U.S. Switches its Power Supply to Wind Energy

2. According to the passage, wind has

   (A) kinetic energy.
   (B) potential energy.
   (C) mechanical energy.
   (D) rotational energy.

3. The purpose of this passage is to

   (A) incite action.
   (B) inform.
   (C) publicize.
   (D) editorialize.

4. Based on information from the passage, a good place to build a wind farm would be

   (A) in a city park.
   (B) within a crowded neighborhood.
   (C) in a valley.
   (D) in a wide-open field.

5. According to the passage, why is the risk in investing in a seaside wind farm low?

   (A) Most residents are not likely to oppose the construction.

   (B) Wind turbines have protection measures to prevent damage from wind.

   (C) Return on investment has been historically high.

   (D) None of the above

6. Wind turbines turn kinetic energy into mechanical energy by

   (A) generators in turbines.

   (B) the rotation of blades.

   (C) the building of turbines.

   (D) none of the above

Use the following passage to answer questions 7 through 12:

Everyone should take an interest in their local government. Not enough people attend their local town council meetings; therefore, they are not informed about the decisions their leaders are making about laws that can affect their lives.

At a town council meeting, an entire agenda of issues is discussed publicly. Members of the council move from item to item, presenting their views on whatever the issue is and eventually taking some kind of action. This can include casting a vote to approve or reject a new law, tabling an issue until more information can be presented, or even making a motion for a new item to be considered immediately or at the next meeting.

There is also usually a public portion of a council meeting. After all of the official business has been handled, comments from the public are heard and entered into the record. This is a rare opportunity for citizens of the town to speak their minds about the issues being discussed. They can also present new issues for the council to address. This is a vital portion of the meeting. It is one of the few chances for the people to question the actions of their elected officials and to ensure that they are being fairly represented.

It's our responsibility as American citizens to monitor the actions of our elected officials and hold them accountable. If we don't, then who will?

7. According to the passage, the average citizen

   (A) is not informed about the actions of their local government.
   (B) attends town council meetings regularly.
   (C) has a good understanding of how local government works.
   (D) pays attention to their surroundings.

8. In the passage, <u>accountable</u> most nearly means

   (A) interested in an outcome.
   (B) has assets at stake.
   (C) responsible for one's actions.
   (D) informed about circumstances.

9. The author of this passage would most likely agree with which of the following statements?

   (A) Too many people come to council meetings.
   (B) Elected officials must answer to the public.
   (C) Council meetings are the best place to air a grievance about the community.
   (D) Town councils should recognize citizens more often.

10. How are elected officials held accountable as a result of public meetings?

    (A) Those who elect them can monitor their official actions.
    (B) The comments and votes that a council member makes is recorded.
    (C) Constituents can directly question council members about their actions.
    (D) All of the above

11. Which of the following statements from the passage is a fact?

    (A) Everyone should take an interest in their local government.
    (B) Not enough people attend their local town council meetings.
    (C) Members of the council move from item to item, presenting their views on whatever the issue is and eventually taking some kind of action.
    (D) It's our responsibility as American citizens to monitor the actions of our elected officials and hold them accountable.

12. This passage is intended to

    (A) inform.
    (B) persuade.
    (C) enrage.
    (D) confuse.

Use the following passage to answer questions 13 through 18:

Most people think of communication in terms of a one-way process where a sender encodes a message that is transmitted to a receiver. However, advancing research in communication studies indicates that most communication is systemic, meaning that conception and transmission of a message is only one part of the equation.

Listener-centric models of communication are taking center stage today. These assert that communication takes place simultaneously through verbal and nonverbal signals from sender to receiver and back again. Furthermore, internal communication, such as thoughts and perception of external stimuli, is also taking place and influencing how both the sender and the receiver interpret messages and form their responses.

It may be better to think of communication as a volleying game of tennis. The sender plans a strategy for executing her game. Speaking is analogous to serving the ball. The receiver then analyzes the message he is receiving and determine the best way to respond, just as the tennis player's opponent needs to analyze the best way to counter the serve.

After the response is formulated, it's sent back to the sender, who will then become the receiver and decide how to counter the message. Just like in tennis, back-and-forth communication is a constant volley between participants.

13. A good title for this passage might be

    (A) Listen Up: Things Are Not What They Seem

    (B) Sender-Focused Communication Is the Future

    (C) Communication as an Interactive Process

    (D) Listener-Centric Communication Models Gain Acceptance

14. According to the passage, thoughts and evaluating perceptions are forms of

    (A) external communication.

    (B) internal communication.

    (C) external stimuli.

    (D) external foci.

15. The sentence that states the main idea of the passage is:

    (A) However, advancing research in communication studies indicates that most communication is systemic, meaning that conception and transmission of a message is only one part of the equation.

    (B) Most people think of communication in terms of a one-way process where a sender encodes a message that is transmitted to a receiver.

    (C) Listener-centric models of communication are taking center stage today.

    (D) It may be better to think of communication as a volleying game of tennis.

16. Which of the following statements from the passage is not a fact?

    (A) Communication takes place simultaneously through verbal and nonverbal signals from sender to receiver and back again.
    (B) Listener-centric models of communication are taking center stage today.
    (C) It may be better to think of communication as a volleying game of tennis.
    (D) Internal communication, such as thoughts and perception of external stimuli, is also taking place and influencing how both the sender and the receiver interpret messages and form their responses.

17. According to the passage, what kind of communication models are becoming more prominent?

    (A) Listener-centric models
    (B) Sender-centric models
    (C) Content-focused models
    (D) Reaction-focused models

18. The tone of this passage is

    (A) exclamatory.
    (B) explanatory.
    (C) incendiary.
    (D) controversial.

Use the following passage to answer questions 19 through 24:

The introduction of electronic devices that keep us constantly connected to work, friends, and family, coupled with an increasingly long workweek, is resulting in chronic exhaustion among U.S. adults. This increases levels of stress the body experiences and thus leads to increased levels of adrenaline. Chemically, our bodies are constantly on edge, which expends a lot of physical and mental energy.

Most adults aren't even aware of the amount of stress they are under during a normal workday because they have become desensitized to its effects in order to get through the tasks they have on their plate. The physical costs of this desensitization, however, are greater than one might imagine.

Chronic stress has been linked to increased levels of stress hormones in the body, specifically cortisol. Prolonged imbalance of this chemical places strain on arteries and organs, which can result in a variety of physical ailments. Metabolic syndrome, high blood pressure (often referred to as "the silent killer"), obesity, and collection of fat in the abdomen have all been linked to cortisol imbalance.

Though completely unplugging may not be an option for most people, a good compromise for many might be to set some limits as to how connected they need to be with the outside world—particularly their jobs. A moratorium on checking emails and answering text messages from 6 to 9 P.M. would enable people to spend more time interacting in person with friends and family or even just to relax for a while.

19. In this passage, the word <u>desensitized</u> most nearly means

(A) more able to physically handle something.

(B) becoming more aware of one's surroundings.

(C) losing the ability to feel or notice something.

(D) more able to remember.

20. According to the passage, a cause of exhaustion is

(A) lack of time away from work.

(B) constant interaction with electronic communication devices.

(C) chemical imbalances caused by external stressors.

(D) all of the above

21. The tone of this passage is

(A) flippant.

(B) concerned.

(C) glib.

(D) bored.

22. The author would most likely support

(A) a stress-awareness campaign being distributed to employees at Fortune 500 companies.

(B) an increase in the number of hours in the standard workweek.

(C) the introduction of computer software that would forward calls to a built-in hands-free phone in your car.

(D) a political candidate whose agenda includes increasing the country's gross national product.

23. This passage

(A) advocates for a paperless society.

(B) advises people to never use electronic devices.

(C) provides an overview of a problem and presents a possible solution.

(D) uses the latest scientific research to make its point.

24. The author's solution to stress caused by constant engagement with electronic media is to

(A) throw out all of your electronic media.

(B) take yoga classes.

(C) get medication to deal with your stress.

(D) unplug for a few hours a day and use the time to relax and enjoy life.

Use the following passage to answer questions 25 through 30:

Vinegar is an extremely versatile substance that can be used all around the house. First, its highly acidic and antibacterial properties make it an excellent natural food preservative. Mixing vinegar with garlic, dill, and other spices produces a brine that can be used to pickle vegetables or marinate meats.

Vinegar is also an effective nonchemical cleaner that can be used on all sorts of surfaces including metal, wood, glass, fabrics, and linoleum. Though its odor is very pungent and distinct, vinegar solutions can be used to clean and deodorize coffeemakers, microwaves, sinks, and bathrooms. This is a great alternative to using chemical-based products and just as effective. You can count on the antibacterial effects of vinegar to help protect yourself and your family against foodborne and other types of bacteria that cause illness.

Vinegar can also be used to treat areas of the house that have been soiled by pets. It even works as a natural way to prevent infestations of fleas and ticks on animals. Fleas don't like the smell or taste of vinegar or the fact that it is so acidic. By bathing your pet in a gentle vinegar solution, these little pests are less likely to bite or to get inside your house.

25. In the passage, the word <u>versatile</u> most nearly means

    (A) having many uses.

    (B) malodorous.

    (C) gentle.

    (D) pleasing.

26. Vinegar might be a good substance to help treat a(n)

    (A) fever.

    (B) coffee stain on the rug.

    (C) heartburn.

    (D) abrasion.

27. One reason you might choose to bathe your pets in a vinegar solution is to

    (A) make their coats shine.

    (B) get them to stop wetting the rug.

    (C) clean paint off of their fur.

    (D) get rid of fleas.

28. Vinegar is an effective food preservative because it

    (A) has antibacterial properties.

    (B) deodorizes.

    (C) repels fleas.

    (D) is a base.

29. The purpose of this passage is to

    (A) promote natural cleaning products.

    (B) inform the reader about uses for vinegar they might not know about.

    (C) get people to give their pets flea baths.

    (D) increase the number of people who use vinegar.

30. Vinegar is an effective flea repellant because of its

    (A) antibacterial properties.

    (B) deodorizing properties.

    (C) acidic properties.

    (D) metallic properties.

Math

Time: 40 minutes

Questions: 40

Directions: Carefully read each question, and choose the answer choice that best answers the question.

1. A doctor prescribes an increase in medication from 75 mg to 125 mg. How much of an increase is this?

   (A) 25%
   (B) 35%
   (C) 50%
   (D) 67%

2. $-14 - 12 + 6 =$

   (A) -26
   (B) -20
   (C) 4
   (D) 8

3. $\frac{6}{15} = \frac{x}{10}$

   (A) $x = 4$
   (B) $x = 6$
   (C) $x = 10$
   (D) $x = 11$

4. If you could wash four loads of laundry at the laundromat for $10.75, how many full loads could you wash for $23.63?

   (A) 6
   (B) 7
   (C) 8
   (D) 9

5. A room measures 16.2 feet long by 8.5 feet wide. What is its area?

   (A) 24.7 ft.²
   (B) 137.7 ft.²
   (C) 321.84 ft.²
   (D) 898.23 ft.²

6. The area of a circle with a diameter of 11 inches is about

   (A) 52 in².
   (B) 95 in².
   (C) 268 in².
   (D) 379 in².

7. What is 287,065,000 equal to in scientific notation?

   (A) 2.87065×10^8
   (B) 2.87065×10^9
   (C) 2.87065×10^{10}
   (D) 2.87065×10^{11}

8. Factor: $42x^2 + 28x$

   (A) $2x(21x + 14)$
   (B) $14x(3x + 2)$
   (C) $14x(3x - 2)$
   (D) $21x(2x + 7)$

9. If Assembly Line A can produce 14 boxes of chocolate per 30 minutes, and Assembly Line B can produce twice as much as that, how many boxes can they produce together in 12 hours?

(A) 168
(B) 336
(C) 672
(D) 1,008

10. What is 22% of 264?

(A) 12
(B) 14.08
(C) 58.08
(D) 132

11. It has been 16 years since Jane has seen a Broadway play. For Max, it has been only one third as long. How many years has it been since he's seen a Broadway play?

(A) $4\frac{1}{3}$
(B) $5\frac{1}{3}$
(C) $5\frac{2}{3}$
(D) $5\frac{7}{25}$

12. Which of these answers is a prime number?

(A) 2
(B) 4
(C) 16
(D) 25

13. What is the mode of the following set of numbers: 2, 1, 2, 6, 5, 6, 3, 6, 2, 5, 6, 1, 6?

(A) 1
(B) 2
(C) 5
(D) 6

14. If for every time your bicycle wheel turns once, you have to pedal three times, what's the ratio of wheel turns to times you have to pedal?

(A) 3:1
(B) 1:3
(C) 2:3
(D) 2:4

15. If the triangles in the figure are equilateral, the area of the square is

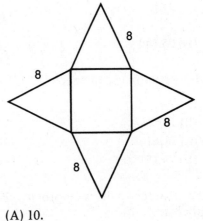

(A) 10.
(B) 16.
(C) 24.
(D) 64.

16. $2 \times 2 \times 2 \times 2 \times 2$ is another way of writing

(A) 2^2.
(B) 2^3.
(C) 2^4.
(D) 2^5.

17. Alex has a plank of wood that is 14 meters long. If Dale wanted to

get a plank of equal length, how many centimeters should he ask the woodshop to cut for him?

(A) 14

(B) 1,400

(C) 14,000

(D) 140,000

18. What is 25.14852 rounded to the nearest thousandth?

(A) 25.14

(B) 25.15

(C) 25.148

(D) 25.149

19. 25 ft = how many meters?

(A) 7.62

(B) 17.62

(C) 71.62

(D) 75.15

20. The answer to a division problem is called a

(A) sum.

(B) product.

(C) difference.

(D) quotient.

21. What is the mode of the following set of numbers: 6, 5, 2, 2, 2, 3, 4, 4, 2, 3, 6?

(A) 2

(B) 3

(C) 4

(D) 5

22. What is 5,253,260,000 equal to in scientific notation?

(A) 5.25326×10^9

(B) 52.5326×10^9

(C) 5.25326×10^{10}

(D) 5.25326×10^{11}

23. The simplest form of $\sqrt{147}$ is

(A) $3\sqrt{4}.$

(B) $7\sqrt{3}.$

(C) $3\sqrt{5}.$

(D) $3\sqrt{7}.$

24. Trixie will be four times as old as Abby on her next birthday which is in two months. If Mark is 15 and Abby is two years older than $\frac{2}{3}$ his age, how old is Trixie now?

(A) 12

(B) 30

(C) 47

(D) 48

Use the following chart to answer questions 25 through 28.

Evening TV Watching Time Begins

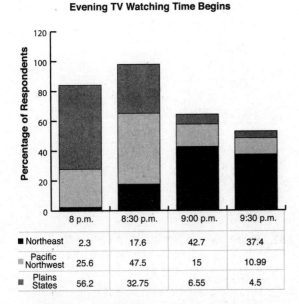

	8 p.m.	8:30 p.m.	9:00 p.m.	9:30 p.m.
■ Northeast	2.3	17.6	42.7	37.4
Pacific Northwest	25.6	47.5	15	10.99
■ Plains States	56.2	32.75	6.55	4.5

25. What is the most common time for respondents in the Plains states to sit down at night to watch TV?

    (A) 8:00 p.m.

    (B) 8:30 p.m.

    (C) 9:00 p.m.

    (D) 9:30 p.m.

26. The most popular time to sit down to watch TV overall is

    (A) 8:00 p.m.

    (B) 8:30 p.m.

    (C) 9:00 p.m.

    (D) 9:30 p.m.

27. If you were planning to run a commercial between 9:00 and 9:30 P.M., in which region(s) would you choose to run it in order to reach the most viewers?

    (A) Plains and Pacific Northwest

    (B) Pacific Northwest and Northeast

    (C) Plains and Northeast

    (D) Plains only

28. About what percentage of respondents indicated that they sit down to watch TV at 9:30 P.M.?

    (A) 40%

    (B) 45%

    (C) 55%

    (D) 65%

29. Solve for x: $23°C = x°F$

    (A) 55.6°F

    (B) 73.4°F

    (C) 93.6°F

    (D) 104.2°F

30. A flight leaves New York City traveling at 520 miles per hour. After three hours in the air, how far will that plane have traveled?

    (A) 1,040 miles

    (B) 1,560 miles

    (C) 1,875 miles

    (D) 2,056 miles

31. You're laying carpet in a room that is 12 feet long by 30 feet wide. You have only half the amount of carpet needed to complete the job. How many more square feet of carpet do you need to get?

    (A) 50 ft.².
    (B) 80 ft.².
    (C) 95 ft.².
    (D) 180 ft.².

32. In the following diagram, what is the value of angle 3?

    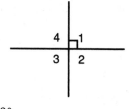

    (A) 30°
    (B) 45°
    (C) 90°
    (D) 180°

33. A single number, variable, or combinations thereof is a(n)

    (A) expression.
    (B) term.
    (C) constant.
    (D) equation.

34. What part of the following expression would you evaluate first according to order of operations: $[2 \times 4 + (3^2 - 3)^4] + (-6) - 9$?

    (A) $(32 - 3)$
    (B) 2×4
    (C) $(32 - 3)4$
    (D) $[2 \times 4 + (32 - 3)4]$

35. In the following expression, which number is a base?

    $5^2 + 6 - 25 + 2$

    (A) 5
    (B) 16
    (C) –25
    (D) 3

36. $24.45\overline{)794.3}$

    (A) 24.6578
    (B) 32.4867
    (C) 132.4867
    (D) 324.867

37. Solve for x: $27°F = x°C$

    (A) –8.2
    (B) –2.8
    (C) 2.8
    (D) 8.2

38. Fourteen is what fraction of twenty-four?

    (A) $\frac{1}{7}$
    (B) $\frac{3}{16}$
    (C) $\frac{29}{50}$
    (D) $\frac{36}{57}$

39. Reduce the following to lowest terms: $\frac{6x+9}{2x+6}$

    (A) $1\frac{1}{2}$
    (B) $\frac{3(2x+3)}{2(x+3)}$
    (C) $\frac{2}{3}$
    (D) $\frac{2(2x+3)}{2(x+3)}$

40. In scientific notation, 6,538,900,000 is:

    (A) 6.5389×10^9

    (B) 65.389×10^8

    (C) 653.89×10^7

    (D) 6538.9×10^6

Life Science

Time: 35 minutes

Questions: 30

Directions: For each of the following questions, choose the best answer out of the choices given.

1. The lithosphere includes the
    (A) lower mantle of the Earth.
    (B) crust and upper mantle of the Earth.
    (C) crust and the asthenosphere.
    (D) crust and the inner core of the Earth.

2. Natural selection is also sometimes known as
    (A) evolution.
    (B) mutualism.
    (C) survival of the fittest.
    (D) commensalism.

3. A cell is the basic unit of
    (A) life.
    (B) measure.
    (C) matter.
    (D) a chemical compound.

4. The most common system for taxonomic classification is the
    (A) Darwinian system.
    (B) Linnaean system.
    (C) Rivinus system.
    (D) de Tournefort system.

5. Which type of organism needs to eat carbon-based substances to survive?
    (A) organelles
    (B) autotrophs
    (C) heterotrophs
    (D) plants

6. A habitat is considered a desert if it
    (A) experiences less than 50 cm/ year of rain.
    (B) has bodies of water with a high concentration of salt.
    (C) is found on mountains that go above an altitude that can sustain the growth of trees.
    (D) all of the above

7. The layer of Earth that is the hottest and under the most pressure is the
    (A) mantle.
    (B) inner core.
    (C) outer core.
    (D) lower mantle.

8. When barometric pressure rises, it signals
    (A) a cold snap is coming.
    (B) a tornado is coming.
    (C) a hurricane is coming.
    (D) fair weather is coming.

9. Relationships among organisms within any given ecosystem are

    (A) hostile.
    (B) punitive.
    (C) symbiotic.
    (D) antibiotic.

10. Fossils are usually found in which type of rock?

    (A) igneous
    (B) sedimentary
    (C) metamorphic
    (D) none of the above

11. Natural selection is driven by

    (A) sexual reproduction.
    (B) genetic mutation.
    (C) both A and B
    (D) none of the above

12. Most meteorites burn up in which layer of the atmosphere?

    (A) troposphere
    (B) stratosphere
    (C) mesosphere
    (D) thermosphere

13. The development of antibiotic resistance is the result of

    (A) the body's increasing ability to fight infection.
    (B) the body's decreasing ability to fight infection.
    (C) deliberate changes in bacteria.
    (D) natural selection.

14. What happens when the moon moves between the Earth and the sun?

    (A) solar eclipse
    (B) lunar eclipse
    (C) new moon
    (D) full moon

15. The coldest planet in the solar system is

    (A) Venus.
    (B) Jupiter.
    (C) Neptune.
    (D) Uranus.

16. Plants reproduce

    (A) asexually.
    (B) sexually.
    (C) semiannually.
    (D) annually.

17. The two main differences between prokaryotic and eukaryotic cells are that prokaryotes have

    (A) no defined capsule but have organelles.
    (B) no defined organelles but have proteins.
    (C) no defined nucleus but have a cell membrane.
    (D) no defined nucleus but have organelles.

18. The products of light-dependent reactions during photosynthesis are

    (A) adenosine triphosphate (ATP).
    (B) nicotinamide adenine dinucleotide phosphate (NADPH).
    (C) oxygen.
    (D) all of the above

19. The main structural component of a plant is the

    (A) root.
    (B) shoot.
    (C) stem.
    (D) leaves.

20. A relationship with an ecosystem where one or a group of organisms benefits while another is harmed is called

    (A) mutual.
    (B) parasitic.
    (C) commensal.
    (D) none of the above

21. The movement of heat through which layer of Earth is believed to be responsible for the movement of tectonic plates?

    (A) inner core
    (B) outer core
    (C) mantle
    (D) lithosphere

22. An organelle that is responsible for housing the cell's genetic information and controlling how the genetic coding is expressed by the cell is called

    (A) the nucleus.
    (B) a protein.
    (C) cytoplasm.
    (D) the plasma membrane.

23. All of the following are functions of the atmosphere except one:

    (A) It protects the Earth from space debris that might otherwise pelt the planet.
    (B) It transports energy from region to region around the planet.
    (C) It filters and disposes of waste gases.
    (D) It keeps the planet in orbit around the sun.

24. While the Earth orbits the sun, the moon

    (A) eclipses the sun.
    (B) eclipses the Earth.
    (C) orbits the Earth.
    (D) none of the above

25. Anaerobic respiration

    (A) needs oxygen for ATP production.
    (B) does not need oxygen for ATP production.
    (C) needs water for ATP production.
    (D) needs hydrogen for ATP production.

26. Which of the following planets orbits the sun in the shortest amount of time?

    (A) Uranus
    (B) Saturn
    (C) Neptune
    (D) Jupiter

27. Fossils are

    (A) skeletons of living organisms that have been preserved over time by rock.

    (B) live animals trapped in sedimentary rock.

    (C) forgotten artifacts from previous civilizations.

    (D) recorded histories of evolution.

28. Cumulus clouds look like

    (A) a blanket in the sky.

    (B) cotton balls.

    (C) wispy shreds of cotton.

    (D) tall, thick clouds.

29. Cumulonimbus clouds are also known as

    (A) thunderheads.

    (B) fair-weather clouds.

    (C) tornado heads.

    (D) gale force clouds.

30. The Continental crust is

    (A) part of the asthenosphere.

    (B) the land under the oceans.

    (C) the land that makes up the continents.

    (D) none of the above

Biology

Time: 35 minutes

Questions: 30

Directions: For each of the following questions, choose the best answer out of the choices given.

1. When molecules move across a membrane from a low to high concentration, they need what to make this happen?

   (A) nucleic acids

   (B) vacuoles

   (C) transport proteins and ATP

   (D) carbohydrates

2. tRNA

   (A) stands for transfer RNA.

   (B) translates the genetic information coded in mRNA into the right sequence of amino acids to replicate DNA.

   (C) has an inverted L structure.

   (D) all of the above

3. Cell walls are made of

   (A) cellulose.

   (B) proteins.

   (C) lipids.

   (D) enzymes.

4. If the concentration of water inside the cell becomes too much for it to handle, the membrane will

   (A) equalize the balance of water.

   (B) use proteins to strengthen itself.

   (C) bulge and then burst.

   (D) dehydrate.

5. Another name for threadlike strands of coiled DNA is

   (A) chromatid.

   (B) chromosome.

   (C) chromatin.

   (D) centriole.

6. Rough ER has

   (A) ribosomes attached to its outer structure.

   (B) ribosomes attached to its inner structure.

   (C) its own spot in the nucleus in a cell.

   (D) vacuoles.

Use the following diagram for questions 7 through 9. "B" indicates an allele for brown eyes; "b" indicates an allele for blue eyes.

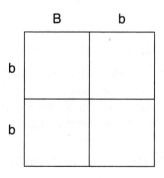

7. The alleles shown at the top of the diagram are

   (A) heterozygous.
   (B) homozygous.
   (C) phenotypical.
   (D) none of the above

8. Based on the data in the square, if this couple had four children, how many would most likely have blue eyes?

   (A) 1
   (B) 2
   (C) 3
   (D) 4

9. What is the probability of these two people having a child that carries a recessive gene for height?

   (A) 1:4
   (B) 2:4
   (C) 3:4
   (D) 4:4

10. Cytokinesis takes place in which phase of mitosis?

    (A) prophase
    (B) anaphase
    (C) metaphase
    (D) telophase

11. Meiosis II produces cells that are

    (A) unable to replicate.
    (B) genetically identical.
    (C) genetically different.
    (D) diploid.

12. Fermentation is a(n)

    (A) anaerobic process.
    (B) step in photosynthesis.
    (C) aerobic process.
    (D) stage in the citric acid cycle.

13. The Law of Independent Assortment states that

    (A) traits are inherited in a ratio of 3:1.
    (B) one inherited allele from each parent is needed for a trait to be expressed.
    (C) gene pairs that result from the union of gametes form independently from each other.
    (D) phenotypes are more common in reproduction than genotypes.

14. Variations in the sequence of synthesized base pairs during DNA replication results in

    (A) variation among a population.
    (B) mutations.
    (C) both A and B
    (D) neither A nor B

15. When meiosis produces sperm, the process is called

    (A) fertilization.
    (B) oogenesis.
    (C) zygotagenesis.
    (D) spermatogenesis.

16. Genes are chemical codes for

    (A) physical traits.
    (B) rates of respiration.
    (C) how many times you will need to blink.
    (D) whether or not you like coffee.

17. Base pairs in DNA are held together by

    (A) one 5-sugar and phosphate spine.
    (B) two 5-sugar and phosphate spines.
    (C) two 6-sugar and phosphate spines.
    (D) two 7-sugar and phosphate spines.

18. Lipids

    (A) are oxidation-reduction molecules used in cellular respiration.
    (B) hold less energy than carbohydrates.
    (C) are long chains of amino acids joined by peptide bonds.
    (D) hold more energy than carbohydrates.

19. Glycolysis breaks down a molecule of glucose from a(n)

    (A) 4-carbon molecule chain into two 2-carbon chains.
    (B) 6-carbon molecule chain into two 3-carbon chains.
    (C) 8-carbon molecule chain into two 4-carbon chains.
    (D) 10-carbon molecule chain into two 5-carbon chains.

20. Glycolysis produces how many total ATP?

    (A) 1
    (B) 2
    (C) 3
    (D) 4

21. What type of organism experiences oogenesis?

    (A) amoeba
    (B) bacteria
    (C) females that reproduce sexually
    (D) males that reproduce sexually

22. During the Krebs cycle, pyruvates

    (A) divide.
    (B) reproduce.
    (C) oxidize.
    (D) coil.

23. The electron transport chain produces how many ATP?

    (A) 34
    (B) 36
    (C) 38
    (D) 40

24. When your body heals a tear in a muscle, the cells in the tissue

    (A) undergo meiosis.
    (B) undergo mitosis.
    (C) fuse together.
    (D) separate.

25. During what stage of cell reproduction can you actually see chromosomes under a microscope?

    (A) G_1 stage
    (B) S stage
    (C) G_2 stage
    (D) prophase

26. G_1 stage, S stage, and G_2 stage all take place during

    (A) metaphase.
    (B) meiosis II.
    (C) interphase.
    (D) cytokinesis.

27. A homologue is

    (A) a centromere.
    (B) a gene pair.
    (C) two sister chromatids connected by a centromere.
    (D) a strand of replicated DNA.

28. How many cells result after mitosis completes?

    (A) 2
    (B) 3
    (C) 4
    (D) 5

29. Gregor Mendel was

    (A) a monk.
    (B) an astronaut.
    (C) a doctor.
    (D) both A and C

30. Thin discs that pack molecules together and either store them for later use or send them out into the cytoplasm for some function are

    (A) ribosomes.
    (B) nucleoli.
    (C) nuclear envelopes.
    (D) golgi.

Anatomy and Physiology

Time: 35 minutes

Questions: 30

Directions: For each of the following questions, choose the best answer out of the choices given.

1. The portion of the peripheral nervous system that includes fibers that connect the CNS (central nervous system) to visceral organs such as the heart, stomach, intestines, and various organs is called the

    (A) somatic system.
    (B) autonomic system.
    (C) brain stem.
    (D) medulla oblongata.

2. How many lobes does the right lung have?

    (A) 1
    (B) 2
    (C) 3
    (D) 4

3. The tibia is located above the

    (A) knee.
    (B) waist.
    (C) ankle.
    (D) humerus.

4. Joints or articulations are junctures between bones that are classified according to the

    (A) bones they connect.
    (B) amount of cartilage.
    (C) number of ligaments.
    (D) amount of movement they make possible.

5. What area of the cerebral hemisphere has sensory areas responsible for sensations of temperature, touch, pressure, and pain from the skin?

    (A) frontal lobes
    (B) parietal lobes
    (C) temporal lobes
    (D) occipital lobes

6. A hematologist specializes in the

    (A) brain.
    (B) bones.
    (C) heart.
    (D) blood.

7. Dorsal means

    (A) pertaining to the back.
    (B) travelling upward.
    (C) front.
    (D) below.

8. Plasma is made up of

    (A) leukocytes.
    (B) erythrocytes.
    (C) both A and B
    (D) neither A nor B

9. Subclavian veins go to the

    (A) stomach.
    (B) arms.
    (C) feet.
    (D) back.

10. Biceps femoris is the anatomical name for the

    (A) hamstring.
    (B) quadriceps.
    (C) gluteus maximus.
    (D) triceps.

11. In the skeletal system, which of the following is a movable bone?

    (A) parietal bone
    (B) frontal bone
    (C) mandible
    (D) maxilla

12. When you cut yourself, you're seeing blood coming from your

    (A) veins.
    (B) aorta.
    (C) arteries.
    (D) capillaries.

13. The duodenum connects what two parts of the digestive system?

    (A) stomach and large intestine
    (B) stomach and esophagus
    (C) stomach and liver
    (D) stomach and jejunum

14. Of the following, which bone is not part of the pectoral girdle?

    (A) clavicle
    (B) scapula
    (C) collarbone
    (D) humerus

15. Ureters move urine to the bladder from the

    (A) renal pelvis.
    (B) renal artery.
    (C) renal vein.
    (D) none of the above

16. Smooth muscle cells

    (A) are narrow.
    (B) have only one nucleus.
    (C) both A and B
    (D) neither A nor B

17. Major events in expiration include having the

    (A) diaphragm and external respiratory muscles relax.
    (B) elastic tissue of the lungs, thoracic cage, and abdominal organs recoil.
    (C) air squeezed out of the lungs into air passages.
    (D) all of the above

18. What bones in children produce red blood cells?

    (A) flat
    (B) long
    (C) finger
    (D) spinal

19. The appendicular skeleton includes all bones except

    (A) arm and leg bones.
    (B) phalanges.
    (C) skull and spinal bones.
    (D) pelvic bones.

20. The knee is an example of what kind of joint?

    (A) sutures
    (B) hinge
    (C) ball and socket
    (D) soft

21. What inorganic salt is stored in the matrix of bone?

    (A) iron
    (B) calcium
    (C) vitamin D
    (D) lead

22. The diaphragm

    (A) is a thin band of fibromuscular tissue.
    (B) separates the chest cavity from the abdomen.
    (C) is controlled by the involuntary nervous system.
    (D) all of the above

23. Alveoli are located in the

    (A) brain.
    (B) heart.
    (C) lungs.
    (D) liver.

24. The formal name for gray matter is

    (A) cerebral cortex.
    (B) basal ganglia.
    (C) occipital lobe.
    (D) temporal lobe.

25. What protects the brain from certain chemicals and toxins that enter the bloodstream?

    (A) cerebral cortex
    (B) cerebrospinal fluid
    (C) the blood-brain barrier
    (D) meninges

26. What are the parts of a long bone?

    (A) epiphysis
    (B) articular cartilage
    (C) diaphysis
    (D) all of the above

27. Maintaining a specific body temperature, blood pressure, and balance of chemicals in the blood and tissues describes

    (A) homeostasis.
    (B) glycolysis.
    (C) peristalsis.
    (D) glomerulus.

28. Vitamin K, B_{12}, thiamine, and riboflavin are

    (A) bacteria found in the colon.
    (B) components in chyme.
    (C) by-products of bacterial processing of chyme in the colon.
    (D) components of feces.

29. The appendix is attached to the

    (A) cecum.
    (B) liver.
    (C) vertebrae.
    (D) gallbladder.

30. What is the number of bones in the human skeleton?

    (A) 152

    (B) 200

    (C) 206

    (D) 306

Chemistry

Time: 35 minutes

Questions: 30

Directions: For each of the following questions, choose the best answer out of the choices given.

1. Which measurement is not part of the Seven Fundamental Units of Measurement (SI)?

    (A) mass
    (B) time
    (C) exponential notation
    (D) electrical current

2. Which of the following is a true statement about acids and bases?

    (A) An acid-base reaction is the transfer of a proton from an acid to a base.
    (B) The weaker an acid is, the greater the base strength of its conjugate base.
    (C) The weaker a base is, the stronger its conjugate acid.
    (D) all of the above

3. How a substance reacts when mixed with other substances describes its

    (A) chemical properties.
    (B) electron configuration.
    (C) physical properties.
    (D) state of matter.

4. A reaction of an insoluble solid that deposits and then settles out of solution is known as

    (A) a precipitation reaction.
    (B) an acid-base reaction.
    (C) a displacement reaction.
    (D) an oxidation-reduction reaction.

5. Chemical reactions involve changing one or more substances into one or more new substances. They use chemical equations to show

    (A) the reactants (substances that react).
    (B) the substances formed (products).
    (C) the relative amounts of the substances involved.
    (D) all of the above

6. What is the molecular mass of 1 mole of CH_4?

    (A) 16.10
    (B) 16.05
    (C) 13.02
    (D) 13.10

7. The following equation shows what type of reaction: $2 C_6H_5COOH + 15 O_2 \rightarrow 14 CO_2 + 6 H_2O$?

   (A) synthesis
   (B) decomposition
   (C) combustion
   (D) double displacement

8. A dipole interaction occurs when

   (A) the covalent bonding is not shared equally between molecules.
   (B) the covalent bonding is shared equally between molecules.
   (C) electrons are transferred from one atom to another.
   (D) none of the above

9. What is an atom?

   (A) the smallest particle of an element that maintains its chemical identity through all chemical and physical changes
   (B) the smallest particle of an element or compound that can have a stable independent existence
   (C) different forms of the same element in the same physical state
   (D) two or more elements in chemical combination in fixed proportion

10. The Law of Conservation of Matter and Energy states that

    (A) heat, light, or electrical energy is converted into chemical energy.
    (B) the combined amount of matter and energy in the universe is fixed.
    (C) chemical energy is converted into heat energy.
    (D) both B and C

11. How many grams does 1 mole of H_2 equal?

    (A) 1 g
    (B) 2 amu
    (C) 2 g
    (D) 4 g

12. What are the states of matter?

    (A) solid, liquid, gas
    (B) chemical, physical, extensive
    (C) color, density, hardness
    (D) extensive, intensive, conductive

13. Express the following number in scientific notation: 3,790,000

    (A) 3.79×10^6
    (B) 37.9×10^5
    (C) 3.79×10^{-5}
    (D) 37.9×10^{-6}

14. Balance the following equation: $Fe + Cl_2 = FeCl_3$

    (A) $2Fe + 3Cl_2 \rightarrow 6FeCl_3$
    (B) $2Fe + 2Cl_2 \rightarrow 2FeCl_3$
    (C) $2Fe + 3Cl_2 \rightarrow 2FeCl_3$
    (D) $2Fe + 6Cl_2 \rightarrow 2FeCl_3$

15. How many protons are found in an atom of neon?

    (A) 5
    (B) 10
    (C) 15
    (D) 20

16. A mixture is considered heterogeneous if

    (A) the mixture has uniform properties throughout and the components are not distinguishable.
    (B) different portions of the mixture have recognizable and different properties.
    (C) the substance can be broken down into a simpler substance by chemical means.
    (D) the substance cannot be broken down into a simpler substance by chemical means.

17. Stoichiometry describes

    (A) a quantitative relationship among elements within compounds.
    (B) a quantitative relationship among substances as they undergo chemical changes.
    (C) the Periodic Table.
    (D) both A and B

18. Intermolecular forces, the attraction between individual particles, include

    (A) hydrogen bonding.
    (B) dipole interactions.
    (C) London forces.
    (D) all of the above

19. The component of an atom that has a negative charge is known as a(n)

    (A) electron.
    (B) proton.
    (C) neutron.
    (D) atomic number.

20. When an acid is mixed with a base, the reactants start to

    (A) multiply.
    (B) neutralize each other.
    (C) combust.
    (D) emulsify.

21. Which of the following is a property of covalent bonding?

    (A) Liquids and molten compounds do not conduct electricity.
    (B) Electrons between two atoms with similar electron configurations are shared.
    (C) Bonds are formed when one or more pairs of electrons are lost.
    (D) both B and C

22. Mayonnaise is an example of a(n)

    (A) dilution.
    (B) tincture.
    (C) emulsion.
    (D) none of the above

23. A liquid-to-gas change of matter is an

    (A) endothermic change called sublimation.
    (B) exothermic change called condensation.
    (C) endothermic change called vaporization.
    (D) exothermic change called deposition.

24. What is the mass composition of hydrogen in the following chemical formula: $Na + 2H_2O$?

    (A) 2.3%
    (B) 6.78%
    (C) 32%
    (D) 59%

25. Which of the following can increase a reaction rate?

    (A) An increase in temperature.
    (B) A decrease in concentration.
    (C) Adding a catalyst.
    (D) Both A and C

26. What is the molarity of the solute in a solution made up of 18 liters of water and 8 moles of salt?

    (A) .44 M
    (B) .49 M
    (C) 1.44 M
    (D) 1.49 M

27. The notation in a chemical equation that indicates a molecule is in liquid form is

    (A) (aq)
    (B) (g)
    (C) (l)
    (D) (s)

28. The chemical symbol for tin is

    (A) Sn.
    (B) Li.
    (C) Ti.
    (D) Ta.

29. The octet rule addresses the

    (A) tendency of atoms to create ionic bonds.
    (B) tendency of atoms to lose and gain valence electrons in order to have a total of 8.
    (C) tendency of matter to convert from one form to another.
    (D) ability of solutes to dissolve in solvents.

30. An element in the seventh row of the Periodic Table has how many electron orbitals?

    (A) 4
    (B) 5
    (C) 6
    (D) 7

Physics

Time: 35 minutes

Questions: 30

Directions: For each of the following questions, choose the best answer out of the choices given.

1. 15 kiloliters =
    - (A) 1,500 liters
    - (B) 1,500 liters^3
    - (C) 15,000 liters
    - (D) 15,000 liters^3

2. How can you increase the pressure of a gas within a container?
    - (A) Lower the temperature of the gas.
    - (B) Increase the temperature of the gas.
    - (C) Both A and B
    - (D) Neither A nor B

3. The metric temperature at which water boils is
    - (A) 100°C.
    - (B) 373.15 K.
    - (C) 212°F.
    - (D) absolute zero.

4. The previous diagram shows a
    - (A) series circuit.
    - (B) power source.
    - (C) parallel circuit.
    - (D) both A and B

5. You're driving a car at a velocity of 28 m/s and accelerate to 38 m/s at a rate of 5 m/s^2. How long did it take you to accelerate to your final speed?
    - (A) 1.85 seconds
    - (B) 2.00 seconds
    - (C) 2.05 seconds
    - (D) 8.05 seconds

6. When you kick a rock,
    - (A) you turn the rock's potential energy into kinetic energy.
    - (B) the rock kicks you.
    - (C) you do work.
    - (D) all of the above

7. When waves bend around an object, they
    - (A) deflect.
    - (B) diffract.
    - (C) disperse.
    - (D) refract.

8. During the course of 10 minutes, a sound wave crests 1,525 times. What is its frequency?
    - (A) .39 joules
    - (B) .39 hertz
    - (C) 2.54 joules
    - (D) 2.54 hertz

9. Nuclear reactors use what to generate power?

   (A) nuclear fission
   (B) nuclear fusion
   (C) both A and B
   (D) neither A nor B

10. Gamma radiation

    (A) emits helium ions and contains two protons and two neutrons.
    (B) is composed of high-energy, high-speed electrons that are negatively charged.
    (C) is composed of high-energy, electromagnetic radiation that has no charge.
    (D) none of the above

11. How much force would you have to exert to push a 1,250-kg motorcycle to accelerate it at a rate of 5 m/s²?

    (A) 6,250 N
    (B) 6,550 N
    (C) 6,650 N
    (D) 6,750 N

12. Sound is what type of wave?

    (A) transverse
    (B) long range
    (C) short range
    (D) longitudinal

13. The volume of a sound wave depends on its

    (A) wavelength.
    (B) wave speed.
    (C) amplitude.
    (D) frequency.

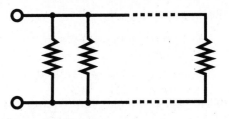

14. The previous diagram shows

    (A) a series circuit.
    (B) a power source.
    (C) a parallel circuit.
    (D) both A and B

15. You have a bag of clothes to donate to the needy. If you drag the bag across a 22.2-m parking lot with a force of 15 N, how much work have you done?

    (A) 111 joules
    (B) 222 joules
    (C) 333 joules
    (D) 444 joules

16. If you drop a 5-kg paper clip, 6-kg bowling ball, and a 15-kg chair off the top of a 105 m building located in a vacuum, which of these objects would hit the ground first?

    (A) the paper clip
    (B) the bowling ball
    (C) the chair
    (D) they would all hit the ground at the same time

17. Ohms are calculated by

    (A) volts divided by amps.
    (B) amps divided by volts.
    (C) volts multiplied by amps.
    (D) volts divided by resistance.

18. Resistance

    (A) converts one form of electricity to another.

    (B) slows the flow of electricity through a conductor.

    (C) speeds the flow of electricity through a conductor.

    (D) all of the above

19. Which of the following objects has greater potential energy: an orange with a mass of 31 g at 4,200 m above Earth or a ball with a mass of 4 kg at 32 m above Earth?

    (A) the orange

    (B) the ball

    (C) their potential energies are equal

    (D) there's not enough information to make a determination

20. Ohms are represented by which Greek letter?

    (A) alpha

    (B) beta

    (C) omega

    (D) zeta

21. $-459.67°F =$

    (A) 273.15 K.

    (B) $-223.15°C.$

    (C) 0°C.

    (D) none of the above

22. Water moving through turbines to create electricity is an example of

    (A) potential energy.

    (B) kinetic energy.

    (C) kinetic energy turning into electricity.

    (D) both B and C

23. In the SI system, temperature is measured in

    (A) Celsius.

    (B) Kelvin.

    (C) Fahrenheit.

    (D) joules.

24. What is the kinetic energy of a bicycle that weighs 20 kilograms when it moves at a rate of 5 kilometers per hour?

    (A) 19.3 joules

    (B) 45.2 joules

    (C) 250 joules

    (D) 250.9 joules

25. Electricity is

    (A) a measure of current.

    (B) the strength with which current flows through a conductor.

    (C) the flow of electrons through a conductor.

    (D) the amount of energy transferred during a specified time.

26. Something that changes an object at rest into an object in motion is

    (A) force.

    (B) work.

    (C) motion.

    (D) energy.

27. To calculate force, you

    (A) multiply the mass of the object by its acceleration.
    (B) multiply the object's mass by the square of its velocity and then multiply that value by half.
    (C) multiply the object's mass by the gravitational force exerted on it and its height above Earth's surface.
    (D) none of the above

28. An object turns because of

    (A) Newton's First Law
    (B) centripetal force
    (C) Newton's Third Law
    (D) centrifugal force

29. How much potential energy does a 42-kg rock have at 175 m above Earth?

    (A) 72,015 joules
    (B) 72,030 joules
    (C) 73,020 joules
    (D) 73,040 joules

30. You live 42 kilometers away from work. How fast would you have to drive from your house to make it to work in 35 minutes?

    (A) 1.2 km/hr
    (B) 52 km/hr
    (C) 62 km/hr
    (D) 72 km/hr

Practice Test 2: Answers and Explanations

Word Knowledge

1. **D.** The context clues of "ideal for those who are not overly fond of extremely cold or hot weather" tell us that we're looking for a word that relates to conditions somewhere in the middle. A and B are out. It could be C, but D is a much better fit because *temperate* means "a range of temperatures that are neither extremely hot nor extremely cold."

2. **B.** *Myriad* means "many" or "a bunch of something." A and C don't make sense. *Myopic* means "short sighted," which also doesn't make sense.

3. **D.** Use roots here to figure out the meaning of the word. *Epi* means "outer" and *derm* means "skin."

4. **B.** Someone who is belligerent is argumentative and abusive. The root *bell* means to "fight."

5. **B.** When you use *goad* as a verb, it means "to spur someone to take action" or "to have some kind of response."

6. **B.** Logic (and history) tells us that a lengthy war drains resources. It would not infuse (increase), sustain (keep steady), or marginalize (keep out of the center of attention) money or manpower.

7. **D.** "Swank" describes something that is classy or fashionable. "Blistering" describes something that is so hot it would blister the skin. "Svelte" describes someone who is tall and thin.

8. **A.** *Minutia* means "small details."

9. **B.** "Staid" and "reticent" are synonyms that mean "restrained." These are the opposite of "vivacious," which means "full of energy." B is the best answer choice.

10. **B.** Someone who is penitent expresses regret. Someone who is awed expresses reverence. A and D show opposite relationships. There really isn't a relationship in Answer C.

11. **B.** In the sentence, you see that the p and b have been switched or transposed.

12. **A.** A bag that's full of liquid is round and plump (taut). When it's drained of that liquid, all you have is the bag, which is limp and expandable.

13. **C.** A perforation is a tear in something.

14. **D.** A capitol is where laws are made. A bakery is where pastries are made. "Foreign : unfamiliar" and "torrent : downpour" are synonyms, while "original" and "trite" are antonyms.

15. **A.** If you swap out the answer choices with the underlined word, you'll find that "apprehensive" is the only one that makes sense in this context.

16. **C.** Halloween is a time for dressing up in costumes. "people in costumes" makes the most sense.

17. **A.** "Oblique" refers to something that is indirect.

18. **D.** A cog is a particle inside of a grandfather clock that makes it work. A microchip is a particle inside of a computer that makes it work. Answer A shows a synonymous relationship. B and C show a "type of" relationship.

19. **C.** Someone who is intrepid takes chances, making them daring.

20. **A.** *Pelted* means "to be hit repeatedly with something."

21. **C.** A murder is a group of crows. A pod is a group of dolphins. There's no relationship in A. B and D show "degree of" relationships.

22. **C.** "Distal" is an anatomical term that refers to something that is as far away as can be from a certain point. Think of "distance" when you see this word.

23. **D.** Someone who is introverted is shy and likes to keep to himself. "Optimistic" and "pessimistic" describe positive and negative attitudes, respectively, which does not fit.

24. **D.** A search that encompasses hundreds of miles is very large. This means the answer you want has something to do with size. Answer D is the only one that addresses size, as "heroic" describes bravery, "fortuitous" describes a chance happening, and "intimate" describes a degree of personal interaction.

25. **A.** Something that is annual happens once per year. Something that is decennial happens once every decade.

26. **A.** *Occlusion* means "a blockage."

27. **C.** This is just a fancy name for a cut.

28. **A.** The prefix *uni* tells us that one side is involved.

29. **B.** Look to the prefix *ex* here, which means "to cut off" or "sever."

30. **D.** Something corrosive eats away at whatever it touches, which makes D the best answer. The other answers don't make sense.

31. **D.** *Inexorable* means "unmoving." Answers A and C don't make sense, and *revered* means "honored."

32. **B.** "Attrition" is the opposite of "gain." "Pass" is the opposite of "fail."

33. **D.** A forge is used to heat metal. A stove is used to heat food. All of the rest of the answer choices show "type of" relationships.

34. **D.** When something is distended, it is abnormally swollen.

35. **C.** *Gratuitous* means "something done for no apparent reason"—it is unwarranted. Answer C makes the most sense.

36. **B.** *Vestige* means "a small part of something." The sentence tells us that Olivia is very old, but you can still see some of what she looked like when she was younger. B is the best choice.

37. **C.** The sentence describes Jane as being inspirational and optimistic. The correct answer will have something to do with this. The only answer that comes close is C. (*Sanguine* has several definitions, and "confident" is one of them.)

38. **B.** *Persnickety* means "fussy" or "someone who pays very close attention to detail." The other answers don't work.

39. **D.** "Lateral" indicates a sideways change. The sentence does not tell us there was any change in rank or pay, so D makes the most sense.

40. **C.** "Laconic" refers to something that is short and sweet—something pithy.

Grammar

1. **D.** Collective nouns name a group and are generally treated as singular, even though they refer to many people or things.

2. **B.** "Potato chips" is the subject; therefore, the verb needs to be plural.

3. **C.** When you're talking distance, it's "farther," not "further." You use "further" to describe more of, or to a greater degree than, something else.

4. **C.** Ben is a singular male name, so the possessive pronoun here needs to be "his."

5. **D.** "Anyone" is a singular noun, so it needs a singular pronoun. Because "anyone" can be of either gender, you would include both male and female pronouns to be grammatically correct. In all of the other answers, it's not clear to whom the pronouns refer, which makes them incorrect.

6. **D.** The plural subject (my girlfriend and I) did something in the past, which makes B and C wrong. A is wrong because it doesn't fit grammatically with the sentence. You wouldn't say "stayed out to the movies."

7. **B.** You want *accept* here, which means "to receive," as opposed to *except*, which means "to exclude."

8. **A.** This is the only one that makes sense with the structure of the sentence.

9. **A.** The predicate shows the action the subject is performing. In this sentence, the subject is implied, because it's an imperative sentence. The subject is "you." What is the action? Listen: "You, listen to the rain fall outside."

10. **A.** Answer B indicates past tense. C indicates present tense. D indicates a plural.

11. **D.** You need a noun to complete this sentence. A is an adverb. B and C are adjectives.

12. **B.** You emigrate *from* one country and immigrate *to* another.

13. **B.** Adjectives modify nouns and pronouns. "Previous" gives more detail about the anatomy professor.

14. **A.** The pronoun in this sentence is reflexive, which means that it refers to its antecedent. In this case, the antecedent is "Jordan," which means A is the only answer that fits.

15. **D.** You have two independent clauses here connected by "and," which means you need a comma at the end of the first clause.

16. **D.** A *principal* is the head of a school. A *principle* is a belief.

17. **A.** The indirect object shows to whom or for what the action is performed. In this case, it was performed on her blog.

18. **C.** The verb *to be* is irregular. Depending on the subject of the sentence, its present tense can be "am," "are," or "is," which are very different from the base form. It can be used in all voices.

19. **C.** "Nor" is always paired with "neither."

20. **B.** "Over" is the only preposition in the sentence and marks the beginning of the prepositional phrase.

21. **C.** This is the only choice that makes sense.

22. **C.** *Illicit* means something "illegal." You want *elicit* here, which means "to get something from someone/something."

23. **A.** Adjectives and adverbs show description. Verbs show action. Direct objects receive action.

24. **B.** A preposition links nouns, pronouns, and phrases to other words in a sentence by describing some kind of relationship. A direct object shows who or what receives the action in the sentence. An indirect object shows to whom or for what the action is performed.

25. **D.** This is the definition of a preposition.

26. **D.** Regular verbs are the ones you're most familiar with, and they show action. Relative pronouns are words that begin a clause that modify an antecedent. A predicate shows the action the subject of a sentence is performing.

27. **A.** "Series" is the only one that makes sense. The others kind of sound like it, but only a series would be released on DVD.

28. **A.** *To set* is "to place something down." The correct word here is *sit*, which means "to place yourself in a seat."

29. **B.** "Sang" is the simple past form of "sing."

30. **C.** The -*ly* suffix here is a dead giveaway. "Amazingly" modifies "easy," which is an adjective. Adverbs modify verbs, adjectives, and other adverbs.

31. **C.** You only use "capitol" in reference to the legislative building of the country or a state. You want to use "capital" here.

32. **D.** "That" is a relative pronoun; "anyone" is an indefinite pronoun; "me" is a personal pronoun.

33. **B.** You have a compound subject here connected with "and," which means you treat it as plural. All of the other answer choices have compound subjects, but incorrect verb agreement: "cars and the vans was," should be "cars and the vans *were*" because "vans" is plural; "either the rides or the cotton candy stand were," should be "either the rides or the cotton candy stand was," because you have "either/or," which means the verb takes the tense of the closest noun. Same with Answer D.

34. **D.** This sentence is correctly punctuated.

35. **B.** The subject performs the action in the sentence. In this case, it's the woman who is looking.

36. **B.** "Group" is a collective noun that takes a singular verb. C is the wrong form of "there" and is incorrect even if it were in the correct form, like A ("their"). D is a contraction that means "it is," which doesn't work for this sentence.

37. **C.** This is the only answer choice that uses there/their/they're correctly. *Their* is a possessive pronoun. *They're* is a contraction of "they" and "are."

38. **A.** Wrong form of there. Use the contraction that means "they are": *They're*.

39. **A.** All of the other answers are using the wrong form of "who." You use "who" as a pronoun that refers to the subject of the sentence. You use "whom" as a pronoun that refers to a direct object. The subjects of answers B through D are you, I, and you, respectively.

40. **D.** A and B don't make sense. "Wait" has to do with time, which people don't use plans to lose. D makes the most sense.

Spelling

1. **B**
2. **C**
3. **A**
4. **B**
5. **C**
6. **A**
7. **C**
8. **A**
9. **A**
10. **B**
11. **A**
12. **B**
13. **C**
14. **A**
15. **A**
16. **B**
17. **B**
18. **C**
19. **C**
20. **A**
21. **C**
22. **B**
23. **C**
24. **B**
25. **C**
26. **B**
27. **B**
28. **A**
29. **C**
30. **B**

31. **A**
32. **C**
33. **C**
34. **A**
35. **B**
36. **C**
37. **A**
38. **C**
39. **A**
40. **B**

Reading Comprehension

1. **C.** This makes the most sense, because the passage describes the scientific process of how wind turbines make electricity. There is no emotion present, which rules out Answer B. And although the passage says that wind farms are a "leading" source of sustainable energy, there's no indication that all of the U.S. power supply comes from this energy source or that this source produces the most energy in the country.

2. **A.** The sentence "this action converts the kinetic energy of the wind into mechanical energy through the rotation of the blades" tells us that the wind has kinetic energy.

3. **B.** Because this passage describes a process without emotion or any call to action, it is clearly intended to inform.

4. **D.** The passage says that "establishing wind farms in areas that experience a steady flow of high-energy wind are a good idea." It also goes on to say that lack of interference from buildings or landforms makes for a good location for a wind farm. Answers A, B, and C have landforms or buildings that can interfere with the flow of wind. Wide-open fields, however, fit the criteria in the passage.

5. **B.** A and C are not mentioned in the passage, whereas the final sentence in the passage says: "With electronic settings that will automatically shut down the blades should high-force winds, such as those in a hurricane, gust and possibly damage the turbine, the risk of damage to an investment in this area is low."

6. **B.** The first paragraph states: "Such farms contain one or more turbines with giant blades that are turned by the wind. This action converts the kinetic energy of the wind into mechanical energy through the rotation of the blades."

7. **A.** This is an inference question. The information in the passage contradicts Answer B, and there is no information to support Answers C and D. Answer A is directly supported by the second sentence in the passage.

8. **C.** Swapping won't work for this Vocab-in-Context question. Look to context clues to tell you how "accountable" is being used in the sentence. "Monitor the actions of our elected officials" tells you that the speaker is urging people to keep an eye on politicians. This sets up the rest of the sentence, which talks about holding them responsible for their actions. The only choice that fits this idea is Answer C.

9. **B.** This is another inference question. The best approach is to go to each answer choice and ask why the author would agree with it:

    (A) "Too many people come to council meetings": the author wouldn't agree because the passage says, "Not enough people attend their local town council meetings."

    (B) "Elected officials must answer to the public": this is a good choice because the author says, "It's our responsibility as American citizens to monitor the actions of our elected officials and hold them accountable."

(C) "Council meetings are the best place to air a grievance about the community": there's no mention of grievances or public speaking in the passage.

(D) "Town councils should recognize citizens more often": there's no reference to citizens being recognized in the passage.

10. **D.** All of these answers can be inferred from the information in the passage.

11. **C.** All the rest of the answers are subjective to someone's point of view, rather than facts that can be proven.

12. **B.** There are too many opinions in the passage for it to be merely informative. C and D don't make sense with the content presented.

13. **D.** This is the best choice because it talks about listener-centric communication and its increased recognition, which is the main idea of the passage.

14. **B.** The passage talks about thoughts and evaluating perceptions as internal communication.

15. **A.** Each of the other answer choices present details, not the overall message being conveyed by the passage.

16. **C.** All of the other answer choices can be proven.

17. **A.** This is stated in the first sentence of the second paragraph.

18. **B.** The other answer choices are too extreme to fit with what's presented in the passage. The passage is more neutral than anything else, and Answer B is the most neutral choice.

19. **C.** The sentence talks about being unaware of physical effects. It doesn't talk about any increased physical ability or memory, which eliminates Answers A and D. Answer B runs contrary to how the word is used in the sentence.

20. **D.** Each of the answer choices is mentioned in the passage. This makes D the best choice.

21. **B.** "Flippant" and "glib" imply an uncaring tone. The author obviously cares about this subject and appears to be concerned with the negative consequences of this lifestyle. This makes B the best choice.

22. **A.** The author would most likely disagree with all of the other answer choices because they run counter to what is written in the passage. Furthermore, the author states that "most adults aren't even aware of the amount of stress they are under during a normal workday because they have become desensitized to its effects in order to get through the tasks they have on their plate." This supports Answer A.

23. **C.** This answer is really the structure of the passage. A and B go against what's stated in the passage. There is no information about the newness of the research to say D is a good answer.

24. **D.** This is the only answer choice that's supported by the passage.

25. **A.** In the sentence, "versatile" describes many uses.

26. **B.** The passage says vinegar is a good cleaner and deodorizer for coffee and fabric.

27. **D.** The passage states that a vinegar solution is good for treating a flea infestation. None of the other choices are supported.

28. **A.** This is stated in the first paragraph. B and C do not apply to food. D contradicts the passage; vinegar is an acid, not a base.

29. **B.** This passage takes more of an informational approach to presenting information, rather than promoting or spurring people to action.

30. **C.** The passage states: "Fleas don't like the smell or taste of vinegar, or the fact that it is so acidic." The only other possible choice might be B, but there is not enough clear information to support this. C is stronger.

Math

1. **D.** The increase in dosage is 50 mg, so what you really want to figure out is how much of an increase 50 mg is in relation to 75 mg. Right off the bat, you know it has to be more than 50% because 50 is more than half of 75. That leaves you with D as your most likely answer. If you wanted to do the math, your equation should be $50 = x \times 75 = \frac{50}{75} = \frac{2}{3} = .6666$. Round up and you have .67, which is the same as 67%.

2. **B.** According to order of operations, solve this from left to right:

    $-14 - 12 + 6 =$

    $-26 + 6 = -20$

3. **A.** Cross multiply and solve for x: $6 \times 10 = 60$; $15 \times x = 60$. Divide 60 by 15 to get $x = 4$.

4. **C.** Divide 10.75 by 4 to find out that one load costs $2.6875. Now divide $23.63 by this amount to get 8.79. Since this number is not nine full loads, you have to round down to eight, because you need to find the number of entire loads the amount will pay for. You'll have change left over, but eight loads in the wash.

5. **B.** Multiply length times width to get the area of a rectangle: $16.2 \times 8.5 = 137.7$ ft.^{2}.

6. **B.** To calculate the area of a circle, use the following formula: $A = \pi r^2$. Because you know the diameter is 11, divide that by 2 and use that value for the radius. Your math should look like this: $A = 3.14 \times 5.5 \times 5.5$. $A = 94.985$ in.^{2}. Round up to 95 and you have your answer.

7. **A.** With 287065000, you'd move the decimal eight places to the left to get 2.87065000. Now drop all of the 0s after the 5 to get 2.87065. Finally, multiply this number by 10 to the eighth power (the number of decimal spaces you moved): 2.87065×10^8.

8. **B.** Start by breaking down each term into prime factors:

    $42x^2 = 2 \times 3 \times 7 \times x \times x$

    $28x = 2 \times 2 \times 7 \times x$

    What do both of these have in common? $2 \times 7 \times x$ (which equals $14x$).

    Next, simplify each of these by crossing out one 2, 7, and x in each expression:

    $42x^2 = 2 \times 3 \times 7 \times x \times x$

    $28x = 2 \times 2 \times 7 \times x$

    Now combine like terms and place the new expression in parentheses with $14x$ outside:

    $42x^2 + 28x = 14x(3x + 2)$.

9. **D.** First, calculate how much Assembly Line A can produce in an hour: $14 \times 2 = 28$. Now multiply that number by 12 to see how much it can produce in 12 hours: $28 \times 12 = 336$. Now multiply that number by 2 to determine how much Assembly Line B can produce in that amount of time: $336 \times 2 = 672$. Add $336 + 672$ to get the total they both make in 12 hours.

10. **C.** $.22 \times 264 = 58.08$

11. **B.** Multiply the number of years (16) by one third to find the answer.

12. **A.** A prime number is one that is only divisible by itself and 1. Each of the other answer choices are divisible by other numbers.

13. **D.** Mode describes the number within a set of numbers that appears the most times. In this case, 6 appears five times. 5, 2, and 1 appear twice. 3 appears only once.

14. **B.** Write this like you would say it: 1 wheel turn equals 3 times you have to pedal, or 1:3.

15. **D.** All sides of an equilateral triangle are equal. Therefore, each of the sides of the square equals 8. To calculate the area of a square, you multiply the value of 2 sides: $8 \times 8 = 64$.

16. **D.** This is an extended way of writing 2^5.

17. **B.** One meter equals 100 centimeters. $14 \times 100 = 1,400$ centimeters.

18. **D.** The third place after the decimal point is the thousandth place. The number is 8, so we look to the number next to it to see if we should round up or down. The number in the hundredths place is 5, which means we round up to 25.149.

19. **A.** 1 foot = 0.3048 meters. Multiply 25 × 0.3048 to find that 25 feet is equal to about 7.62 meters.

20. **D.** A sum is the answer to an addition problem. A product is the answer to a multiplication problem. A difference is the answer to a subtraction problem.

21. **A.** Mode describes the number within a set of numbers that appears the most times. In this case, 2 appears four times. 6, 4, and 3 appear twice. 5 appears only once.

22. **A.** With 5253260000, you'd move the decimal 9 places to the left to get 5.253260000. Now drop all of the 0s after the 6 to get 5.25326. Finally, multiply this number by 10 to the ninth power (the number of decimal spaces you moved): 5.25326×10^9.

23. **B.** Roots can be simplified if the number under the radical sign has a factor that is a perfect square. In this case, we have $\sqrt{147} = \sqrt{49 \times 3} = \sqrt{7 \times 7 \times 3}$. Factor out the square and place it outside as a coefficient. The remaining factor stays inside the radical sign: $7\sqrt{3}$.

24. **C.** First you have to figure out how old Abby is:

$$\left(\tfrac{2}{3} \times \tfrac{15}{1}\right) + 2 =$$
$$\left(\tfrac{30}{3}\right) + 2 =$$
$$10 + 2 = 12$$

If Trixie will be four times as old as Abby on her next birthday, then she will be 48 years old. Today she is 47, because she is still waiting for Abby's birthday to come.

25. **A.** 56.2% of respondents indicated that 8:00 P.M. is the time they sit down to watch TV.

26. **B.** 97.85% of respondents overall indicated that 8:30 P.M. is the time they sit down to watch TV.

27. **B.** In this time slot, the Pacific Northwest and Northeast combined have the greatest number of viewers.

28. **C.** You can get this answer by eyeballing the graph, which tops out not far below 60, but well above 40. You could estimate about 50 to 55 and come out correct. If you add the actual numbers in the table, you'll

find that 52.89% of respondents said 9:30 P.M.

29. **B.** Use the following formula to convert the Celsius measures to Fahrenheit: $°C \times \frac{9}{5} + 32 = F$. Plug in your numbers and use order of operations to solve.

30. **B.** This is a simple rate problem. Use the Distance = Rate × Time formula to solve for the distance: $D = 520 \times 3$.

31. **D.** Calculate the area of the room. Since we know it's a rectangle, multiply the length times the width to get 360 ft.^{2}. Then divide by half to find the missing amount: 180 ft.^{2}.

32. **C.** These angles are perpendicular, which makes them all 90°.

33. **B.** An expression is a mathematical statement that combines terms and operations. A constant is a number that stands by itself in an expression or equation. An equation is a mathematical statement that shows two equal expressions.

34. **A.** Because parentheses come first in order of operations, you should look for those. The only expression in parentheses is inside the brackets. Brackets are a step up from parentheses, so you would look there first anyway. It's logical that among the expressions within the brackets, you would solve $(3^2 - 3)$ first. Exponents are second, so $(3^2 - 3)^4$ is not correct. Answer D, $[2 \times 4 + (3^2 - 3)^4]$, is also not correct because you would not solve the whole expression first, only one smaller part.

35. **A.** The main number or variable in a term is called the *base*, while the raised number is the *exponent*. In this question, the only place this is

applicable is with the term 5^2. Clearly, 5 is the base and 2 is the exponent.

36. **B.** This is division of decimals. Move the decimal point in the divisor two places to the right. Then do the same with the dividend and add a 0 after the 3. Divide down and move the decimal point straight up into the quotient. You'll find that after the first step of division, you'll be able to eliminate all of the answer choices except B.

37. **B.** Use the following formula to convert the Fahrenheit measures to Celsius using the formula $(F - 32) \times \frac{5}{9} = C$. Plug in your numbers and solve.

38. **C.** Start by dividing 14 by 24 to get the percent: .58. You could then convert this to a fraction, by placing 58 over 100 and reducing.

39. **B.** Factor out 3 from the top equation and 2 from the bottom. You should get $3(2x + 3)$ on top and $2(x + 3)$ on the bottom.

40. **A.** With scientific notation, you move the decimal point to the right of the leftmost nonzero digit. With 6538900000, you'd move the decimal 9 places to the left to get 6.538900000. Now drop all the 0s after the 9 to get 6.5389. Finally, multiply this number by 10 to the ninth power (the number of decimal spaces you moved): you then get 6.5389×10^9.

Life Science

1. **B.** The lithosphere encompasses the solid, rocky top layer of the planet (the one on which we live) and part of the upper mantle.

2. **C.** Evolution is the study of how life forms have changed over time through natural selection, not natural selection itself. B and D describe relationships within an ecosystem.

3. **A.** A cell is the basic unit of life. It is an enclosed structure that contains a variety of components that work together to make the cell perform some specific purpose.

4. **B.** Rivinis and de Tournefort are important pioneers of taxonomic classification, but it's the Linnaean system that's most often used.

5. **C.** Heterotrophs are organisms that need to consume carbon-based substances, such as autotrophs and other heterotrophs, to survive. They are known as *consumers*.

6. **A.** B describes marine biomes. C describes alpine-tundra biomes.

7. **B.** Temperatures and pressure in the inner core are higher than anywhere else on the planet, yet the metals that make it up remain solid.

8. **D.** High pressure indicates good or improving weather. Low or falling pressure indicates poor or worsening weather.

9. **C.** Relationships among organisms within any given ecosystem are symbiotic: what affects one affects the others in some way, and there is some benefit to the populations as a result of these interconnected relationships.

10. **B.** Fossils are skeletons of living organisms that have been preserved over time by rock. Soft sedimentary rock, such as shale, often houses fossils.

11. **C.** In addition to random genetic mutations that take place in cells, sexual reproduction plays a big role in natural selection because this process blends genetic information.

12. **C.** This layer extends about 53 miles above the planet. The mesosphere has the opposite effect of the stratosphere in that the higher you go, the colder it gets. But if meteors reach the mesosphere, the friction between the meteor and the air in this layer will cause them to burn up.

13. **D.** The cycle of killing off bacteria that could not fight off antibiotics and the reproduction of bacteria with the genetic changes that enable it to resist the effects of antibiotics is an example of natural selection.

14. **A.** The moon's blockage of the sun's light places the area of the Earth affected by the eclipse in shadow until the Earth revolves enough to move out of the shadow.

15. **C.** Neptune is the coldest planet because it is farthest from the sun.

16. **B.** Plants have both male and female organs for sexual reproduction.

17. **C.** Prokaryotic cells have no defined nucleus, which is the main difference in this type of cell. The contents of a prokaryotic cell are contained within a capsule. A cell membrane is a buffer between the contents of the cell and the capsule, which may also have flagella attached.

18. **D.** Light-dependent reaction products are adenosine triphosphate (ATP), nicotinamide adenine dinucleotide phosphate (NADPH), and oxygen.

19. **C.** Roots anchor a plant underground. The shoot describes the whole of the plant that's above ground. The leaves are where photosynthesis takes place.

20. **B.** In a mutual relationship, all organisms in the relationship benefit. In a commensal relationship, one or a group of organisms benefits while another is not affected at all.

21. **C.** Pressure and temperature in this layer are both very high. In fact, the majority of the Earth's heat comes from this layer, and the movement of heat through the mantle is believed to be responsible for the movement of tectonic plates.

22. **A.** Proteins are chemicals found within a cell that control its metabolism (chemical reactions that occur within the cell) and how the cell interacts with its surroundings. Cytoplasm is the whole of a cell's internal components suspended within cytosol. A plasma membrane is the outer structure that holds everything else inside.

23. **D.** All of the other answers are functions of the atmosphere.

24. **C.** The moon is a satellite of the Earth, like Earth is a satellite of the sun.

25. **B.** The "an" prefix here should be a clue. *An* means "not."

26. **D.** Out of the choices given, Jupiter is closest to the sun, which means it has the shortest trip around the sun to make.

27. **A.** This is the definition of a fossil.

28. **B.** Answer A describes stratus clouds. C describes cirrus clouds. D describes cumulonimbus clouds.

29. **A.** They're sometimes called thunderheads because they often bring thunderstorms.

30. **C.** The Continental crust is part of the Earth's crust, which is part of the lithosphere and lies above the asthenosphere. It is the land that makes up the continents, while the Oceanic crust is the land under the oceans.

Biology

1. **C.** During active diffusion, energy needs to be expended and the molecules need help to get through the membrane. Transport proteins do this.

2. **D.** Each of these is true about tRNA. Its job is to take the information copied by mRNA and translate it into the right sequence of peptides to produce an exact copy of the DNA that's replicating. Its structure is that of an inverted L.

3. **A.** Cellulose is a complex carbohydrate that is used for structural purposes in a cell.

4. **C.** The pressure of the water will first stretch and then break the bonds holding the membrane together.

5. **B.** Chromatids are DNA strands that make up a duplicated chromosome. Chromatin is a substance surrounding the nucleus of a cell and holds the DNA, RNA, and nuclear proteins needed for reproduction. Centrioles are tubelike structures whose only purpose is to assist in cell division.

6. **A.** The ribosomes on the outside of rough ER give it its rough texture.

7. **A.** Heterozygous gene pairs are made up of two different alleles. Homozygous gene pairs are made up of two of the same alleles. Phenotypical refers to phenotype, which is the physical expression of genes.

8. **B.** The brown eye gene is dominant. Only two of the four boxes have a dominant allele for brown eyes in it, which means that it is most likely to be the one expressed. The recessive allele would be carried, not expressed.

9. **B.** The top-left box should have a "Bb." The top-right box should have "bb." The bottom-left box should have "Bb," and the bottom-right box should have "bb." This is a 2:4 split.

10. **D.** Cell division ends when the cells go into cytokinesis, which is just a fancy way of saying that the plasma membrane connecting the two cells breaks off, leaving two completely independent, genetically identical cells.

11. **C.** Cells produced by meiosis II can replicate but are not genetically identical and are haploid.

12. **A.** Glycolysis doesn't need oxygen to take place, but it can take place when oxygen is present. If it is not present, fermentation takes place, which is completely anaerobic.

13. **C.** B is the Law of Segregation. The other answer choices are not laws at all.

14. **C.** The exact transcription of the nucleic acid sequence is vital to DNA replication. Any variation in that sequence results in mutation of the gene.

15. **D.** Fertilization is when two gametes combine. Oogenesis is meiosis for ova. There is no such thing as zygotagenesis.

16. **A.** Genes have nothing to do with the other answer choices.

17. **B.** Base pairs are held together by two 5-sugar and phosphate spines, one on the outside edge of each nucleic acid,

to form a kind of ladder structure if you were to lay a strand of DNA flat.

18. **D.** Lipids are fats. They have a lower concentration of oxygen in their chemical makeup and hold more energy than carbohydrate molecules. Answer A describes $FADH_2$. C describes proteins.

19. **B.** Glucose is a 6-carbon molecule.

20. **D.** This question is asking for total ATP. Each of the two 3-carbon chains produces 2 ATP molecules, 1 NADH molecule, and 1 pyruvate. Net ATP is 2 because 2 ATP is used in glycolysis.

21. **C.** Oogenesis is a process of female sexual reproduction. Answers A and B reproduce asexually. Males that reproduce sexually experience spermatogenesis.

22. **C.** The Krebs cycle begins with the oxidation of one of the pyruvates.

23. **A.** Glycolysis produces 2 ATP. The Krebs cycle produces 2 ATP. The electron transport chain produces 34 ATP. The entire process of cellular respiration produces 38 ATP from one molecule of glucose.

24. **B.** As with skin cells after a cut, muscle cells would go through mitosis to replace the ones that were severed or killed off by the tear.

25. **D.** DNA becomes denser in prophase, which enables chromosomes to be seen by the eye through a microscope during this phase.

26. **C.** The first three steps in mitosis take place during one long phase called interphase.

27. **C.** Homologues contain two chromatids that have similar types of genes. They are connected by a centromere.

28. **A.** In mitosis, cell division ends when the cells go into cytokinesis, which is just a fancy way of saying that the plasma membrane connecting the two cells breaks off, leaving two completely independent, genetically identical cells.

29. **A.** Mendel was an Austrian monk and scientist who, through his studies of genetic traits in pea plants, figured out that the genes we carry are not always expressed.

30. **D.** Ribosomes either make or synthesize proteins for use in the cell; they are involved with the transcription stage of DNA replication. Nucleoli and nuclear envelopes are structures in the nucleus of a cell.

Anatomy and Physiology

1. **B.** The somatic system consists of cranial and spinal nerve fibers that connect the CNS to skin and skeletal muscles. Answers C and D are not part of the peripheral nervous system.

2. **C.** The left lung has two lobes.

3. **C.** The tibia is the shinbone; it runs between the kneecap and the ankle.

4. **D.** Joints are classified according to the amount of movement they make possible: freely movable, slightly movable, and immovable.

5. **B.** Frontal lobes deal with motor areas that control movement of voluntary skeletal muscles. Temporal lobes deal with sensory areas responsible for hearing. Occipital lobes control sensory areas responsible for vision.

6. **D.** The root *hema* means "blood." The root *cerebr* means "brain." The root *cardio* means "heart."

7. **A.** Answer B is "ascending." C is "anterior." D is "inferior."

8. **D.** Blood is made up of three components: white blood cells (leukocytes), red blood cells (erythrocytes), and plasma, which is made up mostly of water, proteins, and dissolved salts.

9. **B.** The superior vena cava connects to the heart at the top of the right atrium and then branches off into two major veins (subclavian) that go into the arms. The subclavian veins then branch off into veins that go into the head.

10. **A.** The word *femoris* indicates the femur is the bone to which it is attached. The femur is the thigh bone. This eliminates C and D as answers because the triceps are in the arms and the gluteus maximus is the buttock muscle. The hamstring is the back-thigh muscle, which is where the biceps femoris is located. The quadriceps are the front thigh muscles.

11. **C.** This is your lower jawbone.

12. **D.** Capillaries are blood vessels that run throughout the tissues. Veins and arteries are larger blood vessels that connect to capillaries from the major blood vessels in the body.

13. **D.** The stomach is not connected to either the large intestine or the liver. The stomach and esophagus are connected by the esophageal sphincter.

14. **D.** The humerus is an arm bone.

15. **A.** The renal artery brings blood to the kidneys. The renal vein brings blood away from the kidneys.

16. **C.** The cells of smooth muscles are narrow and have only one nucleus, whereas striated muscles are made up of long, multinucleated fibers that give them the appearance of being striped.

17. **D.** All of the answers are correct.

18. **B.** Long bones (femur, humerus) in children have marrow that produces red blood cells. Flat bones (pelvis, scapula) in adults have marrow that produces red blood cells.

19. **C.** If it's not a head or spinal bone, it's part of the appendicular skeleton.

20. **B.** Hinge joints are like a door hinge; two bones connect in such a way that only an up-and-down or in-and-out movement is possible. Sutures are only found in the skull and connect the 28 bones that make up this part of the body. Ball and socket joints have a rounded top of a bone that fits into the hollow of a socket to produce circular movement.

21. **B.** Vitamin D is produced by the skin and helps absorb calcium in the small intestines. Lead should not be present in the body.

22. **D.** The diaphragm is a thin band of fibromuscular tissue that is situated below the lungs and separates the chest cavity from the abdomen. When it expands and contracts, it enables the lungs to inhale and exhale.

23. **C.** Alveoli are little capillary-dense sacs that hold air in the bronchioles of the lungs.

24. **A.** The outer layer of the cerebrum is called the cerebral cortex (commonly known as *gray matter*) and is the home of the most neurons in the nervous system.

25. **C.** The blood-brain barrier is a layer of capillaries that cannot accept certain chemicals from the blood, such as certain types of medicines, toxins, and proteins. The cerebral cortex is the outer layer of the cerebrum. Cerebrospinal fluid is found in the meninges, which are three layers of tissue that provide a cushion for the brain.

26. **D.** All of the answers are part of a long bone.

27. **A.** Glycolysis takes place in cellular respiration. Peristalsis takes place during digestion. Glomerulus is the portion of a nephron that removes excess fluid and waste from the blood and turns them into urine.

28. **C.** Intestinal bacteria are prokaryotic microorganisms that serve an important function in turning substances in the colon into vitamins needed by the body. For instance, Vitamin K, B_{12}, thiamine, and riboflavin are all by-products of the bacterial processing of chyme in the colon. These vitamins are absorbed by the blood and used to nourish the body.

29. **A.** The appendix hangs off the bottom of the cecum. It's a fleshy protrusion shaped like an elongated teardrop and serves no known function in the body.

30. **C.** The human skeleton has 206 bones.

Chemistry

1. **C.** Answers A, B, and D are part of the Seven Fundamental Units of Measurement. The others are length, amount of a substance, luminous intensity, and temperature.

2. **D.** All of the answers are true statements about acids and bases.

3. **A.** Answer B describes the number of electrons in each of an element's electron shells. C refers to the physical composition of a substance.

4. **A.** An acid-base reaction is the combination of an acid and a base. A displacement reaction happens when one element displaces another in a compound. Oxidation-reduction reaction transfers electrons from one chemical species to another.

5. **D.** All of the answers are correct.

6. **B.** Take the atomic weight of 1 C and 4 H and add together:

    1 C = 12.01

    H is 1.01 × 4 = 4.04

    12.01 + 4.04 = 16.05

7. **C.** Combustion reactions happen when a compound is combined with elemental oxygen, usually to form water and carbon dioxide. This is exactly what this equation shows. Synthesis combines two reactants that break the existing chemical bonds and form new ones. Decomposition is the opposite of synthesis. Double displacement happens when ionic compounds are added to an aqueous solution—each pair of elements in the compounds separate to become cations and anions and then recombine with the other ion that it was not originally bound to in the reactants.

8. **A.** When a covalent bond is shared equally, it is nonpolar. In ionic bonding, electrons are transferred from one atom to another.

9. **A.** A molecule is the smallest particle of an element or compound that can have a stable independent existence. Allotropes are different forms of the same element in the same physical state. A compound is two or more elements in chemical combination in fixed proportion.

10. **B.** Answer A describes an endothermic reaction. C describes an exothermic reaction.

11. **C.** A mole of one atom of an element is equal to that element's atomic weight. The atomic weight of hydrogen is about 1, and you have two atoms here. The total molecular weight is 2, so 1 mole of H_2 is equal to 2 amu. Because 1 mole is equal to 1 gram, H_2 is equal to 2 g.

12. **A.** Matter is generally classified into these three states, although you may find that some sources point to five states of matter.

13. **A.** Move the decimal six places to the left to place it after the 3. Then drop all the zeroes after the nine and multiply by 10^6.

14. **C.** The iron atoms are even on both sides, so start with the chlorine ones. You have two on the left and three on the right. Because you can only add to these amounts, you need to make the value on the right divisible by 2. Add a 2 as the coefficient, which brings

the value up to 6 atoms of chlorine and 2 atoms of iron. Add a 2 to the iron and 3 to the chlorine on the left and your equation is balanced.

15. **B.** The number of protons is simply the atomic number of the element. In this case the atomic number of Ne is 10.

16. **B.** Homogeneous mixtures have uniform properties throughout and components are not distinguishable. Compounds can be broken down into simpler substances by chemical means. Elements are substances that cannot be broken down into simpler substances by chemical means.

17. **D.** Stoichiometry is the calculation of a relationship between reactants and products in a balanced chemical equation. This includes calculating relationships among elements in compounds and among substances as they undergo chemical changes.

18. **D.** Hydrogen bonding results from the attraction of an H atom and a highly electronegative element. Dipole interactions result from unequal sharing between polar molecules. London forces is the attraction of a positively charged nucleus of one atom for the electron cloud of an atom in a nearby molecule. This happens only over short distances and is stronger for molecules that are larger or have more electrons.

19. **A.** Protons have a positive charge. Neutrons have no charge. The atomic number is the number of protons in an element.

20. **B.** Acids are substances that produce hydrogen ions (H_3^+) when mixed with water. Bases produce hydroxide ions (OH^-) when mixed with water. When these ions come in contact, they react

by neutralizing each other. If an equal number of hydrogen and hydroxide ions are present in a solution, water will be produced.

21. **D.** Covalent bonds happen when two atoms of a similar electron configuration come in contact with each other; they can form a bond by sharing electrons, either equally or unequally.

22. **C.** An emulsion joins two solutes that would not normally mix. A dilution adds volume to the solvent in a solution to reduce the molarity of a solution. Tinctures are solutions made with alcohol and not water.

23. **C.** Answer A describes a solid-to-gas change. B describes a gas-to-liquid change. D describes a gas-to-solid change.

24. **B.** A common chemistry question is to find the mass composition of one element in relation to another within a molecular formula. To find this, calculate the individual masses of the elements that make up a molecule and the molecular mass. Then divide the mass of the element you're solving for by the molecular mass and you'll find the percentage you need.

Na = 23

H = 1 × 4 = 4

O = 16 × 2 = 32

Total molecular mass is 23 + 4 + 32 = 59. Now divide the mass of hydrogen (which is 4) by 59 to find .06779. This translates into about 6.78%.

25. **D.** Choice B, decreasing the concentration, would reduce the rate of reaction.

26. **A.** Divide 8 by 18 to get .44.

27. **C.** Answer A indicates an aqueous solution. B indicates gas form. D indicates solid form.

28. **A.** B is lithium, C is titanium, and D is tantalum.

29. **B.** According to the octet rule, atoms are constantly trying to become more stable by losing or gaining electrons to bring the total number of electrons in their outer orbital up to 8. Hydrogen is the lone exception in which atoms strive to attain two outer electrons.

30. **D.** Each of the elements in a row has the same number of orbitals as the row's number.

Physics

1. **C.** One kiloliter (kL) = 1,000 liters. 15 × 1,000 = 15,000 liters.

2. **B.** When you increase the temperature of a gas, the atoms within the gas move faster, which in turn increases gas pressure in the container. Decreasing the temperature will result in the opposite effect.

3. **A.** Celsius = metric unit of temperature measurement. Kelvin = SI unit of temperature measurement. Fahrenheit = American unit of temperature measurement. Absolute zero is a measure of the absolute coldest that matter can get.

4. **A.** A series circuit provides a single-flow path.

5. **B.** Your formula is $Acceleration = \frac{vf - vi}{time}$. After plugging in your numbers, you have $5 = \frac{38-28}{t}$ To solve for t, multiply both sides by t to get $5t = 10$. Now divide both sides by 5 to get $t = 2$.

6. **D.** The energy you apply to the rock converts the rock's potential energy into kinetic energy through motion. Newton's Third Law states that every motion creates another motion that runs in the opposite direction; therefore, when you kick the rock, it kicks back (so to speak). And when you expend energy to kick the rock, you're doing work.

7. **B.** When waves bounce back from an object, they deflect. When they split up by frequency, they disperse. When a wave's direction changes as a result of passing through a new medium, it refracts.

8. **D.** To measure frequency, divide the number of times a complete wave is made during a given time. Because frequency is measured in hertz, which is a measure of cycles per second, you need to convert 10 minutes into seconds (600): 1,525 ÷ 600 = 2.542. Round down to 2.54 and you have your answer.

9. **C.** The processes of nuclear fission and fusion take place every day in nuclear power plants, which harness the energy created by the reactions and turn it into forms of energy that we can use.

10. **C.** Answer A describes alpha radiation. B describes beta radiation.

11. **A.** Your formula is $F = ma$: 1250 × 5 = 6,250 N.

12. **D.** Electromagnetic waves are transverse. Sound is a longitudinal wave. Either can be long range or short range.

13. **C.** The lower the amplitude, the lower the intensity of the sound. The higher the amplitude, the higher the intensity of the sound.

14. **C.** A parallel circuit provides several flow paths.

15. **C.** Work is calculated using this formula: $W = fd$: 15 × 22.2 = 333 joules.

16. **D.** Gravitational acceleration says that objects that have no other force acting on it besides gravity fall at the same rate of acceleration (9.8 m/s²) regardless of mass. This means that, in theory, a car and a paper clip dropped in an environment with no air friction (essentially a vacuum) would both hit the ground at the same time; the ratio of weight to mass is the same for both the heavy object and the light object.

17. **A.** Answer C is the formula for calculating watts. D is the formula for calculating amps.

18. **B.** Resistance slows the flow of electricity.

19. **A.** Your formula is *PE = mgh*. But before you can compare these two masses, you have to convert the kilograms into grams so that you are comparing the same scales of measure. 1 kilogram (kg) = 1,000 grams, so 4 kg = 4,000 g. Now calculate the potential energy for both:

    Orange: 31 × 9.8 × 4,200 = 1,275,960 joules

    Ball: 4,000 × 9.8 × 32 = 1,254,400 joules

20. **C.** The omega sign looks like this: Ω

21. **D.** The question gives the Fahrenheit equivalent to absolute zero, which is equal to –273.15°C or 0 K. A is the freezing point of water on the Kelvin scale. C is the freezing point of water on the Celsius scale.

22. **D.** Power stations close to sources of running water (such as a dam or waterfall) funnel carefully controlled amounts of water into turbines. As the water moves the turbines, the potential energy is released as kinetic energy. The turbines then harness that kinetic energy and turn it into electricity. This is called hydroelectric power.

23. **B.** Celsius is metric. Fahrenheit is American. Joules measure energy.

24. **A.** First, you have to convert your kilometers per hour to meters per second. Do this by dividing 5 by 3.6 (what you get when you divide the number of total seconds in an hour by the number of meters in a kilometer). This gives you 1.39 m/s as your velocity. Now plug your numbers into the formula for kinetic energy: $\frac{1}{2}mv^2$:

    $\frac{1}{2} \times 20 \times 1.39^2 = \frac{1}{2} \times 20 \times 1.9321 = 1$

    $0 \times 1.9321 = 19.32$ joules.

25. **C.** Answer A describes amperes. B describes voltage. D describes power.

26. **A.** Work is the transfer of energy through force over a distance. Motion describes any change in the position of an object over time. Energy is the amount of work a force can produce.

27. **A.** Answer B is the formula for kinetic energy. C is the formula for potential energy.

28. **B.** Centripetal force is what happens when an object gets pulled into a circular path. Basically, it's an inward force that causes an object to turn. Centrifugal force is an outward motion that results from a rotating motion.

29. **B.** Your formula is *PE = mgh*: 42 × 9.8 × 175 = 72,030 joules.

30. **D.** Your formula is $\text{Speed} = \frac{\text{Distance}}{\text{Time}}$.

$$\text{Speed} = \frac{42}{35}$$

$$\text{Speed} = 1.2$$

Now, you have to multiply 1.2 by 60 because this is the value of kilometers per minute and your answer is in kilometers per hour.

Resources

Boards of Nursing in the United States and U.S. Territories

Rules and regulations regarding nursing are determined by each state's Board of Nursing. It's important for nursing school candidates to become familiar with their state board so that they know what all is required of them in order to be allowed to practice.

For example, some states require student nurses take a course in child or elder abuse to be allowed to practice after licensure. Here is a listing of the Boards of Nursing for all 50 states, as well as 5 U.S. territories.

Alabama Board of Nursing
Mailing Address:
PO Box 303900
Montgomery, AL 36130-3900
Street Address:
770 Washington Ave., RSA Plaza, Suite 250
Montgomery, AL 36104
Phone: 334-293-5201
Phone: 800-656-5318
Web: www.abn.alabama.gov

Alaska Board of Nursing
Mailing Address:
PO Box 110806
Juneau, AK 99811-0806
Street Address:
333 Willoughby Ave., 9th Fl.
State Office Building
Juneau, AK 99801-1770
Phone: 907-465-2550
Web: www.commerce.alaska.gov/web/cbpl/
professionallicensing/boardofnursing.aspx

American Samoa Health Services Regulatory Board
American Samoa Health Services Regulatory Board
Department of Health
Pago Pago, AS 96799
Phone: 684-633-1222
Web: www.ncsbn.org/American%20Samoa. htm

Arizona State Board of Nursing
1740 W. Adams St.
Suite 2000
Phoenix, AZ 85007
Phone: 602-771-7800
Web: www.azbn.gov

Arkansas State Board of Nursing
University Tower Building
1123 South University, Suite 800
Little Rock, AR 72204-1619
Phone: 501-686-2700
Web: www.arsbn.org

California Board of Registered Nursing
Mailing Address:
Board of Registered Nursing
PO Box 944210
Sacramento, CA 94244-2100
Street Address:
Board of Registered Nursing
1747 N. Market Blvd., Suite 150
Sacramento, CA 95834-1924
Phone: 916-322-3350
Web: www.rn.ca.gov

California Board of Vocational Nursing and Psychiatric Technicians
2535 Capitol Oaks Drive, Suite 205
Sacramento, CA 95833
Phone: 916-263-7800
Web: www.bvnpt.ca.gov

Colorado Board of Nursing
1560 Broadway, Suite 1370
Denver, CO 80202
Phone: 303-894-2430
Web: www.colorado.gov/pacific/dora/ Nursing

Commonwealth of Puerto Rico Board of Nurse Examiners
800 Roberto H. Todd Avenue
Room 202, Stop 18
Santurce, PR 00908
Phone: 787-725-7506
Web: www.registerednursern.com/ puerto-rico-board-of-nursing-board-of-nursing-puerto-rico-pr-information-registered-nurse-rn/

Connecticut Board of Examiners for Nursing
Dept. of Public Health
410 Capitol Avenue
MS# 13PHO
PO Box 340308
Hartford, CT 06134-0328
Phone: 860-509-7624; 860-509-7603 (for testing candidates only)
Web: portal.ct.gov/DPH/ Public-Health-Hearing-Office/ Board-of-Examiners-for-Nursing/ Board-of-Examiners-for-Nursing

Delaware Board of Nursing
861 Silver Lake Boulevard
Cannon Building, Suite 203
Dover, DE 19904
Phone: 302-744-4500
Web: dpr.delaware.gov/boards/nursing

District of Columbia Board of Nursing
Department of Health Professional Licensing Administration
899 North Capitol Street NE
Washington, DC 20002
Phone: 877-672-2174
Web: dchealth.dc.gov/node/149382

Florida Board of Nursing
4042 Bald Cypress Way, Bin C-02
Tallahassee, FL 32399
Phone: 850-245-4125
Web: floridasnursing.gov

Georgia Board of Nursing
237 Coliseum Drive
Macon, GA 31217-3858
Phone: 478-207-2440
Web: sos.ga.gov/index.php/licensing/plb/45

Guam Board of Nurse Examiners
194 Hernan Cortez Avenue, Suite 213
Hagatna, GU 96910
Phone: 671-735-7411
Web: www.gbne.org

Hawaii Board of Nursing
Mailing Address:
PVLD/DCCA
Attn: Board of Nursing
PO Box 3469
Honolulu, HI 96801
Street Address:
King Kalakaua Building
335 Merchant Street, 3rd Fl.
Honolulu, HI 96813
Phone: 808-586-3000
Web: cca.hawaii.gov/pvl/boards/nursing

Idaho Board of Nursing
280 North 8th Street, Suite 210
PO Box 83720
Boise, ID 83720
Phone: 208-577-247
Web: ibn.idaho.gov/IBNPortal

Illinois Board of Nursing
100 West Randolph Street, 9th Fl.
Chicago, IL 60601
Phone: 888-473-4858
Web: www.idfpr.com/profs/Nursing.asp

**Indiana State Board of Nursing
Professional Licensing Agency**
402 West Washington St., Room W072
Indianapolis, IN 46204
Phone: 317-234-2043
Web: www.in.gov/pla/nursing.htm

Iowa Board of Nursing
400 SW 8th Street, Suite B
Des Moines, IA 50309
Phone: 515-281-3255
Web: nursing.iowa.gov

Kansas State Board of Nursing
Landon State Office Building
900 SW Jackson, Suite 1051
Topeka, KS 66612
Phone: 785-296-4929
Web: ksbn.kansas.gov

Kentucky Board of Nursing
312 Whittington Parkway, Suite 300
Louisville, KY 40222
Phone: 502-429-3300
Web: www.kbn.ky.gov

Louisiana State Board of Nursing
17373 Perkins Road
Baton Rouge, LA 70810
Phone: 225-755-7500
Web: www.lsbn.state.la.us

**Louisiana State Board of Practical Nurse
Examiners**
131 Airline Drive, Suite 301
Metairie, LA 70002
Phone: 504-838-5791
Web: www.lsbpne.com

Maine State Board of Nursing
161 Capitol Street
Augusta, ME 04333
Phone: 207-287-1133
Web: www.maine.gov/boardofnursing/

Maryland Board of Nursing
4140 Patterson Avenue
Baltimore, MD 21215
Phone: 410-585-1900
Web: mbon.maryland.gov

**Massachusetts Board of Registration in
Nursing**
239 Causeway Street, Suite 500, 5th Floor
Boston, MA 02114
Phone: 617-973-0900; 800-414-0168
Web: www.mass.gov/orgs/
board-of-registration-in-nursing

Michigan/DCH/Bureau of Health Professions
611 West Ottawa, 1st Floor
Lansing, MI 48933
Phone: 517-373-8068
Web: www.michigan.gov/lara/0,4601,7-154-72600_72603---,00.html

Minnesota Board of Nursing
2829 University Avenue SE, Suite 200
Minneapolis, MN 55414
Phone: 612-317-3000
Web: mn.gov/boards/nursing

Mississippi Board of Nursing
713 Pear Orchard Road, Suite 300
Ridgeland, MS 39157
Phone: 601-957-6300
Web: www.msbn.state.ms.us

Missouri State Board of Nursing
3605 Missouri Boulevard
PO Box 656
Jefferson City, MO 65102-0656
Phone: 573-751-0681
Web: pr.mo.gov/nursing.asp

Montana State Board of Nursing
301 South Park, 4th Floor
PO Box 200513
Helena, MT 59620-0513
Phone: 406-444-5711
Web: boards.bsd.dli.mt.gov/nur

Nebraska Board of Nursing
301 Centennial Mall South
Lincoln, NE 68509-4986
Phone: 402-471-3121
Web: dhhs.ne.gov/publichealth/pages/crlNursingHome.aspx

Nevada State Board of Nursing
Las Vegas Address:
4220 S. Maryland Pkwy., Building B, Suite 300
Las Vegas, NV 89119-7533
Phone: 702-486-5800
Reno Address:
011 Meadowood Mall Way, Suite 300
Reno, NV 89502-6547
Phone: 702-687-7700
Web: nevadanursingboard.org

New Hampshire Board of Nursing
21 South Fruit Street, Suite 16
Concord, NH 03301-2341
Phone: 603-271-2323
Web: www.oplc.nh.gov/nursing

New Jersey Board of Nursing
PO Box 45010
124 Halsey Street, 6th Fl.
Newark, NJ 07101
Phone: 973-504-6430
Web: www.njconsumeraffairs.gov/nur/Pages/default.aspx

New Mexico Board of Nursing
6301 Indian School Road NE, Suite 710
Albuquerque, NM 87110
Phone: 505-841-8340
Web: nmbon.sks.com

New York State Board of Nursing
Education Bldg.

89 Washington Avenue, 2nd Floor West Wing
Albany, NY 12234
Phone: 518-474-3817, Ext. 120
Web: www.op.nysed.gov/prof/nurse/

North Carolina Board of Nursing
4516 Lake Boone Trail
Raleigh, NC 27607
Phone: 919-782-3211
Web: www.ncbon.com

North Dakota Board of Nursing
919 South 7th Street, Suite 504
Bismarck, ND 58504
Phone: 701-328-9777
Web: www.ndbon.org

Northern Mariana Islands Commonwealth Board of Nurse Examiners
Mailing Address:
PO Box 501458
Saipan, MP 96950
Street Address:
CHC Bldg., Old Medical Referral Office,
Lower Navy Hill, Saipan, MP 96950
Phone: 670-233-2263
Web: www.nmicbne.com

Ohio Board of Nursing
17 South High Street, Suite 660
Columbus, OH 43215-3413
Phone: 614-466-3947
Web: www.nursing.ohio.gov

Oklahoma Board of Nursing
2915 North Classen Blvd., Suite 524
Oklahoma City, OK 73106
Phone: 405-962-1800
Web: www.nursing.ok.gov

Oregon State Board of Nursing
17938 SW Upper Boones Ferry Road
Portland, OR 97224
Phone: 971-673-0685
Web: www.osbn.state.or.us

Pennsylvania State Board of Nursing
302 North Office Building, 401 North Street
Harrisburg, PA 17120
Phone: 717-787-6458
Web: www.dos.pa.gov/
ProfessionalLicensing/BoardsCommissions/
Nursing

Rhode Island Board of Nurse Registration and Nursing Education
105 Cannon Building
Three Capitol Hill
Providence, RI 02908
Phone: 401-222-5700
Web: health.ri.gov/licenses/detail.
php?id=231

South Carolina State Board of Nursing
110 Centerview Drive, Suite 202
Columbia, SC 29210
Phone: 803-896-4550
Web: www.llr.state.sc.us/pol/nursing

South Dakota Board of Nursing
4305 South Louise Avenue, Suite 201
Sioux Falls, SD 57106-3115
Phone: 605-362-2760
Web: doh.sd.gov/boards/Nursing

Tennessee State Board of Nursing
665 Mainstream Drive
Nashville, TN 37243
Phone: 615-532-5166
Web: www.tn.gov/health/health-
program-areas/health-professional-boards/
nursing-board

Texas Board of Nursing
333 Guadalupe, Suite 3-460
Austin, TX 78701
Phone: 512-305-7400
Web: www.bon.texas.gov

Utah State Board of Nursing
Heber M. Wells Building, 4th Floor
160 East 300 South
Salt Lake City, UT 84111
Phone: 801-530-6628
Web: dopl.utah.gov/nur

Vermont State Board of Nursing
3rd Floor, 89 Main St
Montpelier, VT 05620-3402
Phone: 802-828-2396
Web: www.sec.state.vt.us/professional-
regulation/list-of-professions/nursing

Virgin Islands Board of Nurse Licensure
Mailing Address:
PO Box 304247
St. Thomas, VI 00803
Street Address:
Virgin Islands Board of Nurse Licensure
No. 5051 Kongens Gade, Suite 1
St. Thomas, VI 00802
Phone: 340-776-7397
Web: www.thevibnl.org

Virginia Board of Nursing
9960 Mayland Drive, Suite 300
Henrico, VA 23233-1463
Phone: 804-367-4515
Web: www.dhp.virginia.gov/nursing

Washington State Nursing Care Quality Assurance Commission
Town Center 2
310 Israel Road SE
Tumwater, WA 98501-7864
Phone: 360-236-4703
Web: www.doh.wa.gov/
LicensesPermitsandCertificates/
NursingCommission

West Virginia Board of Examiners for Registered Professional Nurses
90 MacCorkle Ave SW #203
South Charleston, WV 25303
Phone: 304-744-0900
Web: wvrnboard.wv.gov

West Virginia State Board of Examiners for Licensed Practical Nurses
101 Dee Drive
Charleston, WV 25311
Phone: 304-558-3572
Web: www.lpnboard.state.wv.us

Wisconsin Department of Safety and Professional Services
Mailing Address:
PO Box 8935
Madison, WI 53708-8935
Street Address:
4822 Madison Yards Way
Madison, WI 53705
Phone: 608-266-2112
Web: dsps.wi.gov/pages/BoardsCouncils/
Nursing

Wyoming State Board of Nursing
130 Hobbs Ave B
Cheyenne, WY 82002
Phone: 307-777-7601
Web: nursing-online.state.wy.us

Professional Nursing Associations

There are professional associations for just about every nursing specialization. These can be excellent resources for potential nursing students, current students, and practicing professionals since they provide news, information about trends regarding the industry and specific areas, and a sense of community. They are also great resources for networking and job opportunities. Here is a listing of professional nursing associations to get you started:

Academy of Medical-Surgical Nurses: www.amsn.org

Academy of Neonatal Nursing: www.academyonline.org

Air & Surface Transport Nurses Association: www.astna.org

American Academy of Ambulatory Care Nursing: www.aaacn.org

American Association of Nurse Practitioners: www.aanp.org

American Academy of Nursing: www.aannet.org

American Assembly for Men in Nursing: www.aamn.org

American Assisted Living Nurses Association: www.alnursing.org

American Association for the History of Nursing: www.aahn.org

American Association of Colleges of Nursing: www.aacn.nche.edu

American Association of Critical-Care Nurses: www.aacn.org

American Association of Heart Failure Nurses: aahfn.org

American Association of Legal Nurse Consultants: www.aalnc.org

American Association of Managed Care Nurses: www.aamcn.org

American Association of Neuroscience Nurses: www.aann.org

American Association of Nurse Anesthetists: www.aana.com

American Association of Nurse Attorneys: www.taana.org

American Association of Occupational Health Nurses: www.aaohn.org

Academy of Spinal Cord Injury Professionals, Inc.: www.academyscipro.org

American College Health Association: www.acha.org

American College of Nurse-Midwives: www.midwife.org

American Forensic Nurses: www.amrn.com

American Holistic Nurses Association: www.ahna.org

American Nephrology Nurses Association: www.annanurse.org

American Nurses Association: nursingworld.org

American Nursing Informatics Association: www.ania-caring.org

American Organization of Nurse Executives: www.aone.org

American Psychiatric Nurses Association: www.apna.org

American Public Health Association: www.apha.org

American Society of Ophthalmic Registered Nurses: www.asorn.org

American Society of Pain Management Nursing: www.aspmn.org

American Society of Perianesthesia Nurses: www.aspan.org

American Thoracic Society: www.thoracic.org

Association of Camp Nursing: www.acn.org

Association of Child Neurology Nurses: www.childneurologysociety.org/acnn/home

Association of Nurses in AIDS Care: www.nursesinaidscare.org

Association of PeriOperative Registered Nurses: www.aorn.org

Association of Rehabilitation Nurses: www.rehabnurse.org

Association of Women's Health, Obstetric and Neonatal Nurses: www.awhonn.org

Baromedical Nurses Association: hyperbaricnurses.org

Commission on Graduates of Foreign Nursing Schools: www.cgfns.org

Dermatology Nurses' Association: www.dnanurse.org

Developmental Disabilities Nurses Association: ddna.org

Emergency Nurses Association: www.ena.org

Gerontological Advanced Practice Nurses Association: www.gapna.org

Hospice and Palliative Nurses Association: advancingexpertcare.org/HPNA/Default.aspx

Infusion Nurses Society: www.ins1.org

International Association of Forensic Nurses: www.iafn.org

International Council of Nurses: www.icn.ch

International Nursing Knowledge Association: www.nanda.org

International Organization of Multiple Sclerosis Nurses: www.iomsn.org

International Society of Nurses in Cancer Care: www.isncc.org

International Society of Nurses in Genetics: www.isong.org

International Society of Plastic and Aesthetic Nurses: ispan.org

National Association of Directors of Nursing Administration in Long Term Care: www.nadona.org

National Association for Practical Nurse Education and Service, Inc.: www.napnes.org

National Association of Clinical Nurse Specialists: www.nacns.org

National Association of Hispanic Nurses: www.nahnnet.org

National Association of Neonatal Nurses: www.nann.org

National Association of Orthopaedic Nurses: www.orthonurse.org

National Association of Pediatric Nurse Practitioners: www.napnap.org

National Association of Rural Health Clinics: www.narhc.org

National Association of School Nurses: www.nasn.org

National Association of School Nurses for the Deaf: www.nasnd.net

National Black Nurses Association, Inc.: www.nbna.org

National Hospice and Palliative Care Organization: www.nhpco.org

National League for Nursing: www.nln.org

National Nurses in Business Association, Inc.: www.nnbanow.com

National Nurse-Led Care Consortium: nursledcare.org

National Organization of Nurse Practitioner Faculties: www.nonpf.com

National Student Nurses' Association: www.nsna.org

Nurse Practitioner Healthcare Foundation: www.nphealthcarefoundation.org

Nurse Practitioners in Women's Health: www.npwh.org

Oncology Nursing Society: www.ons.org

Society for Vascular Nursing: svnnet.org

Society of Gastroenterology Nurses and Associates: www.sgna.org

Society of Otorhinolaryngology and Head-Neck Nurses: sohnnurse.com

Society of Pediatric Nurses: www.pedsnurses.org

Society of Urologic Nurses and Associates: www.suna.org

Transcultural Nursing Society: tcns.org

Wound, Ostomy and Continence Nurses Society: www.wocn.org

Books

Arnoldussen, Barbara. *Change Your Career: Nursing as Your New Profession.* Kaplan Publishing, 2008.

Atkins, Robert. *Getting the Most from Nursing School: A Guide to Becoming a Nurse.* Jones & Bartlett Publishers, 2008.

Bai, Laura Stark, et al. *301 Careers in Nursing.* Springer Publishing Company, 2017.

Bhatt, Sonal, and Rebecca Dayton. *The Complete Idiot's Guide to Geometry.* Alpha Books, 2014.

Chandler, Genevieve. *The Ultimate Guide to Getting into Nursing School.* McGraw-Hill Professional, 2007.

DePree, Christopher, and Alan Axelrod Ph.D. *The Complete Idiot's Guide to Astronomy,* 4th ed. Alpha Books, 2008.

Fotiyeva, Izolda. *The Complete Idiot's Guide to Algebra Word Problems.* Alpha Books, 2010.

Handwerker, Mark J. *Science Essentials, High School Level: Lessons and Activities for Test Preparation.* Jossey-Bass, 2004.

Hewitt, Paul G., and John A. Suchocki. *Conceptual Physical Science,* 6th ed. Addison Wesley, 2016.

Guch, Ian, and Kjirsten Wayman Ph.D. *The Complete Idiot's Guide to Organic Chemistry.* Alpha Books, 2008.

Guch, Ian. *The Complete Idiot's Guide to Chemistry.* Alpha Books, 2011.

Kavanagh, Robin A. *Vocabulous You! An Interactive Guide to Building Vocabulary for Standardized Tests, College, On the Job and Everyday Life.* Kindle Edition, 2011.

Moulton, Glen E. *The Complete Idiot's Guide to Biology.* Alpha Books, 2004.

Nugent, Patricia M., and Barbara A. Vitale. *Test Success: Test-Taking Techniques for Beginning Nursing Students,* 8th ed. F.A. Davis Co., 2018.

Pancella, Paul V., and Marc Humphrey. *The Complete Idiot's Guide to Physics.* Alpha Books, 2015.

Peterson's. *Nursing Programs 2017,* 22nd ed. Peterson's, 2016.

Seifert, Mark F. *The Complete Idiot's Guide to Anatomy, Illustrated.* Alpha Books, 2008.

Turner, Susan Odegaard. *The Nursing Career Planning Guide.* Jones & Bartlett Publishers, 2006.

Wheater, Carolyn. *The Complete Idiot's Guide to Algebra I.* Alpha Books, 2015.

Websites

AllNurses.com: allnurses.com

C-NET: www.cnetnurse.com

Daily Grammar: www.dailygrammar.com

How Stuff Works.com: www.howstuffworks.com

Khan Academy: www.khanacademy.org/test-prep/nclex-rn

Johnson & Johnson Nursing: www.nursing.jnj.com

Merriam-Webster's Word of the Day: www.merriam-webster.com/word-of-the-day

National Council of State Boards of Nursing: www.ncsbn.org

National League for Nursing: www.nln.org

Nurse.com: www.nurse.com

Nursing Times: www.nursingtimes.net

Occupational Outlook Handbook Report for Licensed Practical/Vocational Nurses: www.bls.gov/ooh/healthcare/licensed-practical-and-licensed-vocational-nurses.htm

Occupational Outlook Handbook Report for Registered Nurses: www.bls.gov/ooh/healthcare/registered-nurses.htm

PrefixSuffix.com: www.prefixsuffix.com

Purdue University Online Writing Lab Resources (for Grammar and Punctuation help): owl.purdue.edu/site_map.htm

Purplemath.com: www.purplemath.com

University of Connecticut Reading Comprehension Resources: www.literacy.uconn.edu/compre.htm

Index

flavin adenine dinucleotide, 144
food web, 132
forest, 131
fossils, definition of, 135
fractions, 90–92
  addition, 91
  basic concepts, 91
  converting decimals to, 93–94
  division, 92
  multiplication, 92
  simplification, 91
  subtraction, 92
freezing, 188
freshwater biomes, 131
fusion, 219

G

gallbladder, 174
gastrointestinal (GI) system, 173
genetics, 153–156
  DNA, 153–154
  gametes, 153
  Mendelian theory, 154–155
  predicting genetic inheritance, 155–156
geometry. see algebra and geometry, 103–121
glands. see endocrine system, 171–172
glycolysis, 148
Golgi apparatus, 146
grammar, 35–51
  answers to practice questions, 51
  common errors, 40–47
    ambiguous pronoun, 43
    commas in compound sentences, 44
    dangling modifier, 44
    misplaced modifier, 43–44
    preposition placement, 45
    run-on sentences, 44
    sentence fragments, 44

spelling, 45
subject/verb disagreement, 42–43
commonly confused words, 45–47
exam approach, 36
exam questions, 36
expectations, 35
parts of speech, 37–40
  adjectives, 39–40
  adverbs, 40
  nouns, 37–38
  prepositions, 40
  pronouns, 38
  verbs, 38–39
practice questions, 48–50
sentence parts, 41–42
spelling rules, 45
subject/verb agreement, 42–43
graphs, charts, and tables, 97–98
grassland, 132
gray matter, 170
greatest common factor (GCF), 90, 109

H

hamstring, 179
haploid, 151
Health Education Systems Exam (HESI) A2, 12–13, 16, 35, 104, 125
Health Occupations Aptitude Examination (HOAE), 19
heart, 164
heterogeneous mixture, 189
heterotrophs, 129
hinge joint, 181
homeostasis, definition of, 171
homogeneous mixture, 189
homologue, 150
human growth hormone (HGH), 172
hydroelectric power, 210
hypertonic solution, definition of, 147

hypothalamus, 172
hypotonic solution, definition of, 147

I

igneous rock, 134
ileum, 174
inequalities (algebra), 106–107
inference questions, 73–74
infinitives, 38
inner core (earth science), 134
integers, positive and negative, 88–89
ionic bonds, 198
irregular verbs, 39
isosceles triangle, 114
isotonic state, 148
isotope, definition of, 192

J

jejunum, 174
job possibilities. see career decision, 3–10
joints, 180
Judgement and Comprehension in Practical Nursing Situations, 18

K

Kelvin temperature, 213
Kepler's Laws, 137
kidneys, 175
kinetic energy, 210
Krebs Cycle, 146, 148

L

larynx, 167
Law of Independent Assortment, 155
law of inertia, 211
Law of Segregation, 155
least common multiple (LCM), 90

mnemonic, 129
order, 129
phylum, 128
species, 129
temperature (physics), 213–214
tense (grammar), definition of, 39
test preparation, 23–32. *see also* exams, 11–22
  final preparations, 31–32
  practice, 29
  practice tests and planning strategies, 23–28
    difficult subjects, 24
    finding the best answer, 26
    guessing, 26–28
    process of elimination, 26
    reading carefully, 25
    rethinking of approach, 24–25
    telltale signs in answer choices, 27–28
    test scores, 24
    your original answer, 25
  smart studying, 30
  studying strategically, 30
  test-specific strategies, 28–29
  timing, 29
testes, 176
testosterone, 172
thermodynamics, 212
thermosphere, 136
thrombocytes, 164
thyroid gland, 172
tinctures, 202
trachea, 167
transcription, 154
trapezoid, 116
triangles, 112–115
  area, 114
  base, 114
  congruent, 113
  equilateral, 114
  isosceles, 114
  perimeter, 114

right, 114
rules, 113
similar, 113
triglycerides, 166
trinomial, 109
troposphere, 135
tundra, 132

U

upper atmosphere, 136
upper GI tract, 173–174
upper respiratory system, 167
urinary system, 175–176
U.S. measurements, 96
uterus, 178

V

vacuoles, 146
vagina, 178
valence electrons, 193
vaporization, 188
vas deferens, 176
vasopressin, 172
veins, 165
velocity, 210
vena cavae, 166
ventricles, 164
verbs, 38–39
vertebrae, 180
vocabulary, 53–66
  analogies, 54
  answers to practice questions, 65–66
  antonyms, 54
  building, 59–62
  expectations, 53
  mnemonic devices, 62
  part of speech, 57
  practice questions, 63–64
  question types, 54
  sentence completion, 54
  strategies, 54–59
    analogies, 59
    clues, 57–58
    connotation, 56
    part of speech, 56
    prefixes, 56

roots, 54–55
swapping of answer choices, 58–59
synonym and antonym questions, 54
words in context and sentence completion, 57
synonyms, 54
voice box, 167
voltage, 215

W–X–Y–Z

waves (physics), 216–218
  amplitude, 217
  cycle, 216
  frequency, 217
  movement, 217–218
  negative amplitude, 217
  trough, 216
  types, 217
  wavelength measurement, 216
  wave speed, 216
websites
  Daily Grammar, 40
  EnglishClub.com, 54
  http
    //grammar.ccc.commnet.edu/grammar, 40
  nursing.jnj.com/specialty, 4
  PrefixSuffix.com, 62
  word-of-the-day, 60
  Word Power, 39
weight, mass and, 208–209
white blood cells (WBCs), 164
words in context, 57–58
work (physics), 210–211

zygote, 151, 178